Vascular Disease of the Gastrointestinal Tract

Pathophysiology, Recognition and Management

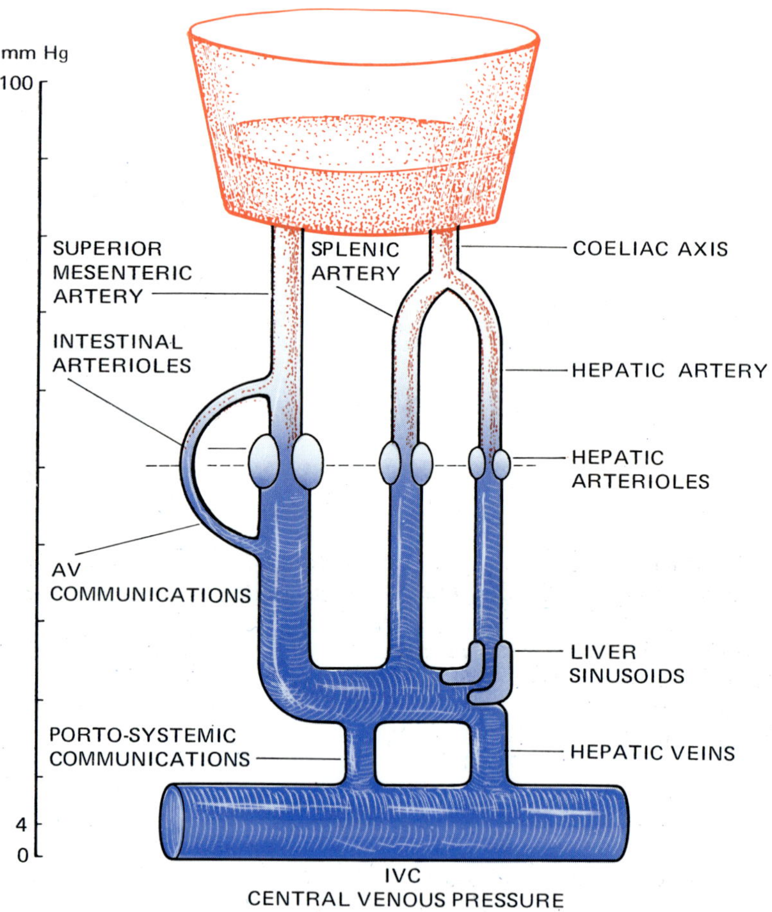

Frontispiece The compartments of the splanchnic circulation, showing pressure relationships.

Vascular Disease of the Gastrointestinal Tract

Pathophysiology, Recognition and Management

Adrian Marston
MA, DM, MCh (Oxon), FRCS (Eng), MD (Hon. Causa, Nice)
Surgeon, The Middlesex and University College Hospital, London;
Senior Lecturer in Surgery, University of London

With Illustrations by
Barbara Hyams, and members of the Department of Photography and Medical Illustration, The Middlesex Hospital and Medical School

Including Chapters by
Ove Lundgren, MD, PhD, Assistant Professor, Department of Physiology, University of Göteborg, Sweden; Member of the Swedish Medical Research Council

Thomas F. Gorey, MCh, FRCSI, Lecturer in Surgery, The Royal College of Surgeons in Ireland; The Charitable Infirmary, The Richmond and James Connolly Memorial Hospitals, Dublin

A.R. Moossa, MD, FRCS, FACS, Professor and Chairman;
Steven Shackford, MD, Assistant Professor of Surgery;
and *Michael J. Sise*, MD, Assistant Clinical Professor of Surgery, Department of Surgery, University of California, San Diego, California, USA

M.R.B. Keighley, MS, FRCS, Professor of Surgery and Consultant Surgeon; and *D.W. Burdon*, M.D., Consultant Microbiologist, University of Birmingham, The General Hospital, Birmingham

D.F.M. Thomas, MA, MRCP, FRCS, Consultant Paediatric Surgeon, St James's University Hospital and the General Infirmary, Leeds; Hunterian Professor, Royal College of Surgeons of England

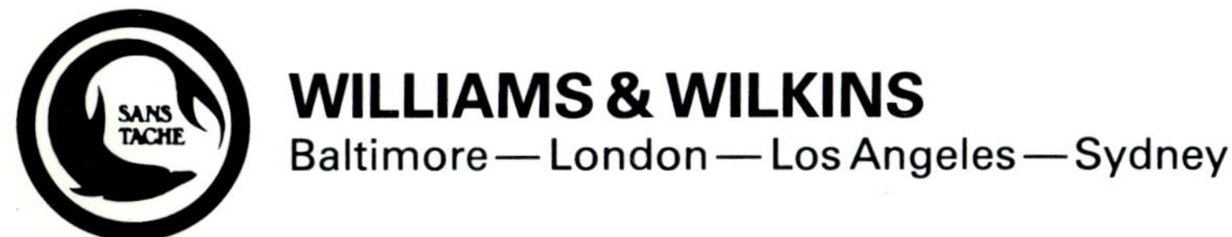

First published 1977 under the title of *Intestinal Ischaemia*
by Edward Arnold (Publishers) Ltd,
41 Bedford Square, London WC1B 3DQ

First published 1977
Second edition 1986

First published by Williams & Wilkins 1986
428 East Preston Street, Baltimore, Maryland 21202
USA

ISBN 0-683-05598-4

Printed and bound in Great Britain

To Sylvie

Preface to the First Edition

This book is the outcome of a personal interest in the clinical and experimental aspects of intestinal ischaemia, which has extended over the last twenty years. It is designed to be a guide to the clinician and a route map for the intending research worker, and represents, I hope, an outline of our present knowledge. It may seem presumptuous for one author to have attempted to cover this field, and in fact the task would have been quite impossible had I not made shameless use of my friends and colleagues. I have studied their patients, adopted their ideas, plagiarized their words and made extensive use of their illustrative material. I hope that I have not misinterpreted them, or anywhere failed to acknowledge my debt. The book is accordingly dedicated to my fellow authors:

Surgeons
John Bergan, *Chicago*;
Scott Boley, *New York*;
Gustav Bounous, *Sherbrook*;
David Cairns, *London*;
Robert Courbier, *Marseille*;
Lucien Deloyers, *Brussels*;
Harold Ellis, *London*;
Richard Gardham, *Enfield*;
Malcolm Gough, *Oxford*;
Mohamed Ahmed Hassan, *Khartoum*;
Leif Hulten, *Göteborg*;
Robert Kieny, *Strasborg*;
John Kinmonth, *London*;
Leslie Le Quesne, *London*;
Lyn Lockhart-Mummery, *London*;
Roger Marcuson, *Manchester*;
James Milliken, *Dublin*;
Francis Moore, *Boston*;
Robert Nevin, *London*;
Alan Parks, *London*;
George Parks, *Belfast*;
Cristobal Pera, *Barcelona*;
Murray Pheils, *Sydney*;
Colin Renton, *Hereford*;
Fredéric Saegesser, *Lausanne*;
Robert Shaw, *Boston*;
Douglas Short, *Glasgow*;
Kenneth Shute, *London*;
Henning Skjoldborg, *Aarhus*;
Michael Solan, *Farnham*;
Rafael Sobregrau, *Barcelona*;
Emeric Szilagyi, *Detroit*;
Gerald Taylor, *London*;
Richard Warren, *Boston*;
Lester Williams, *Boston*;
Colin Windsor, *Worcester*.

Physicians
Francis Avery-Jones, *London*;
Peter Ball, *London*;
Mario de Melos Bernado, *Lisbon*;
Jose Pinto Correia, *Lisbon*;
Elliot Corday, *Los Angeles*;
Peter Cotton, *London*;
Brian Creamer, *London*;
Anthony Dawson, *London*;
Jean-Pierre Delmont, *Nice*;
Peter Dick, *Cambridge*;
Donald Kellock, *London*;
Paul Kestens, *Brussels*;;
Henri Sarles, *Marseille*;
Francisco Villardell, *Barcelona*;
John Vyden, *Los Angeles*.

Pathologists
Peter Antony, *London*;
John Arthur, *Auckland*;
Geoffrey Farrer-Brown, *London*;
Richard Joske, *Perth*;
Vincent McGovern, *Sydney*;
Basil Morson, *London*;
Charles Ross, *Chertsey*;
Henry Thompson, *Birmingham*;
Richard Whitehead, *Oxford*.

Physiologists
Ove Lundgren, *Göteborg*;
Eric Neil, *London*;
Clinton Texter, *Little Rock*.

Radiologists
Malcolm Chapman, *London*;
Jack Farman, *New York*;
Duncan Gregg, *Cambridge*;
Hans Herlinger, *Leeds*;
Michael Lea Thomas, *London*;
Sol Schwartz, *New York*.

My thanks are also due to my secretary, Yvonne Lim, who prepared the manuscript, to Mr R.R. Phillips and the Staff of the Department of Photography of The Middlesex Hospital, and to my younger son, Nicholas, who helped to compile the Index.

A . M .

Preface to the Second Edition

When *Intestinal Ischaemia* was published in 1977, it was possible to write a personal monograph, encompassing the anatomy, physiology, pathology and treatment of arterial disorders of the intestinal tract, without too many important omissions. In the intervening eight years, so much more knowledge has accumulated that a completely new book has become necessary, incorporating chapters by others working in the field. The additional material and the revision of the previous text have been so extensive that it seemed appropriate to use a new title rather than to describe the present work as a second edition. The main changes are as follows.

The chapter on the regulation and distribution of intestinal blood flow always depended heavily on the work of the Swedish School of Physiologists, and Dr Ove Lundgren from Göteborg has now taken over this part of the text.

Additionally, Mr Thomas Gorey, who was Moynihan Travelling Fellow to the United States in 1984 and has made an especial study of the intestinal viability, has contributed an updated section on modern methods of predicting recoverability in ischaemic states.

The term 'acute intestinal failure', which was introduced in *Intestinal Ischaemia* to cover the various syndromes of occlusive and non-occlusive infarction of the bowel, has not gained wide acceptance, and was criticized in review at the time. Furthermore, the same phrase has been used to include a number of other conditions including widespread inflammatory disease and the short bowel syndrome. It seemed wise therefore to abandon it and revert to the more specific term of 'acute intestinal ischaemia'. Dr. A.R. Moossa and his team at San Diego have wide experience in the field and have contributed a completely new chapter on the subject.

Whether pseudomembranous enterocolitis is truly ischaemic in terms of diminished volume flow is still debated. However, the mucosal lesions clearly resemble certain types of ischaemia and it enters strongly into the differential diagnosis. Professor Michael Keighley and Dr Douglas Burdon of the Departments of Surgery and Microbiology at the University of Birmingham are well-known authorities in this area and have given a valuable additional chapter.

Infantile bowel ischaemia, as manifested by necrotizing enterocolitis was a problem which was not touched upon in *Intestinal Ischaemia* but has attained almost epidemic proportions in neonatal units. The omission has been filled by Mr David Thomas from Leeds, who contributes a unique experience. Mr Thomas has recently been awarded a Hunterian Professorship by the Royal College of Surgeons of England for his studies of this condition.

Every section of this book has been updated, and in particular our revised experience at The Middlesex Hospital in the treatment of chronic intestinal ischaemia and our philosophy as regards reconstruction of the visceral arteries are extensively reviewed. While there is no chapter devoted to venous disease, this important aspect of the subject has been expanded in both the clinical and the experimental chapters.

The lists of references have been pruned and modernized, and the expansion of the subject is reflected by a larger format with more detailed illustrations and tables.

In 1977 I expressed gratitude to the many

colleagues who had increased my knowledge of intestinal vascular disease and whose expertise I used. The debt has increased, and to the original list I add the names of Dr M. Brosowic of the Central Middlesex Hospital, Mr N. Carr from Manchester, Dr Arthur Miller of the Department of Chemical Pathology, The Middlesex Hospital Medical School, and Dr J.J. Wenger from the Hospices Civils in Strasbourg. Dr Basil Morson has provided valuable additional photomicrographs, Mr R.R. Phillips and members of his staff of the Photographic Department at the Middlesex Hospital have contributed much work to the illustrations, and I have been fortunate to secure the help of Miss Barbara Hyams who has completely redrawn the diagrams and figures. Finally, I am grateful to my skilled and good-humoured secretary, Patricia Rose, who virtually typed the whole work twice over and who has been of immense help in compiling the manuscript.

1985 A.M.

Introduction

When medical scientists in different disciplines unexpectedly find themselves converging on the same area of study, the result is likely to be a profitable re-examination of previously accepted ideas. Such as been the case with ischaemic bowel disease as the result of three developments in medical thinking over the last forty years.

1. Gastroenterologists suspected for some time that certain disorders of intestinal function were likely to be due to arterial insufficiency, much as happens in the heart, brain, kidney and other circulatory territories. Acute intestinal infarction resulting from mesenteric embolus and thrombosis had been recognized as a cause of death since the development of classic pathology in the mid-nineteenth century. It seemed likely that chronic obliterative disease of the visceral arteries could also occur and the existence of this disorder was speculated upon. However, as often happens, although a subject may have been extensively thought about and discussed in the literature, one observation suddenly illuminates the scene and provides a starting point for scientific advance. In 1936 J.E. Dunphy, who was then a surgical resident at Peter Bent Brigham Hospital, published a paper[1] showing that, of 12 patients dying of acute intestinal infarction, 7 gave a prodromal history of food-related abdominal colic, reminiscent of exercise pain felt in the ischaemic calf. From then on the concept of 'intestinal angina' had a respectable basis in pathology.

2. In the 1950s and early 60s the development of safe water-soluble contrast media and of retrograde arterial cannulation made it possible to map out the living arterial tree and to demonstrate sites of occlusion. The techniques of arterial suture and anastomosis, worked out decades before by Carrel in the experimental laboratory, then came into their own and began to be used on diseased human arteries with, at least in the short term, dramatic success. The first point of attack was the femoral artery, because this vessel is frequently occluded and is accessible to the surgeon. Moreover, the results of treatment are easy to assess because whether or not a patient claudicates, or whether or not a foot pulse is palpable, are recognized end-points which can be expressed in percentage terms of success or failure.

It soon became apparent, however, that to operate unselectively on every patient with claudication was mistaken, because in many cases the symptoms disappeared without treatment, and a failed operation could make the situation much worse, even to the extent of causing someone needlessly to lose a limb. The advent of new and enthusiastically applied surgical techniques provoked a critical re-examination of the natural history of the disease, and indeed it was argued by some that arterial reconstruction had no part to play in the treatment of the ischaemic leg, a concept which today would be quite unacceptable.

It was inevitable that, with new tools for diagnosis and treatment in their hands, surgeons sought to apply them to arteries other than those of the lower limb. The revelation that stroke was often related to lesions in the extracranial circulation, and hypertension to renal artery stenosis, led logically to an assault on the mesenteric circulation. However, the situation there was found to present certain difficulties. There was no clear-cut picture of the symptoms of arterial insufficiency in the gut. Abdominal pain is one of the most commonplace maladies of mankind, with a multitude of causes, many of which are emotionally rather than physically determined, and studies of post-mortem material and of angiograms carried out for reasons other than suspected alimentary disease showed that in fact the visceral arteries are very frequently the site of stenoses and occlusions which bear no discernible relationship to symptoms. Studies of intestinal function performed on patients with such occlusions usually fail to disclose any consistent derangement. In the laboratory animal, also, it was shown that gradual obliteration of the blood supply to the gut was surprisingly well tolerated and could not be linked with any abnormality of structure or function unless a fatal infarct was produced.

Here, then, was an 'illness' with no clear-cut symptoms or physical signs, whose diagnosis depended on the radiographic demonstration of lesions which, it was admitted, were often symptomless, and whose treatment demanded a difficult and dangerous operation. It was scarcely surprising that sceptics poured scorn on the whole idea. However, the fact remained that acute midgut ischaemia was almost always fatal, and that as Dunphy had observed, and others confirmed, many of the victims gave a prodromal history which, if taken seriously, might have led to a timely preventive operation. What is more, each successive year brought a few reports showing how reconstructive arterial surgery could on occasion abolish abdominal pain and to restore lost weight. The dilemma persists.

3. Over roughly the same period, pathologists were engaged in unravelling the tangled classification of inflammatory bowel disease. Apart from specific bacterial infections, two clear-cut 'granulomatous' syndromes were defined: ulcerative colitis (idiopathic proctocolitis) and Crohn's disease (regional enteritis). Although some overlap occurred, it appeared that these were two fundamentally different entities of separate causation, in each case quite undetermined. However, many cases of inflammatory bowel disease refused to fit into either category, and it seemed that some of these might in truth be of ischaemic origin. It was known from experimental studies that minor degrees of infarction could produce an acute inflammatory response in the bowel, but there appeared to be no clinical parallel. Such material was forthcoming in the late 1950s, when reports began to accumulate of the complications of aortic surgery which showed that interference with the visceral arteries could lead to a spectrum of changes in the gut wall which were not only similar to those seen experimentally but also identical to hitherto unclassified types of inflammatory bowel disease. This led to the notion of 'ischaemic colitis' and 'ischaemic enterocolitis' which are now universally accepted diagnostic categories.

However, the logical sequence of arterial blockage–ischaemia–bacterial invasion–inflammation–fibrosis cannot be the whole story, as in many cases of what may appear on clinical and pathological grounds to be ischaemic damage, no arterial occlusion can be found. It is commonplace to encounter lengths of gangrenous ileum and colon at an emergency operation, with vessels pulsating right up to the margin of the bowel. Similarly, selective angiography in the patient who presents the picture of ischaemic colitis may fail to reveal any arterial pathology, even when small vessels are catheterized and magnification techniques used. This has led to the recognition of what has been termed 'non-occlusive' intestinal ischaemia. Why the intestine should on occasion undergo sudden necrosis in spite of a (grossly) normal blood supply is a mystery which has yet to be solved.

The chapters which follow are intended to bring together what is at present known of the ways in which the arterial supply to the alimentary tract can fail, and the clinical effects which result from such failure. There are no separate chapters on radiology or histopathology, although it is of course true that without the help of these disciplines the whole subject of intestinal ischaemia would have remained unexplored. It none the less seemed better to include the radiographs and pathological illustrations along with the clinical experimental material.

REFERENCE

1. Dunphy, J.A. Abdominal pain of vascular origin *Am. J. Med. Sci.* (1936) **192**: 109–11.

Contents

1

Applied anatomy of the intestinal circulation

Introduction

This chapter is concerned with the gross and microscopic structure of the intestinal arteries, veins and lymphatics (lacteals), but mainly with the arteries, upon whose integrity depends the effective function of the alimentary tract as an absorptive, excretory, propulsive and endocrine organ. The basic outlines of this complicated structure were worked out by classic studies over a hundred years ago[1] using the Vesalian techniques of formal cadaveric dissection. Later authors[2, 3, 4] defined the detailed architecture of the system. However, such formal methods tell us little about the working of the living, moving human body, and nothing of the subvisual components of the circulation on which function depends. To conventional dissections have now been added diaphanization techniques[5] and radiological studies using selective arterial catheterization. The microvasculature has been further analysed by means of injection of prepared specimens,[6] by corrosion casts and by induced x-ray fluorescence.[7]

There are three components to the splanchnic arterial tree. First are the *main vessels* arising from the aorta, which are of great clinical importance but, because pressure within them is virtually identical to central (left ventricular) pressure, have little influence on blood flow. Second are the visible, surgically accessible vessels, knowledge of whose anatomy is essential in clinical practice — referred to in this book as the *intermediate vessels*. The *microcirculation* is the final common pathway of arteries, capillaries and venules, and has a lymphatic component. Events here, the actual territory of oxygen exchange, are the true determinants of intestinal function.[8]

The main arteries

The three main visceral arteries correspond to the embryological areas of the gastrointestinal tract: the foregut, midgut and hindgut. Of these, much the largest is the midgut, which is that part of the alimentary system which emerges into the yolk sac during the eighth week of fetal life, on the axis of its main vessel, the superior mesentery artery (SMA). The arteries to the foregut (the coeliac axis, CA) and the hindgut (the inferior mesenteric artery, IMA) convey relatively less blood to the intestine, and, through collateral pathways, their distribution extends over into extracoelomic structures (Figs. 1.1–1.4). Patterns of blood supply to the gut are variable, and in only one-half of cases is the 'classic' arrangement found.[9] For this reason it is sometimes difficult to distinguish between an anatomical difference and an abnormality caused by disease.

The coeliac axis

The coeliac axis runs straight out of the front of the aorta at the level of the first lumbar vertebra. Its origin is crossed by the fibres of the arcuate ligament of the diaphragm and by a network of sympathetic nerves. The vessel may be kinked at this point, and show a poststenotic dilatation below. (The clinical significance of this variant has caused dispute.) Almost immediately, the axis divides into its three branches (Fig. 1.2).

The splenic artery runs upwards and to the left along the upper border of the body and tail of the pancreas, and then enters the hilum of the spleen

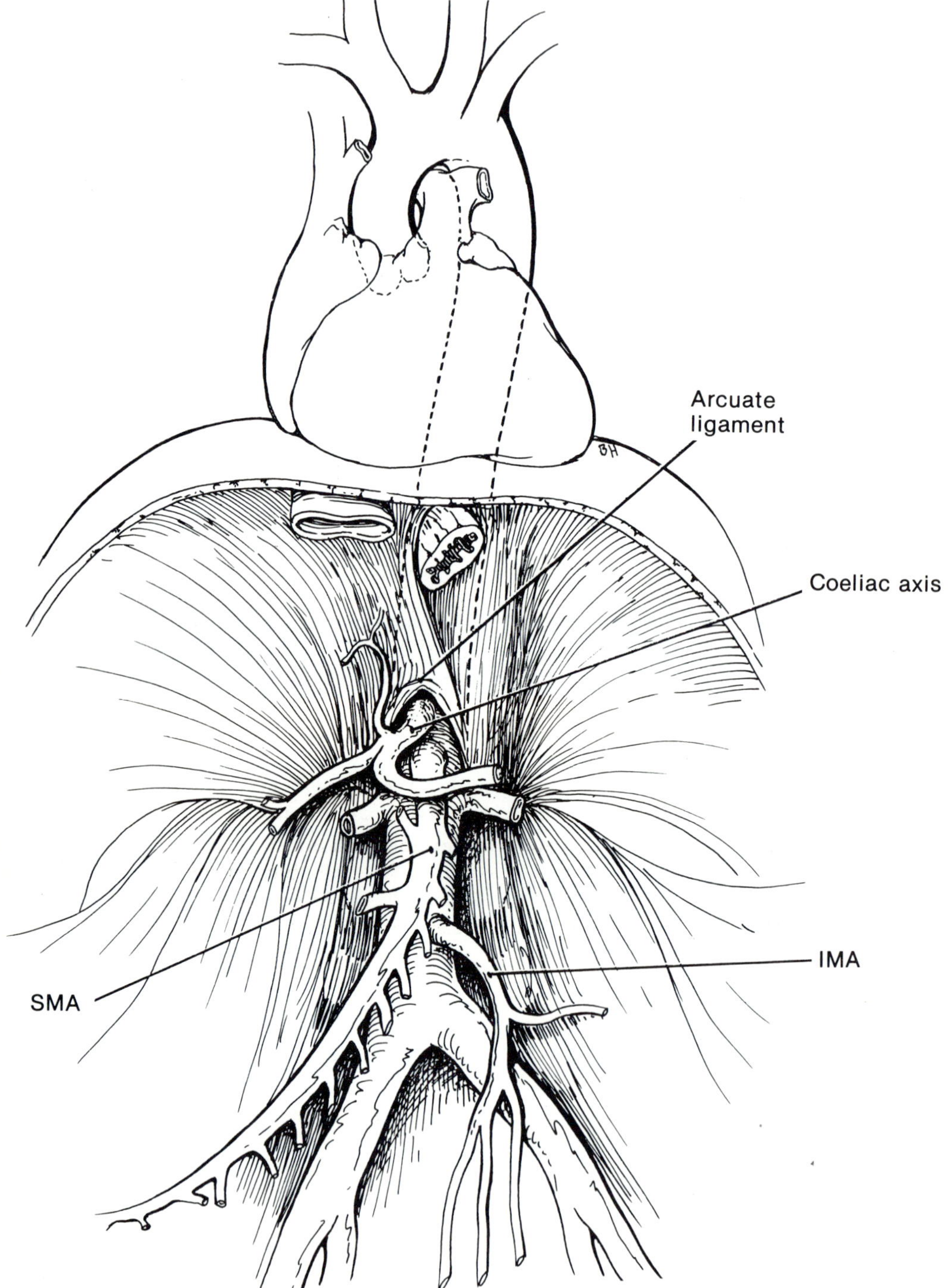

Fig. 1.1 The visceral branches of the aorta.

where it divides into four to twelve branches, some of which supply the spleen substance and others run as the vasa brevia to the greater curve of the stomach, where they anastomose with the left gastroepiploic artery. The splenic artery is unusual in that it does not run a direct course but is wavy and tortuous throughout its length. (This feature can sometimes be put to surgical use, in that the

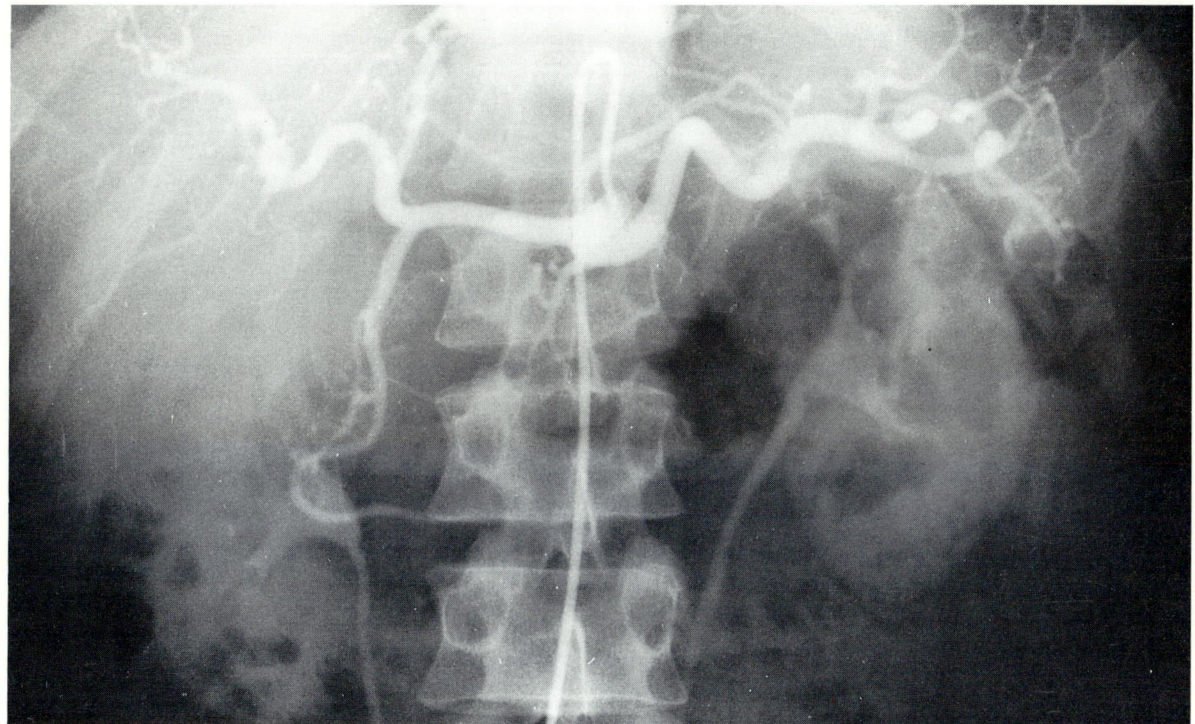

Fig. 1.2 Selective angiogram showing distribution of the CA.

spleen may be removed and the splenic artery mobilized, straightened out and brought down to other parts of the mesenteric circulation to irrigate an ischaemic area.)

The left gastric artery runs directly forwards from the coeliac axis to reach the midpoint of the lesser curve of the stomach. Here it divides into upper and lower branches. The upper branch supplies the upper part of the lesser curve and connects with the oesophageal arteries, the phrenic branches of the aorta and the lower intercostals. The lower branch runs down to anastomose with the right gastric artery around the pyloric antrum. This artery sometimes gives important supply to the liver via a large accessory left hepatic artery which runs across the lesser omentum.

The hepatic artery runs to the right, along the upper border of the head of the pancreas, to the first part of the duodenum. Here it gives off the large and important gastroduodenal artery, which grooves the pancreas as it runs down behind the first part of the duodenum to supply that structure and the head and uncinate process of the pancreas. The main trunk of the hepatic artery turns upwards and to the right to enter the free edge of the lesser omentum, in a variable relationship to the portal vein and common bile duct but usually lying anterior and to the left. It passes up to the hilum of the liver and divides into right and left branches which supply the respective 'lobes' of the liver which do not, however, correspond with the pattern of venous and biliary drainage.

In the non-cirrhotic liver some two-thirds of the oxygen and nutritional requirement are met by the portal vein, so that occlusion of the hepatic artery is relatively well tolerated. It used to be thought that interruption of this vessel led inevitably to necrosis of the liver, but such is not in fact the case, and the hepatic artery is quite frequently tied deliberately, as part of the treatment of metastatic tumours. Conversely, when the SMA is occluded, the hepatic artery may contribute significantly to the blood supply of the gut, without any deleterious effect on liver function.

The superior mesenteric artery

The superior mesenteric artery (SMA) is by far the

most important vessel of the alimentary tract. It arises from the front of the aorta, usually just above the renal arteries and at the level of the L1/2 intervertebral disc. At its origin it is 1–5 cm in diameter. It runs immediately in front of the neck of the pancreas, crosses behind the uncinate process, and then passes in front of the third part of the duodenum to enter the mesentery of the small intestine. This area can sometimes be seen on a barium study as a band of translucency running vertically across the duodenum. If the proximal duodenum appears dilated, this normal finding may be misinterpreted as representing an obstruction, to which clinical symptoms are then attributed. In fact, the syndrome of 'duodenal ileus' has little factual evidence to sustain it, and has never been confirmed by endoscopy. This band of translucency probably also accounts for the mythical 'sphincter of Ochsner' analogous to the high pressure zones at the ileocaecal valve and the rectosigmoid junction.

Just as the left hepatic artery can arise from the left gastric, so the right hepatic artery may originate as the first branch of the SMA, running up under the uncinate process and through the pancreas.[4]

The first branch of the SMA is the inferior pancreatoduodenal artery, which passes up behind the head of the pancreas to join the superior pancreatoduodenal branch of the gastroduodenal artery. These small vessels have considerable clinical importance. In the first place, they provide a major part of the blood supply to the head of the pancreas and the lower part of the common bile duct, and thus must be carefully preserved whenever the pancreas is partially resected. More important, this anastomosis represents the main collateral pathway between the arterial territories of the coeliac axis and the superior mesenteric artery, and is capable of a remarkable degree of dilatation if the SMA becomes occluded (see Figs. 1.16 and 1.17).

The origin of the SMA, lying well back in the

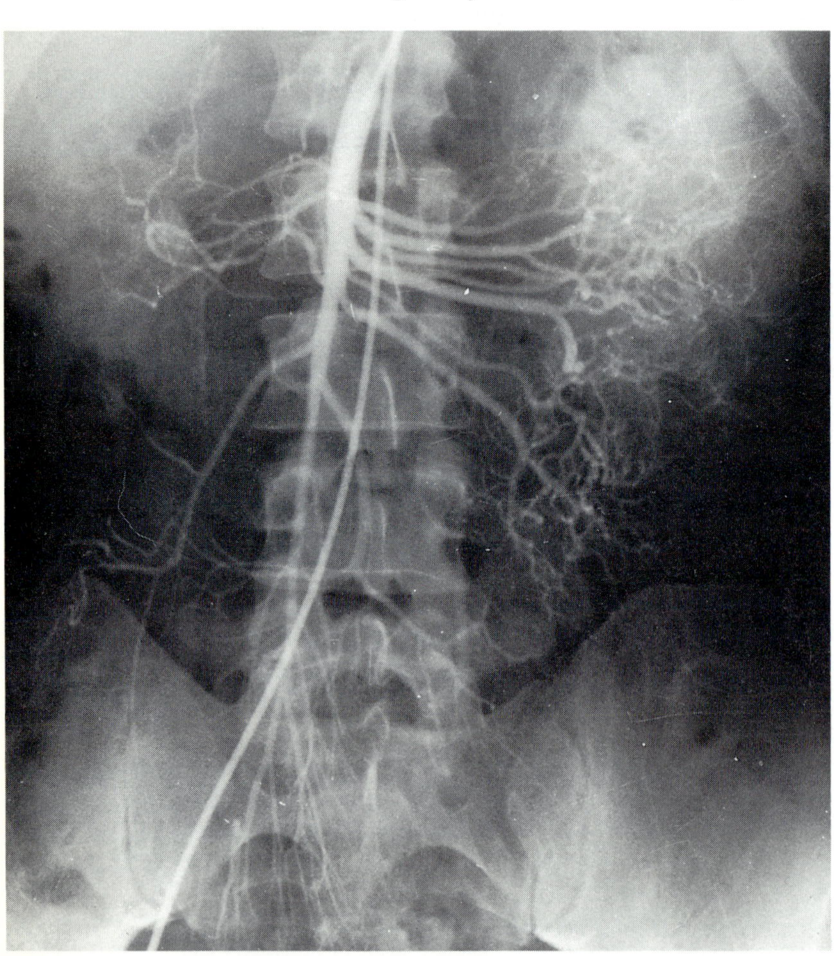

Fig. 1.3 Selective angiogram showing distribution of the SMA.

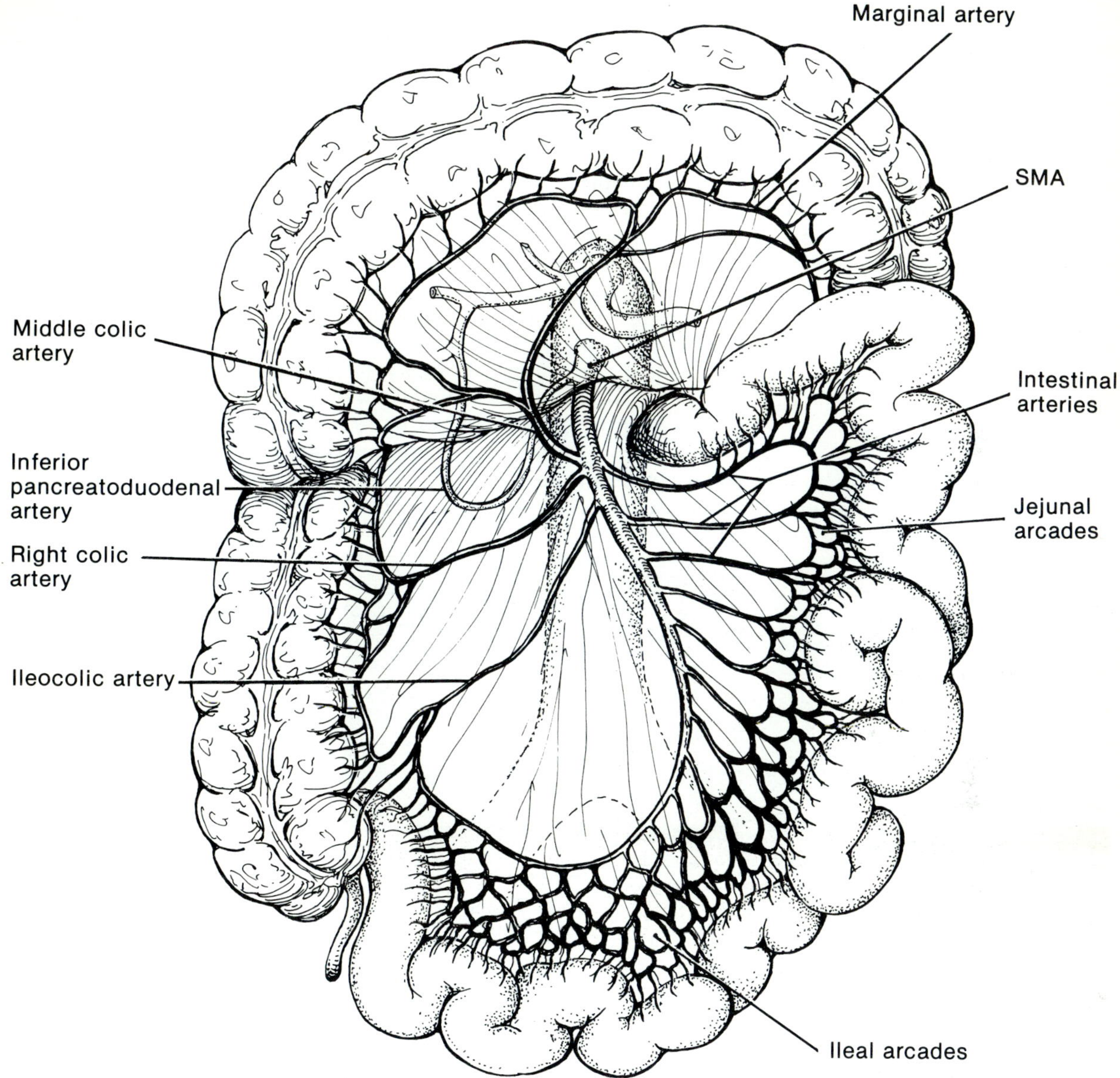

Fig. 1.4 Detailed distribution of the SMA.

upper part of the abdominal cavity and surrounded by pancreas, sympathetic nerve fibres, portal vein and duodenum, is one of the most inaccessible structures in the human body. It is almost impossible to expose it without a full thoraco-abdominal incision, which constitutes a major anatomical insult. For this reason, operations on the area of origin are best avoided, and when possible the vascular problem should be solved by an indirect approach.

Emerging from behind the duodenum, the SMA passes downwards in the root of the small bowel mesentery towards the right iliac fossa, usually with a left-sided convexity. The first branch after the inferior pancreatoduodenal artery is the middle colic artery, which springs from the right side of the vessel, enters the transverse mesocolon and divides into left and right branches, which constitute part of the important marginal supply to the colon (see below). The right colic artery, which is usually quite small, arises some 4 cm further down, and the ileo-colic 4 cm below that. The main trunk of the SMA passes downwards to enter the marginal colonic circulation as the ileocolic artery. Of these three right-sided colonic vessels, the only constant artery is the ileocolic,[4] which supplies the base of the right colon. The right and middle colic arteries have a variable pattern of origin from the main trunk[4] and often arise in common. In 10 per cent of cases the right colic artery arises from the ileocolic.[9]

The small bowel circulation comes from the left side of the SMA via the so-called 'intestinal arteries' which vary in number between three and twenty, and from a series of arcades which increase in number and complexity from above downwards (Fig. 1.4).

The inferior mesenteric artery

The inferior mesenteric artery (IMA) (Figs. 1.5 and 1.6) is a very much smaller vessel than are the coeliac axis and the SMA. It arises from the left anterior face of the aorta some 4 cm above the bifurcation, and for the first 2 cm of its course is buried within the aortic wall. Typically, it then gives off one or two downward-running branches to the sigmoid colon, and an important upward-running left colic artery which gives rise to three or four vasa recta before joining the marginal artery to the colon. It then runs downwards behind the rectosigmoid junction and rectum, and ends as the superior haemorrhoidal artery which divides into three major arterial trunks, one on the left and two on the right. The collateral circulation from the branches of the internal iliac artery (that is to say, the middle haemorrhoidal branch of the pudendal artery) anastomoses freely with this lower territory of the inferior mesenteric (Fig. 1.7).

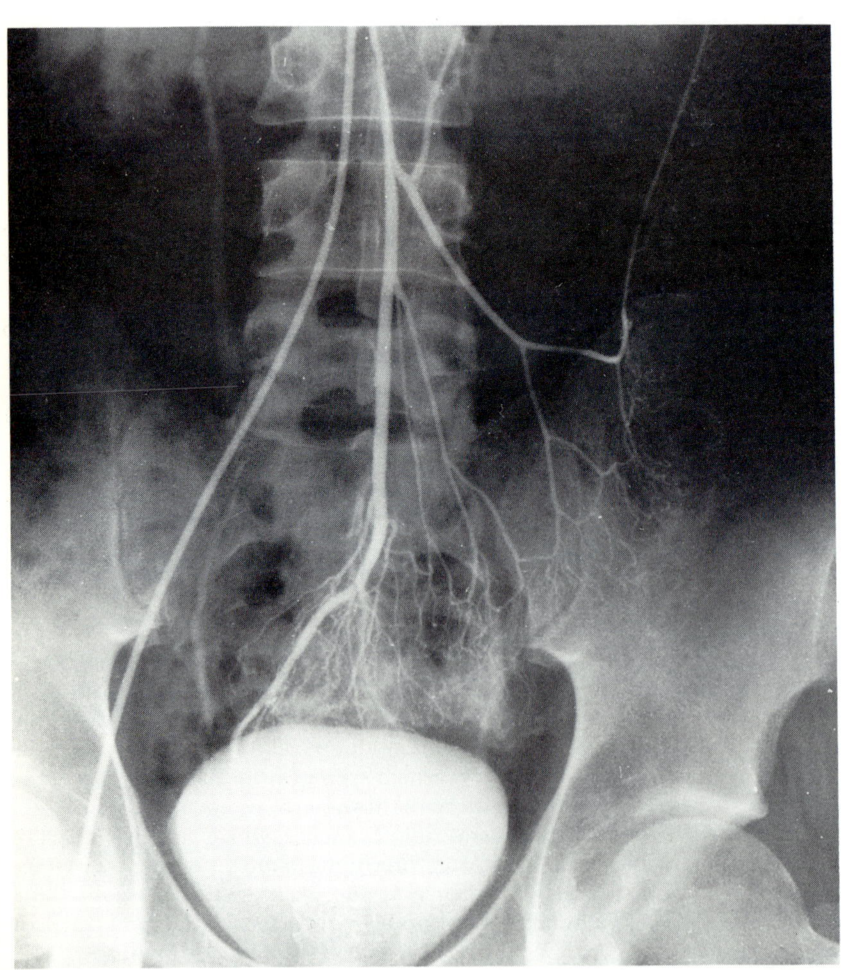

Fig. 1.5 Selective angiogram showing distribution of the IMA.

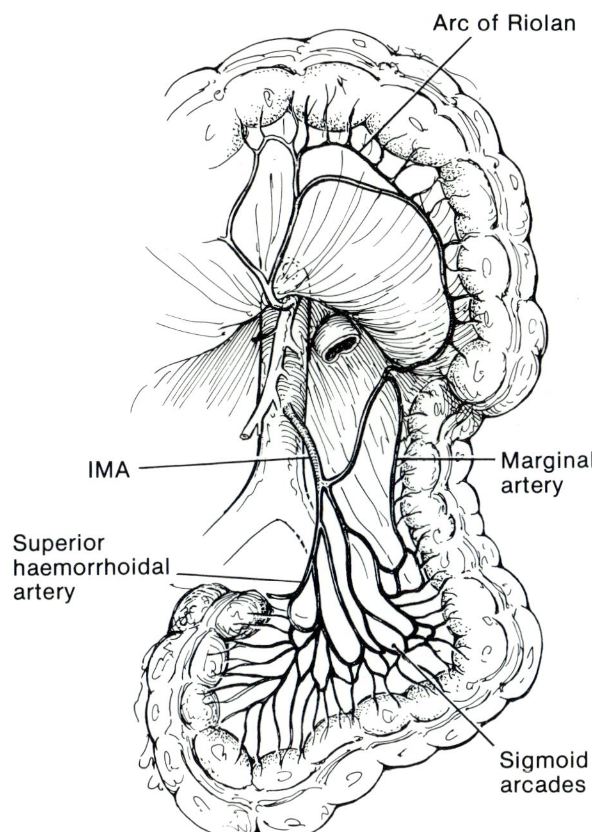

Fig. 1.6 Detailed distribution of the IMA.

The intermediate arteries

Lying between the three major aortic branches and the microscopic plexuses which supply the intimate structures there is a network of anatomically visible trunks which are of clinical importance because they may be the seat of intrinsic disease or may be damaged by incidental or surgical trauma. The intermediate circulation comprises the intestinal vessels and the arcade systems of the small bowel, and the marginal circulation and the vasa recta of the colon. Interruption of an individual vessel in this system produces no damage to the mucosal circulation nor to the function of the bowel. However, if several vessels are involved, as may occur from embolus or atheromatous thrombosis, from a wound or haematoma, or from a badly planned surgical resection, considerable damage to the bowel may follow, even to the extent of complete necrosis. Because of the arrangement of the vessels, injuries which occur at right angles to the long axis of the bowel are less dangerous than those which run parallel to it.

At its beginning, the branches of the SMA to the small bowel are narrow, spaced at intervals of 1–2 cm and do not form an arcade system. Proceeding downwards along the small bowel, the system becomes more complicated and a series of three to four parallel arcades develops (see Fig. 1.4). A sort of anatomical watershed exists at the terminal ileum, which is reflected in embryology.

At the 17 mm stage the most distal right-sided branch of the SMA (the future ileocolic artery) vascularizes the ensemble formed by the caecum, the appendix and the terminal ileum. This vessel forms the only collateral to the distal portion of the umbilical loop.

Thus, in the course of development, two different vascular territories of the SMA appear:

1. The proximal segment of the umbilical loop, which comprises the third and fourth parts of the duodenum, the whole of the jejunum and most of the ileum, is supplied by a network of collaterals arising from the left side of the artery.
2. The distal segment of this loop, formed by the terminal ileum, the caecum, the ascending colon and the greater part of the transverse colon, is vascularized by two or three branches originating from the right side of the artery.

This explains why the region between these two segments of the ileum, one belonging to a territory receiving numerous vessels and the other supplied by few branches, has gained the reputation of having a poor blood supply. In fact, recent studies[5] have demonstrated that this view is incorrect as regards the adult anatomy. The vasa recta are the same in number and disposition up to the last 5 cm of ileum, after which they become more sparse. However, the terminal ileum segment receives some recurrent blood supply from vessels to the caecum (Fig. 1.8).

The overall pattern of distribution of the intermediate vessels to the small bowel is represented in Fig 1.4. Of greater clinical importance, however, are the intermediate vessels to the colon (see Fig. 1.6).

The marginal artery to the colon

This is formed by the union of the three main colonic branches, which arise from the right side of the SMA and then continue around the splenic

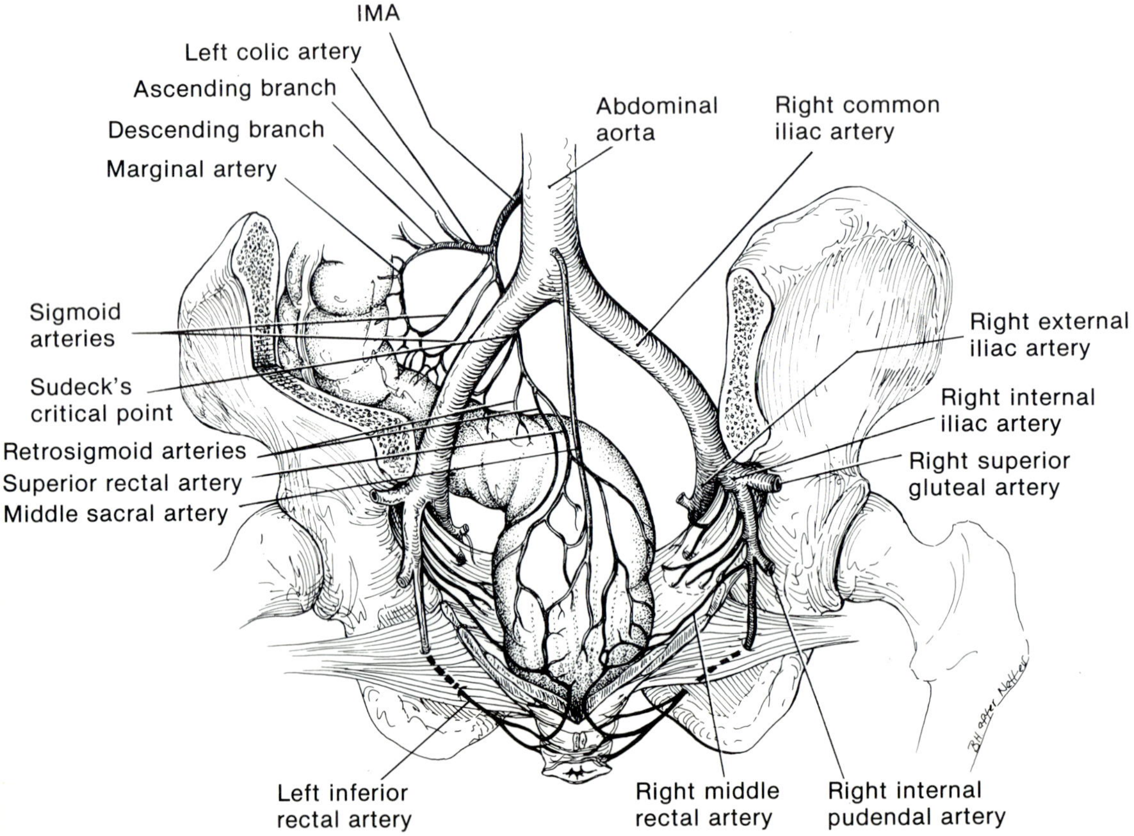

Fig. 1.7 The arteries to the recto-sigmoid showing anastomosis between IMA and internal iliac systems (seen from behind).

flexure to join the upward-running left colic branch of the IMA. This is a very important vessel, whose detailed anatomy is now precisely known.[4, 10, 11]

The arrangement of vessels along the right colon is fairly constant, there being one marginal artery giving off vasa recta and vasa brevia which occasionally communicate, although the anastomoses are less developed than in the arcades of the small bowel. It is at the point of junction of superior and inferior mesenteric systems (at the splenic flexure) that confusion and variability occur.

The IMA divides into two or three branches, the uppermost of which (the left colic) almost always reaches the splenic flexure. Here it bifurcates, the slender outer branch joining the left branch of the middle colic to form the marginal artery (of Drummond) of the colon, the inner (large) branch running back into the trunk of the middle colic artery to form an additional arcade, the arc of

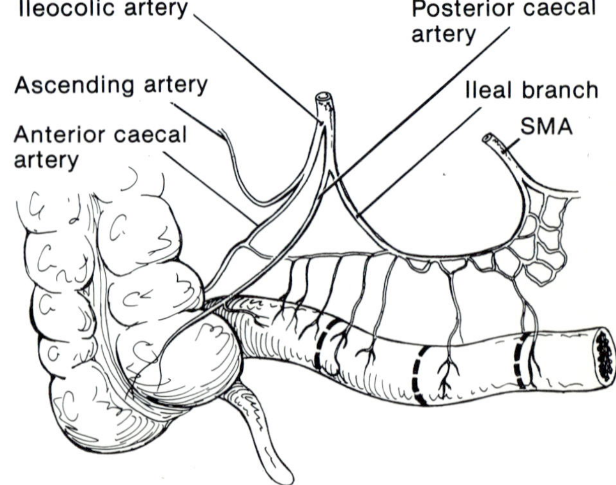

Fig. 1.8 The arteries to the ileocaecal region.

Riolan (Fig. 1.9). The outer anastomosis is here often small or incomplete, so the continuity of the marginal artery is broken. If the arc of Riolan is not well developed, there exists here a critical area of anastomotic supply, so impairment of flow in either the SMA or the IMA will not be compensated, and may result in ischaemic damage. This concept is confirmed by the frequency of ischaemic lesions at the splenic flexure (see Chapter 9).

Where there is a requirement for collateral flow, the arc of Riolan will dilate according to a number of well-established radiological patterns (see below). There are also a number of aberrant arteries which supply this area of the colon, arising as primary anatomical variations or forming extracoelomic pathways. Gross dilatation of this artery (Fig. 1.10) suggests a haemodynamically significant obstruction of the SMA.[9]

The detailed lower anatomy of the IMA is subject to many variations, but is of less clinical significance than the arrangements higher up in the bowel because of the rich communication with the internal iliac system. It used to be taught that a critical point[12] existed between the last sigmoid branch and the superior haemorrhoidal arteries, but more detailed anatomical studies[6, 9, 10] have shown that this is not the case.

The terminal vessels to the hindgut are the middle and inferior rectal arteries (see Fig. 1.7).

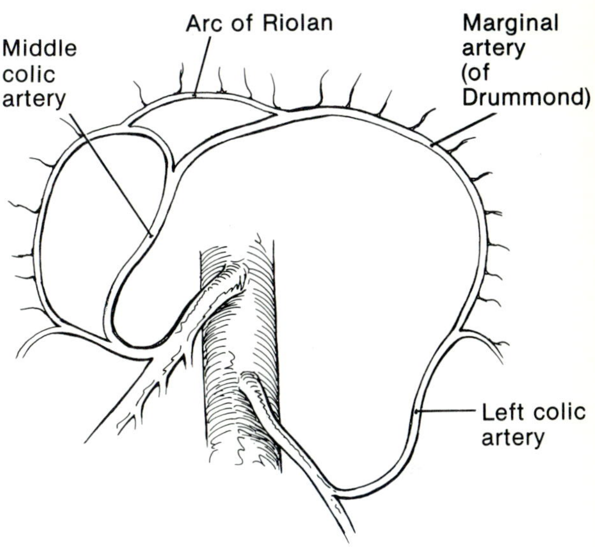

Fig. 1.9 The arc of Riolan and the arc of Drummond.

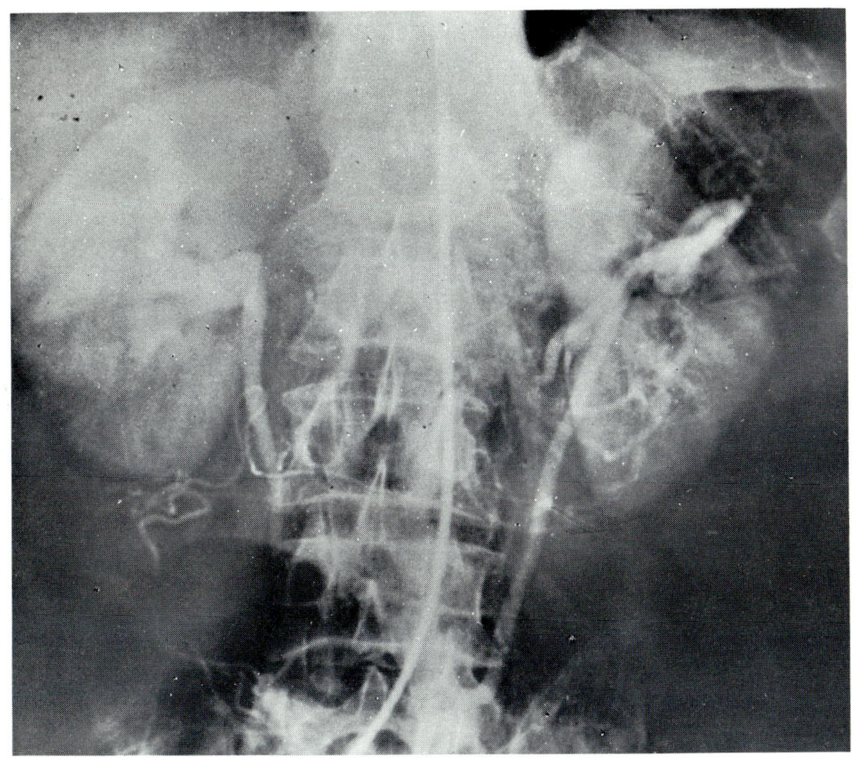

Fig. 1.10 Dilatation of the marginal artery of the colon.

The middle rectal artery arises either directly from the internal iliac or from one of its main divisions, and usually anastomoses with the lower branches of the IMA outside the rectal wall.

The inferior rectal artery arises constantly from the inferior pudendal, below the origin of the levator ani muscle, and supplies blood to the lower, non-endodermal parts of the alimentary tract (i.e. the anal canal with its intrinsic and extrinsic muscles) and the ischiorectal fossa. It anastomoses freely with the superior and middle rectal arteries and also with the median sacral artery (vestigial in man but of great importance in caudate animals) (see Fig. 1.7).

As in the small bowel, the colonic arcade gives rise to vasa recta which pass round alternate aspects of the colon, then divide into anterior and posterior branches which run to the edges of the antimesenteric taeniae, where they again divide, and pierce the circular muscle. From the origins of the vasa recta the vasa brevia run to the mesenteric attachment, anastomose there, and finally pierce the muscle on either side of the mesenteric taeniae (Fig. 1.11).

The microcirculation

The intramural vessels

Small branches arise from both vasa recta and vasa brevia which run outwards to supply the peritoneal coat and (in the case of the colon) the appendices epiploicae. Beneath the serosa is formed an external muscular plexus. Having pierced the muscle, the arteries unite into a rich *submucosal plexus* (with a few backward-running branches into the external plexus) which extends as a continuous layer over the length of the bowel, composed of a coarse meshwork arranged in roughly rectangular pattern. Between the vessels in this network there lies a smaller fine mesh from which spring the arterioles running up the villi, or between the crypts, to supply the mucous membrane itself. The submucosal plexus is richer and better developed in the small intestine than in the colon,[13] which helps to explain the former's capacity to withstand ischaemic insult.

More recent studies[7, 14] have shed light on the ultrastructure of the intimate circulation to the bowel, making use of γ-ray-induced x-ray fluorescence of specimens injected with barium, a technique which provides an index of comparative blood flow throughout the layers of the bowel. The use of this medium is convenient as it allows confirmatory visualization of the small vessels by conventional radiography. Uniform perfusion with contrast medium was observed in all bowel wall layers. Variations in luminal diameter and vessel irregularities were infrequent. The measurements appear well reproducible.

It was confirmed that vascular density is most pronounced in the mucosal and submucosal layers of the bowel wall (Fig. 1.12): the large tortuous

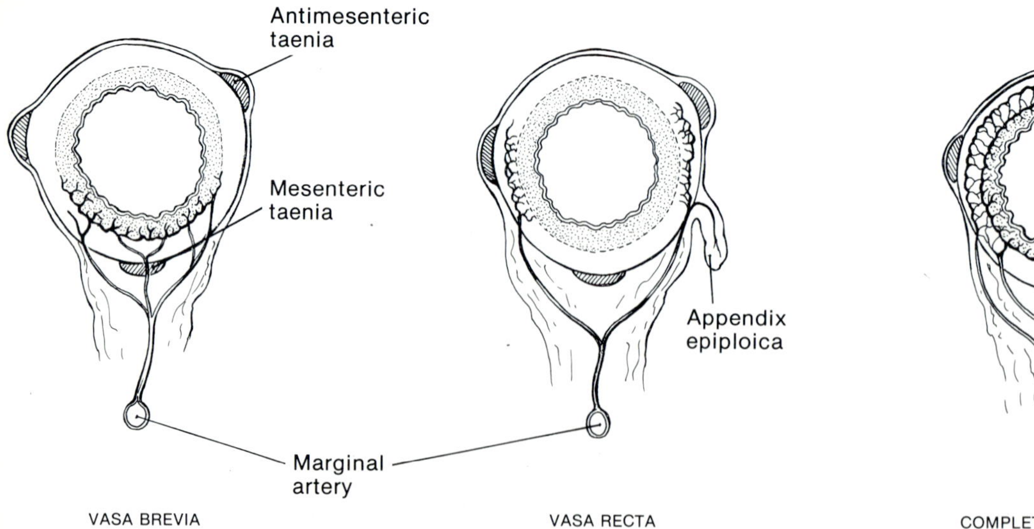

Fig. 1.11 The vasa recta and the vasa brevia.

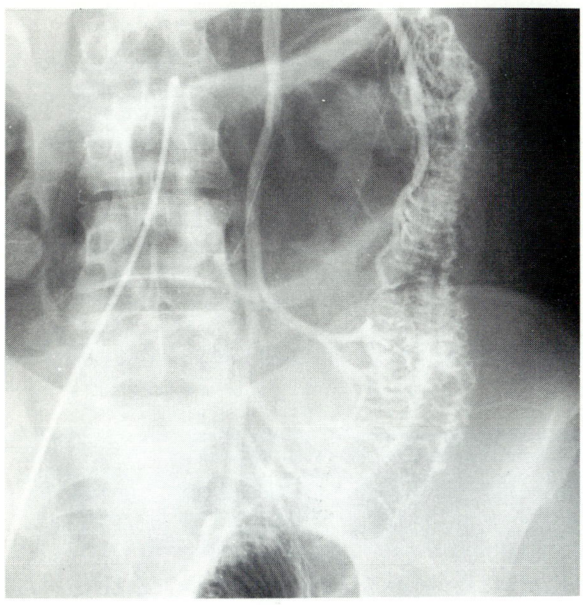

Fig. 1.12 Angiogram showing the termination of the IMA. (By courtesy of Professor F. Tongio and Dr J.J. Wenger.)

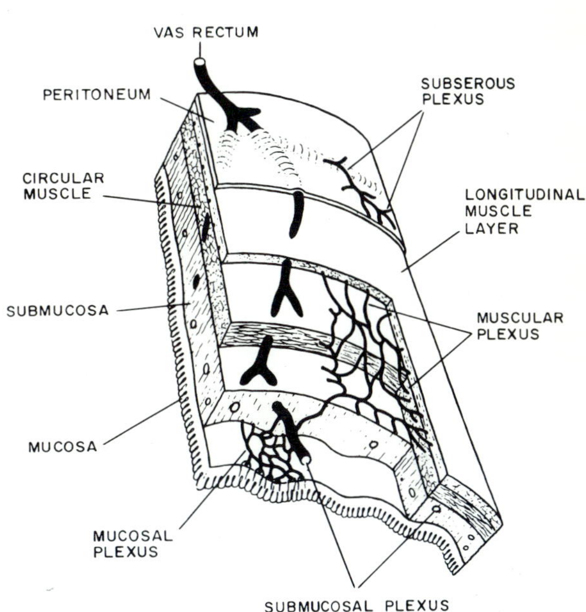

Fig. 1.13 The intramural plexuses.

vessel in the submucosa gives rise to smaller vessels which supply the mucosa and muscularis propria; in the muscle layer there lies a freely anastomosing network of vascular channels. In the colon the mucosal capillaries were closely packed together and regularly arranged. The vascular pattern of the villi observed in the ileum consisted of a central arteriole which branched at the tip into several capillaries which formed a rich anastomotic network on the surface.

However, there are considerable age differences. The incidence of fibrous intimal hyperplasia of the small intramural arteries and arterioles is greater in older patients and in those with hypertension or diabetes. The degree of this change was in general mild, but produced some narrowing of the lumina of these small vessels (Figs. 1.13 and 1.14).

A highly significant negative correlation was found between barium concentration and age in the samples of the whole bowel, the muscularis propria and the mucosa/submucosa, but no significant correlation exists between the distribution of barium between the mucosa/submucosa and muscularis propria and the age of the subject.

The authors concluded that, although the degree of fibrous intimal hyperplasia may not be severe in any individual vessel, these lesions cause an overall reduction in microvascular space and a redistribution of blood flow, factors which, particularly during low perfusion, may predispose the bowel to ischaemia.

Arteriovenous anastomoses

The significance of arteriovenous anastomoses (AVA) is disputed. Although Spanner[15] was confident of his demonstration of arteriovenous connections in the submucous plexus of the gut wall, later authorities are less certain.[16] Such anastomoses are not easy to identify. Most authors seem to agree that they are few and far between, and probably not of great functional importance. These communications are more easily demonstrated in the stomach than in the small bowel, although their existence even here has been disputed.[17]

The circulation to the villus

Vessels from the submucosal plexus contribute a single arteriole to each villus, about 20 μm in diameter, which runs up the central stroma and becomes capillarized (in other words, loses its smooth muscle coat) at a short distance beyond its base. As the tip of the villus is approached, the

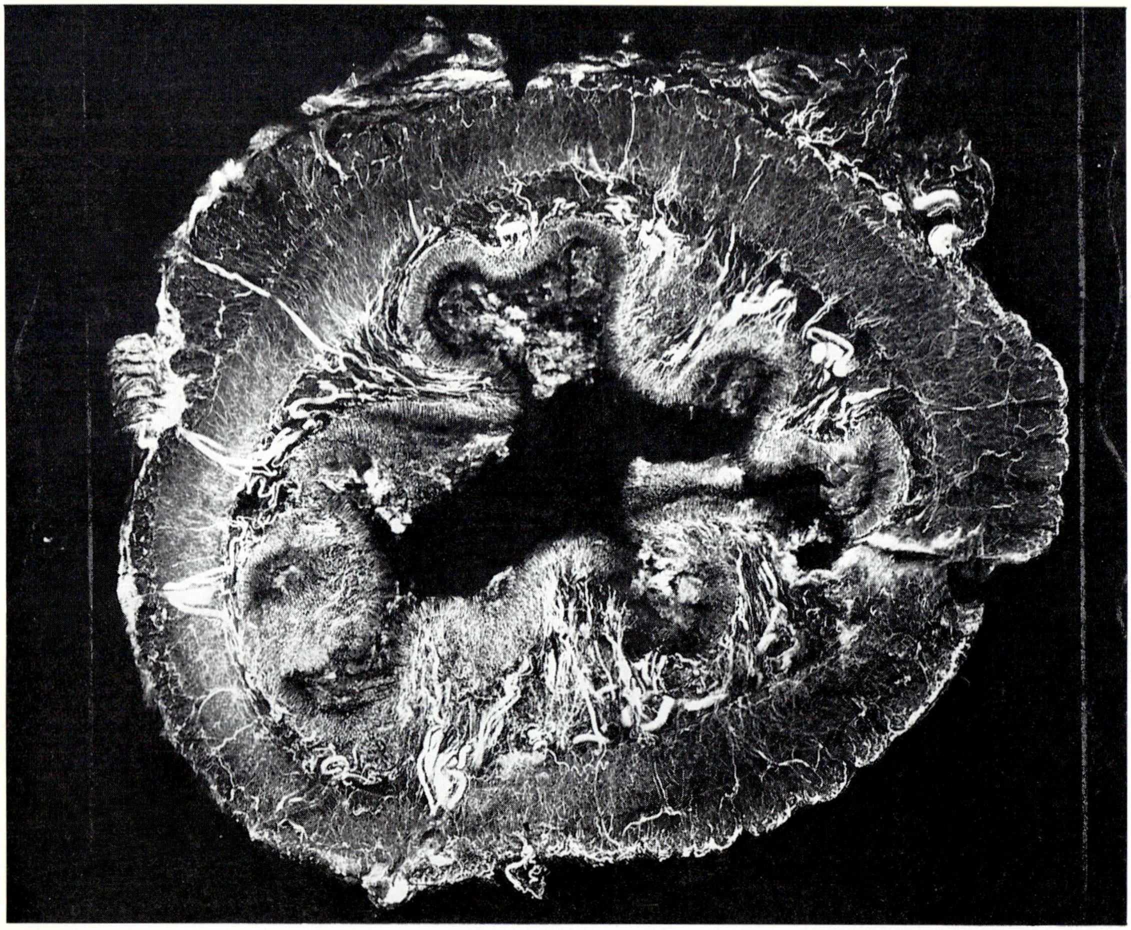

Fig. 1.14 Injected specimen demonstrating the pattern of microcirculation to the colon. (By courtesy of Mr N.D. Carr and Mr P.F. Schofield.)

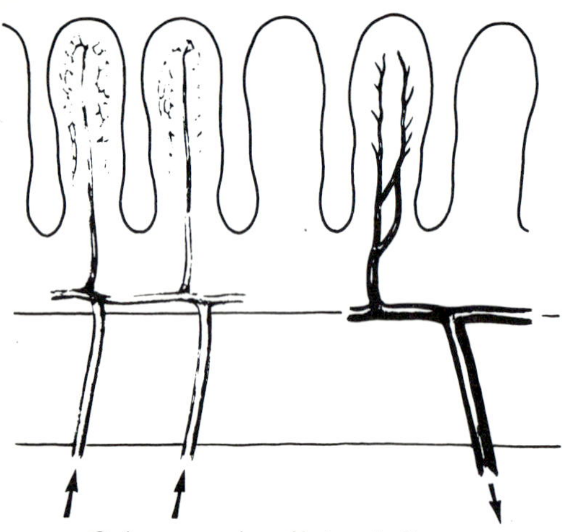

Submucosal collateral flow
3x nutritional needs
Redistribution
Countercurrent exchange

Fig. 1.15 Plan of the microcirculation to the villus.

arteriole begins to arborize, and eventually divides into a very complicated system of fine subepithelial channels, which eventually drain into a central vein (Fig. 1.15). (See also Chapter 2).

The relationship between the minute arteries and minute veins in the villous circulation is extremely close, and how much actual anatomical shunting takes place has for long been a matter of debate. This is of crucial importance in the maintenance of the mucosal circulation in hypotensive states and in the production of pseudomembranes.

The arterial and venous loops in the villi are arranged in the same 'hairpin' pattern as is seen in the nephron, which is the basis of countercurrent exchange of oxygen and nutrients. The aspect of the capillary which faces the epithelium is thin and contains pores, whereas the opposite side which bears the cell nucleus is thicker and without pores. This question of porosity is discussed in Chapter 2.

Pathological anatomy: the importance of collateral pathways

The coeliac axis

The CA may be occluded by atheroma, by fibromuscular hyperplasia or by a malignant tumour, but the usual anatomical lesion is compression by the fibres of the arcuate ligament of the diaphragm, which may or may not give rise to symptoms.[18] The distal branches of the coeliac axis are rarely affected by disease.

The territory irrigated by the coeliac axis has a rich collateral supply from:

1. The lower intercostal branches, via the abdominal wall.
2. The phrenic branches of the aorta.
3. The lower oesophageal arteries, which perfuse the fundus and upper part of the body of the stomach via the mucosal and submucosal plexuses.

Occlusion of the CA results in comparatively little disturbance in blood supply to the upper abdominal organs. The few flow studies[18] which have been carried out in cases of coeliac axis compression do not suggest that this causes any major degree of ischaemia, such as would interfere with function.

The superior mesenteric artery

It used to be thought that the SMA was either totally or partially occluded in most subjects over the age of 55, as determined by random autopsy and radiological studies.[19, 20] However, recent work has shown the incidence to be much less.[21]

Because of its angle of emergence from the aorta, it accepts emboli with readiness, and mesenteric embolus has been a classically recognized complication of atrial fibrillation, mural thrombosis of the left ventricle and aortic atheroma. In the last decade, however, because of the decline in rheumatic heart disease and the better control of

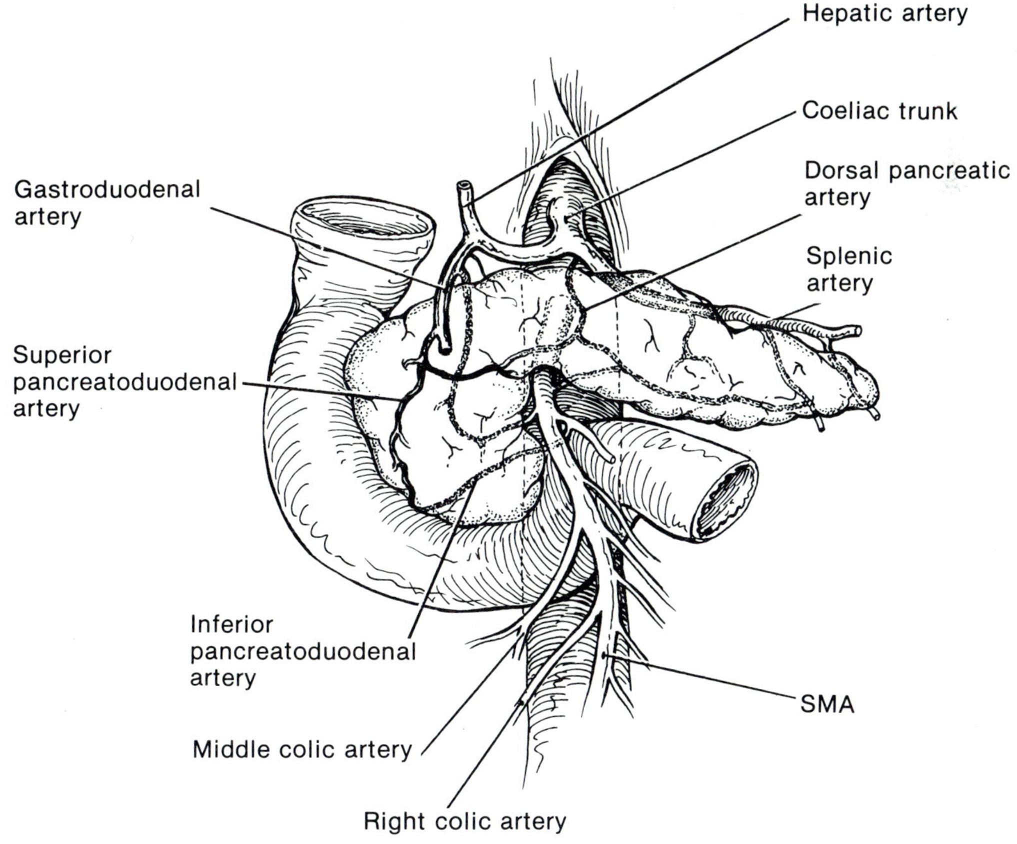

Fig. 1.16 Detail of the pancreatic arcades.

acute endocardial ischaemia, all types of arterial embolism have become rare, and the gut is no exception. Nevertheless, in contrast to what obtains in the coeliac axis, the upper and lower routes of collateral supply to the main midgut loop are ill developed and precarious, and if the main vessel is occluded the results are serious. The midgut can be perfused from above via the mucosal plexuses of the duodenum, which are supplied by the gastric and gastroepiploic arcades, and also from extracoelomic vessels. The most obvious route of supply is via the pancreatic vessels which can enlarge very considerably if required (Figs. 1.16 and 1.17). There may be a single or a double connecting channel between the SMA and the CA depending on the configuration of the superior and inferior pancreatoduodenal arteries. Less conspicuously, the dorsal pancreatic artery, which may originate from either SMA or CA, can carry blood backwards if either main trunk is blocked.

These routes of perfusion, when combined, may allow as much as 50 cm of jejunum to remain viable when the SMA has been abruptly blocked. Indeed, it is unusual for the whole midgut loop to die following a mesenteric embolus, given early diagnosis (see Chapter 6). When the blockage occurs more gradually, development of other anastomotic channels may support a small intestine which shows no structural abnormality whatever (see Chapter 7).

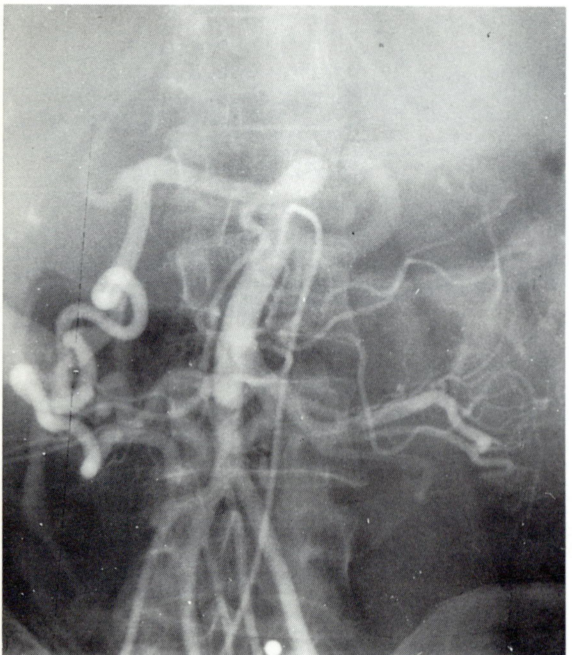

Fig. 1.17 Dilatation of the pancreatic arcade, following obstruction of the SMA.

From below, the contribution of the SMA is augmented by blood arriving from the marginal and intramural circulations of the colon. The main route of supply here is, of course, the inferior mesenteric artery, via the anastomotic circulation already described, but the large intestine also obtains a variable quantity of arterial blood from the abdominal wall. Occlusion of the SMA, therefore, affects the colon when (1) the block has occurred proximal to the origin of the middle colic artery, or (2) the IMA is occluded.

The inferior mesenteric artery

The IMA is often atherosclerotic[19, 20] but does not often receive emboli. Occlusion close to its origin is well tolerated. The main surgical importance of the artery lies in its involvement in atheromatous lesions of the aorta, and in the need to find the correct site of its ligation in the course of colonic resections.

The IMA is almost always interrupted during the repair of an abdominal aortic aneurysm, since it arises from the sac. The artery will often have been already blocked but, even if still patent, it can usually be safely tied provided that the ligature is applied in the intra-aortic part of the vessel, thereby preserving the vital sigmoid branches and the marginal circulation to the colon. Nevertheless, there is a certain incidence of ischaemic damage to the large bowel following aortic reconstruction, which is discussed in Chapter 9, and in case of doubt the IMA should be reimplanted into the prosthesis (see Fig. 10.2).

The rich route of collateral supply to the anal canal and lower rectum via the internal iliac arteries has already been described.

Comparative anatomy

There are enormous species differences, related in the main to dietary habit. These should be borne in mind by any researcher who aims to resolve a clinical problem related to the mesenteric circulation, in the animal laboratory. For example, it was shown forty years ago[22] that, whereas the SMA is the sole route of supply to the midgut loop in all mammals, there are considerable differences where the distal circulation is concerned. On the whole the chimpanzee, the opossum and, to a lesser extent, the rabbit resemble man, but the dog, cat and other carnivores are quite different. Nevertheless, almost all experimental work in this field has been carried out on dogs and cats.

The main differences between the dog and man are:

1. The dog has a common colic artery which arises above the inferior pancreatoduodenal and supplies the whole colon.
2. The vasa recta intercommunicate in the dog.
3. The number of arcades in the dog remain few and fairly constant from jejunum to ileum.
4. The subserosal plexus is much less well developed.

The veins and lymphatics

The anatomy of the effluent vessels of the intestinal tract has received little study, as they follow so closely the paths of the arteries. The alimentary veins are notable in that they contain no valves so that flow can take place in either direction and changes in portal pressure are communicated directly to the gut wall. In other words, tissue pressure in the intestine is influenced by events in the liver rather than in the systemic circulation. The portal system of veins is of large capacity and in many species can expand and 'pool' a considerable proportion of the blood volume. This probably does not take place in man.

The lymphatics here have a special role to play in that, rather than simply draining tissue fluid, they are a major route of absorption of nutrients. The osmotic effect of chyle is much greater than that of lymph, and the effect on intestinal function of chylous ascites (as may occur from congenital lymphatic abnormalities) is an unexplored area.

References

1. Heller, A. Über die Blutgefässe des Dünndarmes. *Berliner Sächsige gesamte Wissenschaft* (1872) **24**: 165–171.
2. Lardennois, G., Okinczyc, J. La véritable terminaison de l'artère mésentérique supérieure *Bull. Mem. Soc. Anat. Paris* (1910) **85**: 12–23.
3. Corsy, E., Aubert, A. Artères de l'intestin grêle et des colons. *Bibliogr. Anat.* (1913) **23**: 221–54.
4. Michels, N.A. *Blood Supply and Anatomy of Upper Abdominal Organs, with Descriptive Atlas.* Philadelphia: J.B. Lippincott (1955).
5. Chevrel, J.P., Guéraud, J.P. Arteries of the terminal ileum. *Anatomia Clinica* (1978) **1**: 95–108.
6. Reiner, L., Rodriguez, F.L., Jimenez, F.A., Platt, R. Injection studies on mesenteric arterial circulation. *Arch. Path.* (1962) **73**: 461–72.
7. Carr, N.D., Schofield, P.F. The colonic microcirculation. In Givel, J.-C., Saegesser, F., eds. *Colo-Proctology*, Berlin, Heidelberg, New York, Tokyo: Springer, (1984): 11–25.
8. Marston, A. Basic structure and function of the intestinal circulation. *Clin. Gastroenterol.* (1972) **1**: 429–41.
9. Baum, S. Normal anatomy and collateral pathways of the mesenteric circulation. In: Boley, S.J., ed. *Vascular Disorders of the Intestine*, New York, London: Appleton-Century-Crofts (1971): 3–18.
10. Griffiths, J.D. Extramural and intramural blood supply of the colon. *Br. Med. J.* (1961) **1**: 323–6.
11. Bernardo, M.O. de M. *Alguns aspectos da vascularizacào parietal do colon.* Thesis, University of Lisbon (1974): 46–47.
12. Sudek, P. Über die Gefassversorgung des Mastdarmes im Hinsicht auf die Operative Gangrän. *Münch. Med. Wochenschr.* (1907) **54**: 13–14.
13. Spjut, H.J., Margulis, A.R., McAlister, W.H. Microangiographic study of gastrointestinal lesions. *Am. J. Roentgenol.* (1964) **92**: 1173–87.
14. Carr, N.D., Schofield, P.F., Pullen, B.R. A method for the determination of microvascular volume in tissue samples. *Clin. Phys. Physiol. Meas.* (1984) **5**: 21–7.
15. Spanner, R. Neue Befende über die Blutwege der Darmwand und ihre funktionelle Bedeutung. *Morphol. Jahrbuch* (1940) **69**: 394–434.
16. Boulter, P.S., Parks, A.G. Submucosal vascular patterns of the alimentary tract and their significance. *Br. J. Surg.* (1960) **47**: 546–9.
17. Delaney, J.P. The paucity of arteriovenous anastomoses in the stomach. *Surgery* (1975) **78**: 411–13.
18. Marston, A., Kieny, R., Szilagyi, D.E., Taylor, G.W. Intestinal ischemia — a panel by correspondence. *Arch. Surg.* (1976) **111**: 107–12.
19. Carucci, J.J. Mesenteric vascular occlusions. *Am. J. Surg.* (1953) **85**: 47–51.
20. Derrick, J.R., Pollard, H.S., Moore, R.M. The patterns of arteriosclerotic narrowing of the celiac and superior mesenteric arteries. *Ann. Surg.* (1959) **149**: 684–9.
21. Croft, R.J., Menon, G.P., Marston, A. Does intestinal angina exist? — a critical study of obstructed visceral arteries. *Br. J. Surg.* (1981) **68**: 316–18.
22. Noer, R.J. The blood vessels of the jejunum and ileum — a comparative study of man and certain laboratory animals. *Am. J. Surg.* (1943) **73**: 293–6.

2

The regulation and distribution of intestinal blood flow

Ove Lundgren

Introduction

The vascular bed supplied by the mesenteric arteries represents one of the major circuits of the body and accepts about one-fifth of the cardiac output during 'rest'. This compartment of the circulation has to adapt to the functions of propulsion, secretion and absorption, and is supplied with an independent (enteric) nervous system.

The description which follows of the physiology of the intestinal vasculature reflects these complexities. For obvious ethical reasons, most studies have been based on animal experiments, but where clinical knowledge is available this is indicated. All major topics related to the intestinal circulation are covered, with an emphasis on those which are of importance in intestinal ischaemia. More detailed information is available in recent review articles, referred to below.

Functional characteristics of the intestinal circulation

A detailed description of the anatomy of the intestinal vascular bed was given in the previous chapter. From a functional point of view this area can be looked upon as consisting of a number of parallel-coupled and series-coupled vascular sections.[1] The parallel-coupled circuits supply the various layers of the bowel wall. Most studies confirm that these vascular circuits (i.e. the nutritional vessels of the mucosa, submucosa and muscularis) are linked in such a way. Observations using microspheres suggest that in the small intestine the mucosal and submucosal vascular beds are coupled in series.[2] This is, of course, true in the sense that the blood diverted to the mucosa must pass through the submucosal vascular network of fairly large vessels. However, no anatomical observation in the small intestine suggests that the capillaries of the connective tissue in the submucosa are series-coupled with those in the mucosa.

Each parallel-coupled vascular bed is made up of several anatomically and functionally different series-coupled (consecutive) vascular sections (Fig. 2.1). The *precapillary resistance vessels* consist of muscular vessels, that is the arterioles and met-arterioles. These vessels are the main determinants of blood flow to a particular region, and are the site of the local and remote control systems which regulate the rate of blood flow from moment to moment by changes of tone in the vascular smooth muscle. The *precapillary sphincters* are a specialized section of the smallest precapillary resistance vessels. This section usually contributes little to total regional vascular resistance, but it is of paramount importance as regards the control of the numbers of perfused capillaries and, hence, the mean blood–tissue diffusion distance and the time available for transcapillary exchange. It should be stressed, however, that the term 'precapillary sphincter', as used here, is a functional concept which corresponds to the anatomical arrangements found in different organs. The anatomical counterpart in the intestine to the precapillary sphincter seen elsewhere is as yet not known.

The capillaries or the *exchange vessels* constitute the key section in any vascular circuit. It is across their thin endothelial lining that the all-important exchange takes place between intra- and extra-

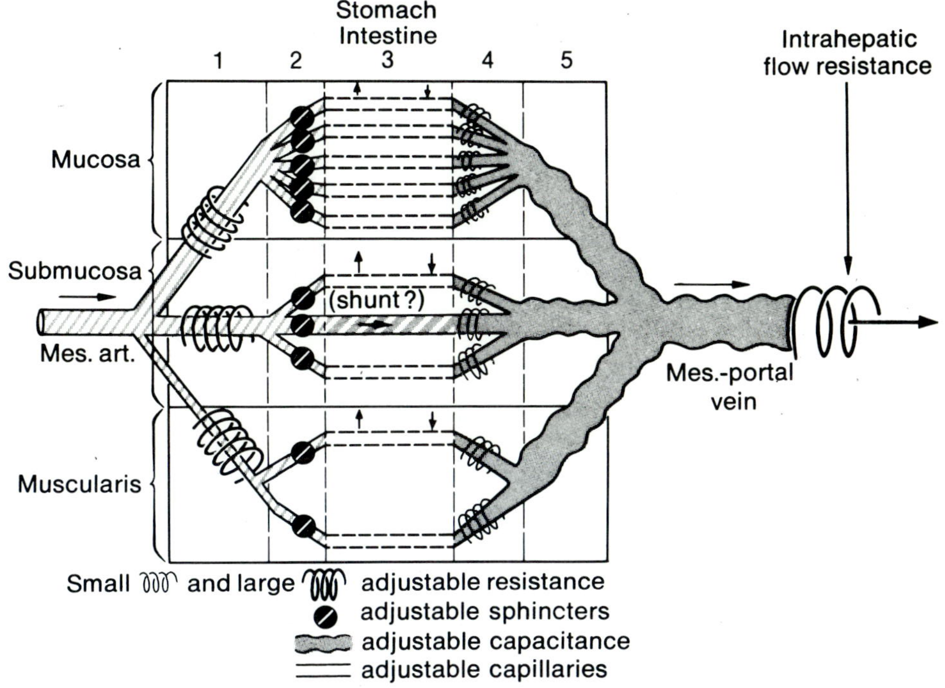

Fig. 2.1 Schematic illustration of the different parallel-coupled vascular circuits of the intestines with their consecutive vascular sections. 1: precapillary resistance vessels; 2: precapillary sphincters; 3: exchange vessels; 4: postcapillary resistance vessels; 5: capacitance vessels. (From Folkow,[2] by permission.)

vascular compartments.

Distal to the capillaries are the venules and veins, called *postcapillary resistance vessels* from a flow resistance point of view. The tonus of this vascular section is one of the main determinants of mean hydrostatic capillary pressure and of the rate of fluid exchange across the capillary wall. An isolated constriction of these vessels, for example, increases hydrostatic pressures proximally, thus producing a capillary filtration of fluid into the interstitial tissue. The postcapillary resistance section overlaps anatomically with the *capacitance vessels* composed of the venous compartment as a whole. Changes in the smooth muscle tone of these vessels may markedly alter regional blood volume, without significant changes in the total regional vascular resistance.

The presence of arteriovenous shunts in the submucosa of the gastrointestinal tract has been a subject of great controversy. Although such shunts have been described in all parts of the alimentary tract, their functional significance seems to be small. Thus, to judge from experiments on the small intestine, only 3 per cent of blood flow passes through vessels with a diameter greater than 20 μm.[3, 4]

Methodology

Qualitative methods

Simple observation of the colour of a loop of bowel, or of the arteries supplying it, gives a rough-and-ready guide to the adequacy of its nutrition, and in fact forms the basis of many crucial surgical decisions in situations where exact measurements cannot be made. Likewise, the state of a mucosal circulation can be assessed by observing the colour of an accessible surface directly, endoscopically via a gastroscope or colonoscope, or by looking at a surgically constructed stoma.

The reliability of such simple tests is not very high, and it is difficult to judge by eye whether or not an ischaemic loop of bowel is able to recover. More accurate prediction can be made by measuring surface temperature during reactive hyperaemia or by recording action potentials from the muscle layers. Although these methods do not measure absolute levels of flow, they are of use in estimating gross changes under different physiological circumstances or following the administration of drugs (see Chapter 4).

Recent developments in laser technology have made it possible to estimate flow on the surface of organs, at least in a qualitative way, by measuring the change of Doppler laser light caused by the movement of red cells in living tissue.[5] The technique is non-invasive and easy to use. In animal experiments a good quantitative correlation has been demonstrated between intestinal blood flow and the output signal from the laser Doppler flowmeter (Ahn and colleagues, in preparation). It seems probable that this method may soon be introduced into clinical medicine.

Quantitative methods

Total blood flow

The direct method of measuring total intestinal blood flow consisted simply in recording the output of the cannulated superior mesenteric vein (SMV) over a standard time, using a beaker and a stopwatch. The method is of mainly historical interest and is applicable to acute animal experiments. The method has, however, also been used in human studies during surgery.[6] Furthermore, suitably modified, it forms the basis of an accurate method of blood flow measurements in which the SMV output is passed in drops through silicone oil, recorded photoelectrically and returned to the animal. This is frequently used in academic physiology.

Most researchers have preferred to replace venous outflow measurements by extravascular flowmeters based on ultrasound or (more usually) electromagnetic principles in which a probe is placed around the vessel and the current induced in the electromagnetic field by the moving stream of blood is amplified and calibrated in terms of volume flow. Such probes can be implanted around the superior mesenteric artery (SMA) and left in position for long periods so that chronic experiments can be carried out or responses in splanchnic flow to varying stimuli observed in the conscious animal.[7, 8] In man, they have been used to measure flow during surgical operations, and are particularly useful in assessing the immediate result of an arterial reconstruction.[9] The two main disadvantages of such flowmeters are the cost of having a sufficiently wide range of probe diameters to fit accurately around arteries of varying size and the complexities involved in their calibration.

One recent development in the study of intestinal and/or portal blood flow in conscious man is the technique which involves reopening the umbilical vein.[10] Through this vessel up to three catheters can be introduced, and, by infusing the appropriate radioactive isotope (or 'heat') upstream, flow can be estimated by measuring the extent of dilution from a 'downstream' sample. The umbilical vein can also be used for access to the portal system so that a tracer injected into the SMA can be collected and blood flow measured using the indicator dilution principle.[11]

Clearances of bromosulphthalein (BSP) or indocyanine green (ICG) have been used extensively in hepatic blood flow measurements, using the Fick principle, as the hepatic veins are easily cannulated. Total hepatic blood flow closely approximates to total splanchnic flow, but of course gives little information regarding the intestinal component, due to the large and unpredictable contribution made by the hepatic artery and splenic vein.

Blood flow distribution

In animals it is possible to study the distribution of blood flow between the different intestinal wall layers by a variety of methods. For full coverage of the different techniques available the interested reader should consult a recently published book on the subject.[12] Here only a few methods are briefly described. One of those currently most popular involves the injection of radioactive microspheres into the left ventricle (so as to obtain optimal mixing) and subsequently measuring their distribution between the different layers of the intestinal wall. However, several recent reports (for discussion, see ref. 12) have pointed out that caution is required when using this method.

Other techniques make it possible to study the mucosal or villous circulation separately. One such involves the use of radioactively labelled blood cells or plasma particles.[13] They are injected into an artery close to the bowel and their passage through the mucosa monitored with an appropriate detector. Using a tracer with a 'weak' β-emission, it is possible to quantify red cells or plasma flow in the villi.

Another method makes use of the affinity of carbon monoxide to haemoglobin. Due to the high rate of diffusion of CO, its elimination from the intestinal lumen is flow limited above a certain luminal pCO_2.[14] It would seem possible to use the same technique in man, but this has not so far been attempted.

Mucosal blood flow in conscious man has been estimated quantitatively by following the

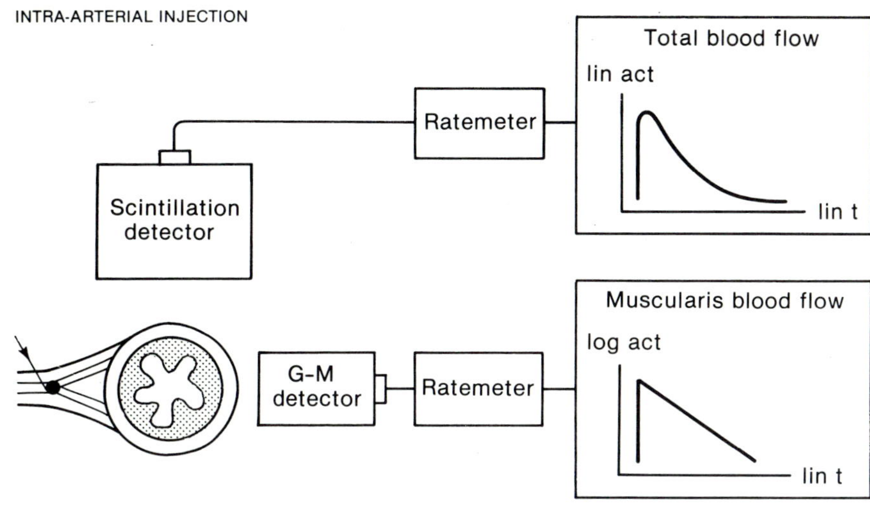

Fig. 2.2 The ^{85}Kr washout method for determining intestinal blood flow distribution as described by Hultén et al.[6] (Reproduced by permission.)

elimination of small amounts of ^{125}I 4, iodoantipyrine injected into the mucosa of colostomies.[15] This radioactive compound is lipid soluble and highly diffusable, and flow can be calculated, according to Kety,[16] as described for krypton (Fig. 2.2).

During surgery, total intestinal blood flow has been estimated using the method illustrated in Fig. 2.2.[6,17] The elimination of the tracer is followed with a scintillation detector placed above the organ and a Geiger–Muller tube at the antimesenteric border. The scintillation detector records γ-radioactivity from the whole organ, and the recorded curve can be analysed by the height : area formula proposed by Zierler[18] to determine total blood flow. This method also makes it possible to estimate blood flow distribution within the human intestine, since the Geiger–Muller tube records only the low-energy β-radiation emitted from the tracer located in the muscularis. The registered exponential decay of β-radiation thus reflects flow in the muscularis, which can be calculated according to the Kety equations.[16] Knowing the weight relationship between mucosa–submucosa and muscularis (determined from histological sections) and the total and muscle layer flow, mean blood flow in the mucosa-submucosa can be calculated.

Basic haemodynamic data

Total intestinal flow

'Resting' blood flows in the intestines of man, cat and dog are given in Table 2.1. Blood flow in the

Table 2.1 Resting blood flow in the small intestine and the colon of man, dog and cat

	Small intestine	Colon
Man[17, 44]	20–75	10–35
Dog[4]	20–60	35
Cat[4]	20–50	15–30

The animal studies were performed on anesthetized animals using a venous flowmeter.
Blood flow in man was determined during surgery using an inert gas elimination method.
Flow is expressed in ml/100 g of the respective tissue per minute.

small and large intestines in man is about 40 and 20 ml/100 g per minute, respectively. The total weights of the small and large bowel are about 1300 and 1200 g, respectively. Hence, during 'rest' 10 per cent of total cardiac output is distributed to the small intestine and about 5 per cent to the colon. After a meal, gastrointestinal blood flow increases approximately twofold. Intestinal blood flow in man is several orders of magnitude higher than that of resting skeletal muscle. In all probability these differences reflect the different nutritional demands of the organs.

The potential flow range of the intestinal vasculature is high indeed, as illustrated by investigations in the cat showing that blood flow can be increased approximately ten times by infusion of a potent vasodilator drug. This probably mainly reflects an extraordinary vasodilatation in the mucosa, as discussed below. In man a colonic blood flow of similar magnitude has been measured in fulminant cases of ulcerative colitis[19] implying that total colonic blood flow is around 1500 ml per minute, which represents about 30 per cent of the resting cardiac output. Hence, even if cardiac output is doubled, the fraction diverted to the colon is still high in this clinical disorder.

Blood flow distribution

Most investigators studying the haemodynamics of the intestines have recorded total blood flow. However, blood flow is not homogenous throughout the intestinal wall and when considering the relationship between flow and function it is important to obtain detailed information on the regional distribution of flows. There are several functional reasons for the uneven distribution of blood within the intestinal wall. In part it reflects the varying demands for oxygen and other nutrients of the different functions of the bowel. Thus, secretion and absorption, two metabolically demanding tasks, are localized to the mucosa, where blood flow is comparatively high. Nevertheless, functional demands other than those of nutrition must be of importance, since mucosal blood flow provides not only the solutes for cell metabolism but also the fluid necessary for the secretory activity.

A quantitative survey of the intramural blood flow and its distribution is given in Table 2.2, based on studies made on human, canine and feline intestines. It is evident from the Table that mean flow in the mucosa is about three times greater than in the muscularis, expressed per unit of tissue weight. As total blood flow increases there is a steady augmentation of the proportion diverted to the mucosa.

In Table 2.2 the intestinal wall is divided into three anatomical regions. There are reasons to believe that some of them may not be homogenously perfused. For example, the nerve plexus situated between the circular and longitudinal muscle layers may be perfused at a rate different from that of the muscular coat, and the cell renewal zone at the base of the crypts appears to be preferentially well supplied with blood.

Consecutive vascular sections

Apart from the studies of resistance vessels described above, few investigations of the consecutive intestinal vasculature have been performed on humans. Thus our knowledge of the functions of the exchange vessels is based on animal work. In the cat it has been calculated that the capillary length in 100 g mucosa is approxmiately 100 km, corresponding to a capillary surface area of about 2 m^2.[20, 21] The overall hydraulic (water) conductivity in the intestinal capillaries has been estimated in the cat by determinations of the capillary filtration coefficient (CFC). In the resting situation this measured 0.05–0.1 $ml \cdot mmHg^{-1} \cdot 100\ g^{-1}$ per minute. The corresponding values for resting and maximal CFC in skeletal muscle capillaries are about 0.01 and 0.04 $ml^{-1} \cdot mmHg^{-1} \cdot 100\ g^{-1}$ tissue, per minute, respectively. The difference in CFC between intestinal and skeletal muscle in all probability reflects both varying capillary density and capillary 'porosity'. The so-called fenestrated capillaries in the intestinal mucosa are probably more porous than those in skeletal muscle capillaries, simply because of a difference in the number of their pores.

The large hydraulic conductivity of the mucosal capillaries in the intestines represents a potential risk, since a small increase of mean hydrostatic capillary pressure could induce a massive shift from the intravascular to the extravascular compartment,

Table 2.2 Blood flow and flow distribution in the wall layers of the small and large bowel at 'rest'

	Small intestine			Colon		
	Man[17]	Dog[44]	Cat[17]	Man[6]	Dog[44]	Cat[6]
Total blood flow (ml/100 g/min)	38	79	28	18	74	22
Regional blood flow (ml/100 g/min)						
Mucosa–submucosa	51	87	37	28	109	31
Muscularis	21	27	14	11	48	10
Blood flow distribution (%)						
Mucosa-submucosa	75	85	80	66	49	80
Muscularis	25	15	20	34	51	20

an event of major haemodynamic importance. Mean capillary pressure is particularly sensitive to changes in venous pressure, since the postcapillary flow resistance is smaller than the precapillary. Two mechanisms exist which counteract fluid losses induced by increased capillary hydrostatic pressure. Firstly, the precapillary sphincters constrict in response to a rise in transmural pressure, thus reducing the number of perfused capillaries and the potential area for fluid exchange. Secondly, a sustained rise in venous outflow pressure results in a new Starling equilibrium, due to an increased interstitial hydrostatic pressure and/or a decreased interstitial colloid osmotic pressure.

The blood volume, mainly contained in the capacitance vessels, amounts to 7–10 ml/100 g.[22] A large portion of this is localized in the veins of the delicate mesenteric tissue, and the blood volume in the intestine *wall* is about 5 ml/100 g tissue. These regional blood volumes are two to four times larger than that reported for skeletal muscle. This difference is at least in part explained by the denser vascularization of the intestines. In the intestinal wall proper the blood content of the submucosa is comparatively great, owing to the presence of a dense vascular plexus. Thus in the cat some 15–20 per cent of the submucosal tissue volume is blood, mainly localized in veins.

Local control mechanisms

Chemical

The local chemical milieu in the tissue is believed to be of great importance for the control of flow resistance in many vascular territories.[23] Thus, the cerebral and the coronary circulation are assumed to be under the constant influence of such factors, so that they can adapt blood flow to the prevailing metabolic needs. With regard to the splanchnic circulation, it has been shown repeatedly that blood flow increases after a meal.[4, 24] This functional hyperaemia is partially located in the intestines. An accumulation (or possibly a deprivation) of certain key substances may be one mechanism underlying this postprandial hyperaemia. However, it should be emphasized that virtually nothing is known about the true nature of vasodilating metabolites in relation to the intestines. There is also no information concerning the metabolites that are released into venous blood during vascular occlusion. It seems likely that the compound, or compounds, responsible for the local control of the intestinal microcirculation is among such released substances.

Based on observations made in other vascular beds, a number of proposals have been made with regard to the intestinal circulation. For each proposed mechanism, experimental support from animals is at hand. However, it is difficult to judge whether the observed vasodilator effect of any compound studied occurs at concentrations achieved under physiological circumstances.

Two obvious dilator candidates are oxygen deprivation and carbon dioxide accumulation, both of which result from tissue metabolism. Adenosine, a metabolite of ATP, has been postulated as being important in the local control of muscle tissues, and in accord with this it has been shown that adenosine may be also involved in the functional hyperaemia of the muscle layer of the small intestine. Finally, hyperosmolality and potassium ions are also vasodilator 'agents' that have been suggested as playing a role in the functional hyperaemia of the gut.

The intestines are unique in the body in that a chemical environment other than that of the tissue itself may influence blood flow; that is, the composition of material within the lumen. Experimental efforts have been made to elucidate the substances involved in that response. All the major constituents of food, as well as bile, have been studied. These animal experiments suggest that breakdown products of carbohydrates and lipids, together with bile, are the important luminal stimuli for hyperaemia after food intake.[4,24] This effect has been ascribed to several mechanisms, including nervous and hormonal.

Nervous

It has been shown that mechanical stimulation of the mucosa of a denervated intestinal segment increases blood flow in the small bowel, often more than twofold.[25] This vascular response was not mediated by adrenergic or cholinergic receptors but was blocked by tetrodotoxin, and it was thus concluded that the vascular response is elicited via an intramural nervous reflex arc. A nervous dilator reflex of the same type has been shown in colon. Biber and colleagues[25] suggested that these local nervous vasodilator reflexes are evoked during digestion as the food bolus moves along the intestinal tube. It may also be that a similar vascular reflex is in part responsible for the vasodilatation evoked by different substances in the lumen.

Autoregulation of blood flow

Many vascular beds in the body exhibit autoregulation — that is, the capacity to maintain constant flow in the face of large variations in perfusion pressure. Several studies performed on animals indicate that the intestinal vascular beds also exhibit autoregulation, although the extent of this may vary from one experiment to the other. In the feline small intestine, attempts have been made to estimate the autoregulatory ability of the different parallel-coupled vascular circuits. It was found that the villous circulation exhibited a more pronounced autoregulatory capacity than did total intestinal blood flow. Blood flow in the absorptive parts of the intestinal wall stayed fairly constant in the face of a perfusion pressure reduction to 30–40 mm Hg. This haemodynamic readjustment was accomplished by a concomitant increase of perfused blood volume (i.e. increased number of perfused villi) and mean transit time through the hairpin vascular loops of the villi. This change of intestinal haemodynamics may be of importance in the development of the villous ulcerations seen in hypotensive states, as discussed later in this chapter.

The mechanism underlying autoregulation of flow is much debated.[4, 23] There are two main schools of thought. According to one, the constancy of blood flow is secondary to myogenic properties of the intestinal vascular smooth muscle. An increased transmural pressure induces a contraction of the vascular smooth muscle and vice versa. Such a mechanism is suggested by experiments showing that increasing venous outflow pressure induces a constriction of the precapillary vessels. It may also be supported by the observation that increasing the pressure in the intestinal lumen abolishes autoregulation, since such a procedure would increase tissue pressure and hence decrease transmural pressure.

According to the other hypothesis, autoregulation of flow reflects a relaxation of vascular smooth muscle secondary to an accumulation of vasodilating metabolites. In some vascular beds the major metabolite responsible for flow autoregulation is known. In the cerebral circulation, for example, it is probably an accumulation of hydrogen ions. In the intestine we do not yet know which metabolites are concerned in autoregulation.

Both autoregulatory mechanisms discussed above probably exist in most tissues. The relative importance of transmural pressure and the influence of tissue metabolites may, however, vary between vascular beds and may even vary in the same vascular bed during different functional states, as suggested by recent observations in the small intestine.

The phenomenon of autoregulation is usually discussed in terms of blood flow. However, autoregulation may also be designed to keep mean capillary hydrostatic pressure constant. Functionally, such a mechanism is of great importance, since the vascular beds with great ability for autoregulation, such as kidney and intestine, are also provided with extensive capillary networks. Hence, small changes in capillary pressure may provoke sudden and large shifts between intra- and extravascular compartments.

Nervous control of the intestinal circulation

Vasoconstrictor fibres

Nervous vasoconstrictor control is mediated via fibres in the sympathetic nervous system, running partly via the splanchnic nerves and partly via the lumbar colonic nerves. In man the boundary between the areas of distribution of these two nerves is located in the *transverse colon*.

The distribution of adrenergic fibres has been studied in detail by use of the Falck–Hillarp fluorescence method. A strong adrenergic fluorescence can be seen around the nerve cells in the nervous plexuses of the intestine. Nerve fibres are also found around blood vessels in all layers of the intestinal wall. In the mucosa, sympathetic fibres are especially frequent in the deeper layers. The vascular sympathetic fibres make contact with the smooth muscle cells in the outer layers of the vessels, indirectly controlling also the rest of the smooth muscle cells via the intercellular nexuses.

Activating the sympathetic outflow to the intestinal vasculature evokes a characteristic flow pattern which has been investigated most thoroughly in the cat[26, 27] (Fig. 2.3), and to some extent in man.[22] When the nerve fibres are stimulated a fairly intense vasoconstriction is observed initially, particularly at the higher frequencies (above 4 Hz). However, within 2–4 minutes blood flow begins to rise, despite continued stimulation, reaching a new steady state only slightly below control level. During the steady state phase of nervous vasoconstriction, the increase in blood flow resistance seldom exceeds 100 per cent, even when the rate of stimulation is high. The secondary increase of flow in the face of continued nerve activity has been called 'autoregulatory escape from vasoconstrictor fibre influence' in the small intestine and is also seen in the colonic, gastric, hepatic and renal vascular beds. It is not due to fatigue of nervous transmission, since the intestinal veins remain constricted throughout the stimulation period. This constriction of the capacitance vessels expels approximately 20 per cent of the regional blood content when the nerves are activted at a frequency of 2 Hz, and 30–50 per cent at 8 Hz. It can be calculated that a venous constriction of this order in man would mobilize about 50–150 ml blood from the intestine. The corresponding volume calculated for the whole splanchnic region amounts to 250–500 ml.

Stimulation of the sympathetic nervous fibres to the intestine does not significantly change mean capillary hydrostatic pressure, to judge from recordings of total organ volume. However, the sympathetic nerves control the number of perfused capillaries, and this is decreased during the steady state phase of vasoconstriction. Quantitatively, nerve stimulation at 4 Hz reduces the CFC to about 60 per cent of control. This may be explained if we assume the existence of 'precapillary sphincters' whose response to nervous stimulation is to constrict.

Blood flow distribution between the different layers of the intestines during the steady state phase of sympathetic vasoconstriction has been investigated with several techniques, most thoroughly in the feline small bowel. A summary of the results in cat is given in Table 2.3. These studies in the small intestine strongly indicate that the villous circulation is maintained at the pre-stimulatory control level, even when total intestinal blood flow is reduced by one-half. Since muscle

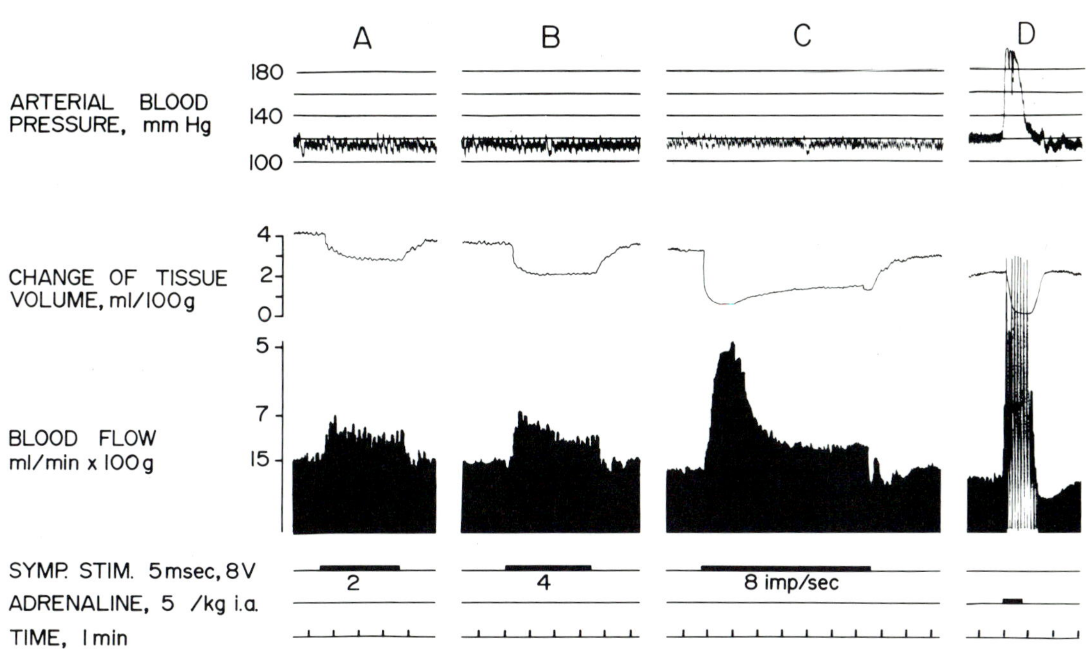

Fig. 2.3 The effect of graded stimulation of the regional vasoconstrictor fibres on arterial blood pressure, tissue volume and blood flow of the cat large bowel (panels A, B and C). The changes in tissue volume reflect variations in regional blood volume. As a comparison the effect of a large dose of intra-arterial (i.a.) adrenaline is illustrated in panel D. (From Hultén, Jodal and Lundgren,[27] by permission.).

Table 2.3 Blood flow (F) and flow distribution (D) in the feline small intestine during control and during sympathetic nervous vasoconstriction[22]

	Villi		Crypts		Muscularis–submucosa	
	F	D	F	D	F	D
Control	40	30	50	40	17	30
Sympathetic influence	40	35	25	30	10	25

Flow is expressed in ml/100 g of the respective tissue per minute. Distribution in percentage of total blood flow.

blood flow is reduced by roughly the same extent as total flow, this suggests that flow in the crypts is markedly reduced by sympathetic influence (Table 2.3), which thus gives rise to a pronounced redistribution of blood from the crypts towards the villi. These observations are interesting with regard to localization of the mucosal damage in the intestine in shock. The characteristic feature of these lesions is that they always start at the tips of the villi, i.e. in a region where flow is apparently unaltered by sympathetic influence.

In man, blood flow distribution has been investigated during the steady state phase of nervous vasoconstriction by inert gas washout techniques.[22] Vasoconstriction is observed in both muscle and mucosa upon electrical activation of the sympathetic nerves, although this seems to be more pronounced in the muscularis since a larger portion of total blood flow is distributed to the mucosa–submucosa in the experimental group than in the controls. The technique used does not allow for any detailed analysis of the mucosal haemodynamics in the way described above for the feline studies (Table. 2.3).

The mechanisms underlying 'autoregulatory escape' (see Fig. 2.3) have been investigated in great detail. The phenomenon is most probably of multifactoral origin, and several hypotheses have been devised.[4,21] According to one school of thought, the escape reflects an inherent property of vascular smooth muscle. Somewhat in line with this, it has also been suggested that autoregulatory escape is secondary to an adaption of the α-receptors on the vascular smooth muscle of the gastrointestinal canal. Another proposal involves the concomitant activation of adrenergic α-receptors, causing vasoconstriction, and adrenergic β-receptors, inducing vasodilatation. Finally, one obvious explanation is the accumulation of vasodilating metabolites during the initial intense vasoconstriction. The relative importance of these mechanisms in explaining autoregulatory escape in the gastrointestinal tract remains to be determined.

Vasodilator fibres

Earlier it was usually assumed that most vascular beds in the mammalian organism are innervated by both vasoconstrictor and vasodilator fibres, considered sympathetic and parasympathetic, respectively. In the small intestine this general view was not substantiated by the thorough investigations of Kewenter,[28] who was unable to demonstrate any vasodilator fibres in the vagi, using a wide range of modalities of nerve stimulation.

However, the possible presence of external vasodilator fibres in the sympathetic supply to the small intestine has been demonstrated in studies in which the sympathetic outflow to the small intestine was stimulated electrically after an α-adrenergic blocking agent was administered.[29] This vascular response was neither abolished by atropine nor enhanced by physostigmine, and is apparently mediated via non-adrenergic, non-cholinergic nerves. The functional significance of the vasodilatation is not known.

The autonomic innervation of the colon is more complex than that of the small intestine. The parasympathetic supply to the colon consists of two main nerves, the vagal and the pelvic. The distribution areas of the two nerves meet in the transverse colon.

Electrical stimulation of the vagal fibres to the colon does not elict any flow changes apart from those caused by an increase in colonic motility. Stimulating the pelvic nerves, on the other hand, induces marked changes in colonic haemodynamics. A fairly detailed analysis of this has been performed in the cat.[27, 30] On pelvic nerve stimulation, blood flow increased transiently followed by an oscillating blood flow accompanied by an increased secretion. After atropinization the initial increases in flow and tissue volumes were observed, but the oscillations and the secretion were abolished. It was concluded from this and similar experiments that two vasodilator mechanisms are involved in the pelvic nerve response in the colon: an initial, atropine-resistant hyperaemia and an atropine-sensitive flow increase which may be secondary to the increase in net secretion.

The intramural flow distribution during nervous vasodilatation has been studied in the cat with local microinjections of inert tracers. These studies demonstrated that the initial marked vasodilatation is accompanied by an increase of blood flow exclusively to the colonic mucosa, particularly the superficial layers. Blood flow in the mucosa at rest increases from 25–40 to 150–200 ml/100 g mucosal tissue per minute at a total colonic blood flow of 60 ml/100 g colonic tissue per minute.

Hormonal control

The number of known gastrointestinal hormones has increased greatly during the last two decades, due to more refined ways of isolating peptides from tissues. Several of these new hormone 'candidates' have haemodynamic effects, but usually at concentrations that are considered to be greater than the 'physiological' plasma concentration seen, for example, after a meal. Therefore, no hormone produced in the gastrointestinal tract has, as yet, been convincingly shown to participate in the physiological control of intestinal blood flow.

On the other hand, in abnormal circumstances, observations suggest that hormones may be of importance in the control of intestinal blood flow. Pronounced haemorrhage evokes a vasoconstriction which, at any rate in the cat, is in part hormonally mediated.[31, 32] Experimental observations suggest that the hormones involved may be circulating catecholamines, angiotensin and possibly also vasopressin.

The intestinal countercurrent exchanger

Evidence is accumulating for the presence of a countercurrent exchanger in the villi of the small intestine.[33] The experimental evidence for this mechanism has largely been obtained in cats, but evidence also exists for an exchanger in rats, dogs and man. The anatomical basis for the exchanger consists of the characteristic vascular arrangements in the villi (Fig. 2.4). According to the classic studies performed by Heller,[34] Mall[35] and Spanner,[36] the arteriolar supply to the villi of most species consists of one or two vessels branching off from the extensive vascular network in the submucosa. These vessels, located in the central core of the villus, lack vascular smooth muscle in their upper two-thirds. At the tip, these supplying vessels branch into a close-meshed capillary network just beneath the epithelial lining, with the capillaries collecting into venules at various levels. Spanner[36] called this vascular arrangement the 'fountain type'. A similar vascular architecture has been reported in the human villus (Fig. 2.4), although in man the number of supplying vessels seems to be related to the size of the villus, large villi more often having two such vessels. Their position in the villus is sometimes central sometimes peripheral, and in

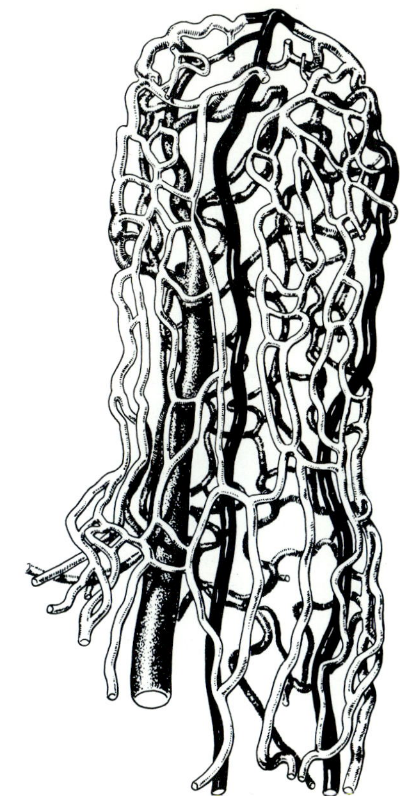

Fig. 2.4 Vascular anatomy of a human villus according to Spanner.[36] Black vessels denote arterial vessels, grey a venous one. (Reproduced by permission.)

close approximation to capillaries and/or veins.

The vascular anatomy described above strongly suggests that the main direction of blood flow in the subepithelial capillary network is opposite to that of the central arteriole (or venule). Hence the anatomical prerequisites for a countercurrent exchanger do exist. The efficiency of such an exchanger depends on the distance between the two limbs in the exchanger and their length. Information concerning this distance is sparse. I made calculations based on histological observations reported by Schriever that the intervascular distance in the slender, finger-like feline villi is only 15–20 μm.[37]

A countercurrent exchanger may exhibit three fundamental functional properties. These will be discussed below.

1. An easily diffusible solute may be delayed in its net blood absorption by diffusing from the extensive subepithelial network to the ascending arterial vessel provided a concentration gradient exists. This bring the compound back toward the villus tip, delaying its absorption ('trapping'). Thus, lipid-soluble compounds, such as antipyrin and several inert gases, have been demonstrated to be very efficiently hindered in their net blood absorption by the exchanger (Fig. 2.5).

2. A solute may diffuse from the central artery to the subepithelial capillary network provided that a concentration gradient exists between these vessels and that the solute can easily diffuse between them (Fig. 2.5). This mechanism tends increasingly to impair net blood transport of the solute towards the tips of the villi. Because the vascular wall is a diffusion barrier to water-soluble but not to lipid-soluble solutes, the latter compounds should be most efficiently excluded from the villi when they are approached through the blood.

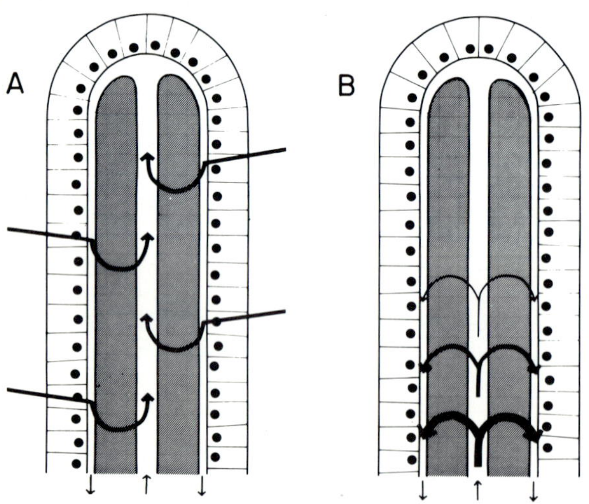

Fig. 2.5 Functional implications of the intestinal countercurrent exchanger. Intervascular distances are grossly exaggerated for sake of clarity. (From Lundgren,[38] by permission.)

Experimental support for such extravascular shunting in the villi was reported in the cat for the lipid-soluble solutes oxygen, krypton and antipyrin, and to some extent for the water-soluble solutes urea and rubidium. (The experimental approaches of these studies vary and the reader is referred to the survey of Lundgren[38] for a summary.) Oxygen appears 1–2 seconds earlier on the venous side than do labelled red cells after intra-arterial injection during resting conditions. Because red cells pass faster along a vascular bed than does plasma, due to their axial position in the vessels, the early appearance of oxygen is evidence for its short-circuiting the vessels in the villous exchanger. Such shunting of oxygen in the intestinal countercurrent exchanger implies that the pO_2 of the villus decreases from the base toward the tip, as can be demonstrated in the rat.[39] Hence the villous tips are relatively hypoxic, a fact that may be important for transport mechanisms which depend on cellular metabolism. In the author's studies, however, little countercurrent exchange of oxygen seemed to occur when intestinal blood flow was increased above 60 ml/100 g per minute in the cat.

This functional implication of the intestinal countercurrent exchanger is of particular importance in intestinal hypotension. The efficiency of the exchanger is greatly increased during arterial hypotension for two reasons. Firstly, the number of perfused villi increases at low perfusion pressure, thus increasing the area of the exchanger. Secondly, the transit time for red cells and plasma is greatly prolonged. In feline villi plasma mean transit time in the whole villus increases from 5 to 15–20 seconds.[40] Hence, area and time for exchange are increased. The greater effectiveness of the villus exchanger, due to an increase both in area and in time available, implies that the low pO_2 already present at normal perfusion pressure is lowered even further during hypotension. An increased countercurrent exchange of oxygen may therefore explain the development of the mucosa ulceration at the villus tips seen in intestinal ischaemia.

3. The countercurrent exchanger may also function as a countercurrent multiplier. In the small

intestine we have provided experimental support for the view that the intestinal multiplier creates the tissue hyperosmolality necessary to explain the absorption of water from the intestinal lumen. The reader interested in this functional implication of the intestinal countercurrent exchanger is referred to the reports by Jodal and Hallbäck and their colleagues.[41, 42]

Intestinal blood flow and function

The three major functions of the intestine comprise motility, secretion, and absorption. Their relationship to blood flow is discussed below.

Motility

Motility may affect total blood flow of the intestine in two ways. Firstly, it may increase blood flow owing to enhanced metabolism, leading to an accumulation of metabolites in the same way as exercise causes hyperaemia in skeletal muscle. Secondly, the muscular movements may mechanically interfere with blood flow. In animal experiments designed to study the relationship between flow and motility in the small intestine, a prolonged increase of total intestinal blood flow has never been demonstrated. This seems to rule out the first possibility. However, a slight increase in muscularis blood flow might be easily missed by conventional methods of measuring total flow.

The way in which motility interferes with blood flow has been studied in several investigations.[4] The expected results were obtained; that is, during strong intestinal contractions flow transiently decreased, to increase again when the muscles relaxed.

The contractions of the gastrointestinal muscle layer may influence blood flow, not only by their direct effects on the intramural vessels but also by increasing luminal pressure. There are several reports devoted to the question of how luminal pressure influences blood. The results vary, but most researchers report a decreased blood flow confined to the mucosa. A linear relationship between intraluminal pressure above 20–30 mm Hg and intestinal blood flow has been shown. If luminal pressure is high enough, it may induce gangrene of the intestinal wall due to ischaemia.

Secretion

The current discussion concerning physiological mechanisms underlying secretion across epithelial centres around transcellular 'active' transport of solutes via carrier molecules or changes in epithelial permeability, and transcapillary filtration is not believed to contribute to any significant extent. Mucus secretion occurs via exocytosis. Blood flow is considered to be of importance only for delivery of nutrition and raw material. In situations of increased secretion the vessels supplying the glands dilate in response to the altered metabolic demands, as shown in the colon during pelvic nerve stimulation.

Absorption

Blood flow fulfils two functions with regard to intestinal absorption: it represents the major transport vehicle for the absorbed material, and it provides the necessary nutrients for the cellular metabolism underlying active transport across the intestinal epithelium. All our knowledge on the flow–absorption relationship has been gained in studies on the small intestine, most of them being performed by Winne.[43] This relationship becomes fairly complicated for an actively absorbed solute, since it may be difficult to decide to what extent an altered absorption rate, induced by a blood flow change, is caused by flow *per se* and/or by an indirect effect on cell metabolism. Passively absorbed solutes are more easily studied, and Winne[43] has explored the effect of variations in total intestinal blood flow on the absorption rate of such solutes. The results demonstrate that the absorption rate of lipophilic compounds increases with blood flow. Water-soluble substances, with the exception of water itself, are on the other hand largely unaffected by the rate of flow, probably because the rate of the absorption of hydrophilic compounds is limited by their passage across the intestinal epithelium. The importance of the countercurrent exchanger in intestinal absorption has already been discussed.

References

1. Greenway, C.V., Murthy, V.S. Effects of vasopressin and isoprenaline infusions on the distribution of blood flow in the intestine; criteria for the validity of microsphere studies. *Br. J. Pharmacol.* (1972) **46**: 177–88.
2. Folkow, B. Regional adjustments of intestinal blood flow. *Gastroenterology* (1967) **52**: 423–32.

3. Grim, E., Lindseth, E.O. Distribution of blood flow to the tissues of the small intestine of the dog. *Univ. Minn. Med. Bull.* (1958) **30**: 138–45.
4. Lundgren, O. The microcirculation of the gastrointestinal tract and the pancreas. In Renkin, E., Michel, C., eds. *Handbook of Physiology*, Washington DC: American Physiological Society (1985) In press.
5. Tenland, T. *On laser doppler flowmetry. Methods and microvascular applications.* Linköping University Medical Dissertations no. 136. Linköping (1982).
6. Hultén, L., Jodal, M., Lindhagen, J., Lundgren, O. Colonic blood flow in cat and man as analyzed by an inert gas wash-out technique. *Gastroenterology* (1976) **70**: 36–44.
7. Burns, G.P., Schenk, W.G. Jr. Effect of digestion and exercise on intestinal blood flow and cardiac output. *Arch. Surg.* (1969) **98**: 790–4.
8. Vater, S.F., Franklin, D., Van Citters, R.L. Mesenteric vasoactivity associated with eating and digestion in the conscious dog. *Am. J. Physiol.* (1970) **219**, 170–4.
9. Edwards, A.J., Taylor, G. Experience with the coeliac axis compression syndrome. *Br. Med. J.* (1970) **1**: 342–5.
10. Strandell, T., Erwald, R., Kulling, K.G., et al. Measurement of dual hepatic blood flow in awake patients. *J. Appl. Physiol.* (1973) **35**: 755–61.
11. Norryd, C., Dencker, H., Lunderquist, A., et al. Superior mesenteric blood flow in man studied with a dye dilution technique. *Acta Chir. Scand.* (1975) **141**: 109–18.
12. Granger, D.N., Bulkley, G.B., eds. *Measurement of blood flow. Applications to the splanchnic circulation.* Baltimore: Williams & Wilkins, (1981).
13. Biber, B., Lundgren, O. Stage, L., et al. An indicator-dilution method for studying intestinal hemodynamics in the cat. *Acta Physiol. Scand.* (1973) **87**: 433–47.
14. Micflikier, A.B., Bond, J.H., Sircar, B., et al. Intestinal villus blood flow measured with carbon monoxide and microspheres. *Am. J. Physiol.* (1976) **230**: 916–19.
15. Forrester, D.W., Spence, V.A., Walker, W.F. The measurement of colonic mucosal–submucosal blood flow in man. *J. Physiol.* (1980) **229**. 1–11.
16. Kety, S.S. The theory and applications of the exchange of inert gas at the lungs and tissue. *Pharmacol. Rev.* (1951) **3**: 1–41.
17. Hultén, L., Jodal, M., Lindhagen, J., et al. Blood flow in the small intestine of cat and man as analyzed by an inert gas washout technique. *Gastroenterology* (1976) **70**: 45–51.
18. Zierler, K.L. Equations for measuring blood flow by external monitoring of radioisotopes. *Circ. Res.* (1965) **16**: 309–21.
19. Hultén, L., Lindhagen, J., Lundgren, O., et al. Regional intestinal blood flow in ulcerative colitis and Crohn's disease. *Gastroenterology* (1977) **72**: 388–96.
20. Biber, B., Lundgren, O., Svanvik, J. Intramural blood flow and blood volume in the small intestine of the cat as analyzed by an indicator-dilution technique. *Acta Physiol. Scand.* (1973) **87**: 391–403.
21. Svanvik, J., Lundgren, O. Gastrointestinal circulation. In: Crane, R.K., ed. *Gastrointestinal Physiology*, vol. 2. Baltimore: University Park Press (1977) 1–33.
22. Hultén, L., Lindhagen, J., Lundgren, O. Sympathetic nervous control of intramural blood flow in the feline and human intestines. *Gastroenterology* (1977) **72**: 41–8.
23. Folkow, B., Neil, E. *Circulation.* Oxford University Press (1971).
24. Granger, D.N., Richardson, P.D.I., Kvietys, P.R., et al. Intestinal blood flow. *Gastroenterology* (1980) **78**: 837–63.
25. Biber, B., Lundgren, O., Svanvik, J. Studies on the intestinal vasodilatation observed after mechanical stimulation of the mucosa of the gut. *Acta Physiol. Scand.* (1971) **82**: 177–90.
26. Folkow, B., Lewis, D.H., Lundgren, O., et al. The effect of graded vasoconstrictor fiber stimulation on the intestinal resistance and capacitance vessels. *Acta Physiol. Scand.* (1964) **61**: 445–7.
27. Hultén, L., Jodal, M., Lundgren, O. Local and nervous control of the consecutive vascular sections of the colon. *Acta Physiol. Scand.* (1969) suppl. 335 51–64.
28. Kewenter, J. The vagal control of the jejunal and ileal motility and blood flow. *Acta Physiol. Scand.* (1965) suppl. 251: 65.
29. Ross, G. Vascular effects of periarterial mesenteric nerve stimulation after adrenergic neurone blockade. *Experientia* (1973) **29**: 289–90.
30. Hultén, L., Jodal, M., Lundgren, O. Nervous control of blood flow in the parallel-coupled vascular sections of the colon. *Acta Physiol. Scand* (1969) suppl. 335: 65–76.
31. McNeil, R.J., Stark, R.D., Greenway, C.V. Intestinal vasoconstriction after hemorrhage: role of vasopressin and angiotensin. *Am. J. Physiol* (1970) **219**: 1342–7.
32. Redfors, S., Sjövall, H. The importance of nervous and humoral factors in the control of vascular resistance, blood flow distribution and net fluid absorption in the cat small intestine during hemorrhage. *Acta Physiol.Scand.* (1985) In press.
33. Jodal, M., Haglund, U., Lundgren, O. Counter-

current exchange mechanisms in the small intestine. In: Shepherd, A.R., Granger, D.N., eds. *Physiology of the intestine circulation.* New York: Raven Press (1984) 83–96.

34. Heller, A. Uber die Blutgefässe des Dünndarmes. *Berliner Sächsiger gesamte Wissenschaft* (1872) **24**: 165–71.
35. Mall, J.P. Die Blut- und Lymphwege im Dünndarm des Hundes. *Abhandlung Sächsiger gesamte Wissenschaft* (1888) **14**: 153–89.
36. Spanner, R. Neue Befunder über die Blutwege der Darmwand und ihre funktionelle Bedeutung. *Morphol. Jahrbuch* (1932) **69**: 394–454.
37. Schriever, O. *Die Darmzotten der Haussäugetiere.* Giessen. Thesis (1899).
38. Lundgren, O. Studies on blood flow distribution and countercurrent exchange in the small intestine. *Acta Physiol. Scand.* (1967) suppl. **303**: 1–42.
39. Bohlen, H.G. Intestinal tissue P and microvascular responses during glucose exposure. *Am. J. Physiol.* (1980) **238**: H164–71.
40. Lundgren, O., Svanvik, J. Mucosal hemodynamics in the small intestine of the cat during reduced perfusion pressure. *Acta Physiol. Scand.* (1973) **88**: 551–63.
41. Jodal, M., Hallbäck, D.-A., Lundgren, O. Tissue osmolality in intestinal villi during luminal perfusion with isotonic electrolyte solutions. *Acta Physiol. Scand.* (1978) **102**: 94–107.
42. Hallbäck, D.-A., Hultén, L., Jodal, M., et al. Evidence for the existence of a countercurrent exchanger in the small intestine in man. *Gastroenterology* (1978) **74**: 683–90.
43. Winne, D. Influence of blood flow on intestinal absorption of drugs and nutrients. *Pharmacol. Ther.* (1979). **6**: 333–93.
44. Chou, C.C., Grassmick, B. Motility and blood flow distribution within the wall of the gastrointestinal tract. *Am. J. Physiol.* (1978) **235**: H34–9.

3

Laboratory studies of intestinal ischaemia

Introduction

It is easy to interfere with the arterial supply to the intestine in the experimental animal, and there exists a large body of information as to methods and results. Thus ligation of the SMA and later release of the ligature has been used for years as a standard shock model, the ischaemic loop preparation is the recognized model for the study of strangulation–obstruction, and chronic occlusion by means of Ameroid cylinders has shed some light on the pathophysiology of chronic ischaemia.

Because, however, of different patterns of evolution of the alimentary tract, there are enormous species differences in the behaviour of the ischaemic intestine, so care must be taken when extrapolating animal data to human beings. This particularly applies to the role played by the splanchnic circulation in shock and low flow states.

The three principal techniques which have been used in the study of the ischaemic bowel are:

1. Acute occlusion of the SMA, with or without subsequent release.
2. Chronic obliteration of the main arteries
3. Occlusion of the IMA and the smaller segmental vessels.

Additionally, the ways in which the damage caused by ischaemia can be mitigated (by drugs, by mechanical means and by removal of toxic by-products) have been extensively examined.

Acute occlusion of the superior mesenteric artery

Effects on the bowel

The effects of ligation of the superior mesenteric artery have now been studied for over a hundred years, as 1975 marked the centenary of Litten's original experiments.[1] He found that ligation of the artery in 40 dogs resulted in every case in death within 12–48 hours, accompanied by vomiting, bloody diarrhoea and fever.

The immediate effects of tying the SMA were as follows. All pulsations disappeared and the bowel became blue-white and spastic, with collapsed arteries and prominent veins. Contractions initially increased, but eventually disappeared and after some hours the loops became relaxed and distended. After 8–10 hours frank haemorrhage began to occur and finally at autopsy the bowel from the duodeno-jejunal flexure to the transverse colon was dark red, without sheen, and soaked in bloody oedema. The serosal coat was raised in blebs, and there was bleeding into the muscular layers. The mucosa was swollen by a massive secretion of serosanguinous fluid. The mesenteric lymph nodes were haemorrhagic. The veins were engorged with blood but not thrombosed. These appearances are identical to those later described by Hertzler[2] and Boyd[3] in human subjects following mesenteric embolus. The histological appearances were those of progessive necrosis from the mucosa outwards, with oedema and haemorrhage; microscopy of the mesentery and bowel wall showed a backward-running venous stream and gradual filling of the veins.

The source of the haemorrhage was a matter of dispute among the early workers.

Litten clearly believed that it came from the veins. He excluded the possibility of its arriving via the arterial collateral by injecting various dyes into the left heart following SMA ligation and demonstrating that particles were present in every tissue except the infarcted bowel. This was later confirmed by our group[4] (Fig. 3.1).

Welch,[5] in his studies on haemorrhagic infarction, took the opposite view and concluded that the bleeding occurred from arterial collateral to the infarct. His studies, however, were of short loops of intestine, which in the dog have an abundant arterial collateral from either end. Welch measured the arterial and venous pressures following SMA occlusion and showed that a pressure of 30 mm Hg persists in the SMA beyond the point of ligature, and a pressure of 30–50 mm Hg is recordable in the portal vein. As the SMA pressure was gradually reduced, haemorrhagic infarction occurred when it reached a value of a quarter of normal.

Later studies on the effect of SMA ligation in rats by Khanna[6] confirmed the presence of an outward-spreading mucosal necrosis (which is apparent within a few minutes of ligation) and suggested that, at any rate in this animal, haemorrhage occurs from the arteries, as intraortic dye was found to enter the bowel through collaterals. No oedema and no evidence of altered capillary permeability in the serosa were observed. (The origin of the haemorrhagic infarct may well vary with species.)

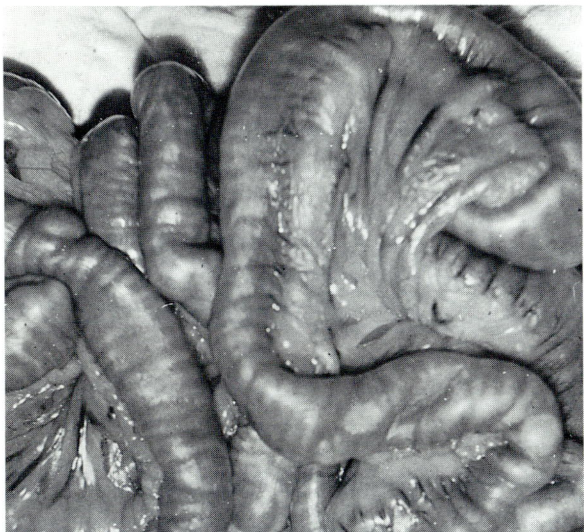

Fig. 3.1 Initial effects of SMA ligation — spasm and concentric pale stripes.

We re-examined the effects of acute occlusion of the SMA some twenty years ago[4] and largely confirmed Litten's observations. The initial reaction is of spasm, with empty arteries, and the appearance of concentric pale stripes at sites of maximum ischaemia (Fig. 3.2). After 3–4 hours tone disappears and the bowel becomes cyanotic, flabby and oedematous. Over the next few hours the swelling increases, and areas of discoloration appear, most obviously at the region of the ileocaecal junction, which is that part most distant from the embryological origin of the blood supply. A sharp demarcation appears between healthy and infarcted tissue, above, at the duodenojejunal flexure (Fig. 3.3) and, below, at the descending colon. These areas represent the junction of territories irrigated by the SMA and the other two great vessels. Although the bowel becomes progressively damaged and areas of greenish and even black gangrene appear, frank perforation is unusual. Areas of quite healthy intestine may persist, and the animal usually dies before the whole of its alimentary tract has succumbed. Disappearance of peristalsis is a capricious and unreliable sign, and indeed movement may be evoked in segments of bowel in an animal which has already died.

Destruction of the bowel is patchy because blood flow is sensitive to many factors, some of them mechanical, others biochemical and hormonal. The diameter and position of an individual loop, although unimportant in the healthy individual, becomes crucial when the arterial input pressure is drastically reduced, and under these circumstances small alterations in intraluminal tension, due to areas of spasm and obstruction, may have drastic effects on intramural flow. Furthermore, the bacterial and chemical contents of the bowel have been shown to have important effects on the speed of necrosis following SMA occlusion.[7, 8, 9]

Two other constant features are the appearance of a moderate quantity of turbid offensive fluid in the peritoneal cavity, and the appearance of bubbles of gas in the mesenteric veins, presumably derived from bacterial activity within the lumen and wall of the gut (Fig. 3.4).

Histological appearances

The very earliest change seen following SMA occlusion is lifting of the epithelium and formation of a space (Grunhagen's space) between the

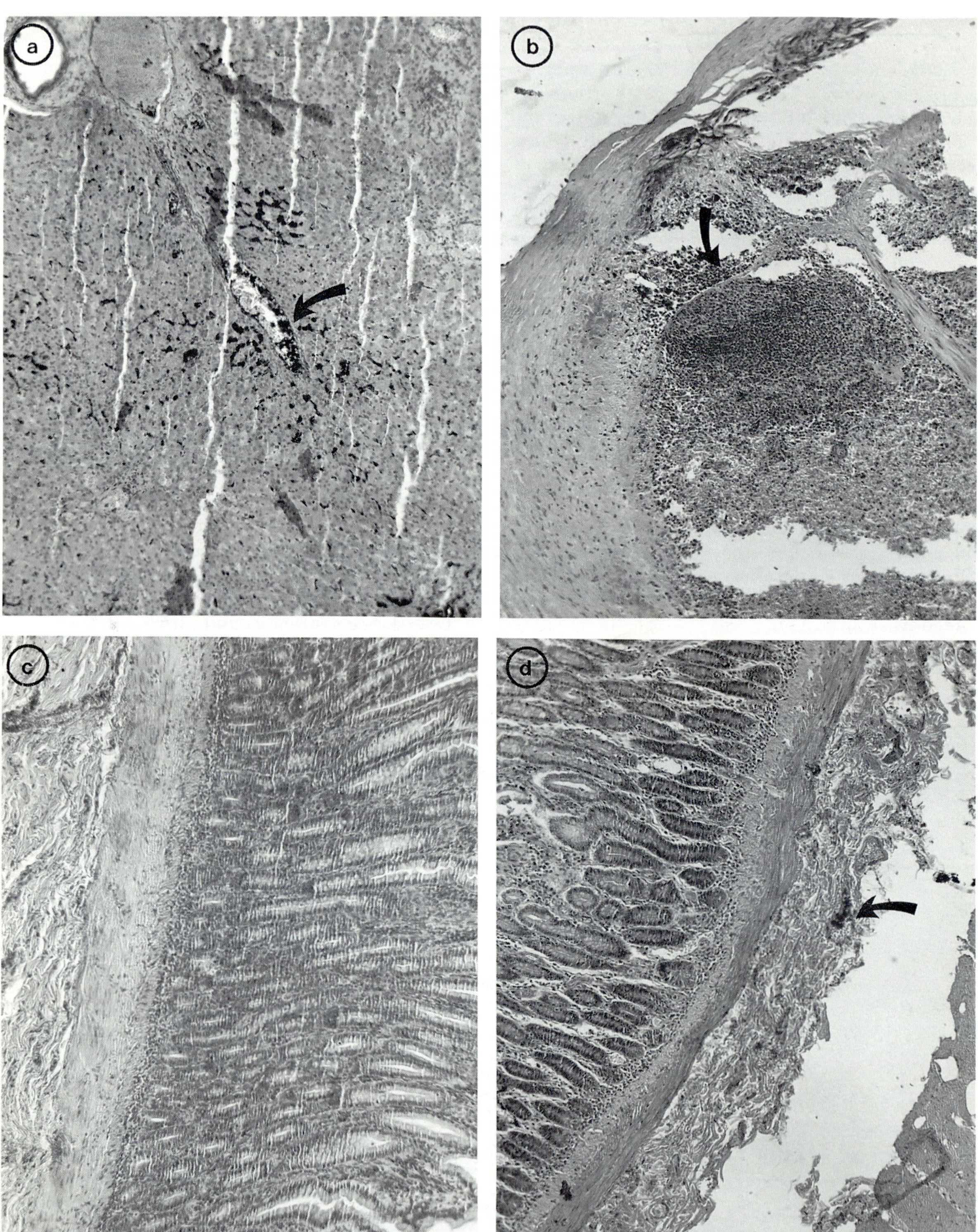

Fig. 3.2 Intra-arterial injection of graphite following SMA occlusion: (**a**) liver, (**b**) spleen, (**c**) terminal ileum and (**d**) terminal ileum following injection of graphite into the portal vein.

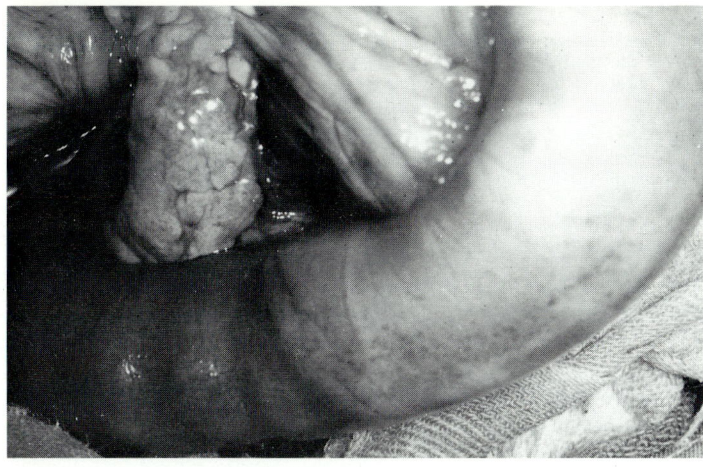

Fig. 3.3 Appearance of duodenojejunal flexure following occlusion of the SMA.

glandular cells and basement membrane.[10,11] The tips of the villi then begin to slough and a membrane of necrotic epithelium, fibrin, inflammatory cells and bacteria accumulates. Later on, oedema appears, with haemorrhage into the submucosa, while there is a steady progression of necrotic change from the lumen outwards until, in the worst-affected area, no trace of mucosal detail remains (Figs. 3.5–3.7). While these events occur in the mucosa, there is progressive emptying of the arterial tree with simultaneous engorgement of the veins, some of which thrombose (Fig. 3.8).[4] The initially brisk inflammatory response in the wall of the bowel gradually recedes, presumably due to depletion of cell numbers by anoxia, with no corresponding replacement from the arterial circulation. The bowel wall becomes progressively thinned as the mucosa separates and sloughs into the lumen, and at 9–10 hours (see Fig. 3.7) perforation may occur.

General effects of SMA occlusion

Until the advent of effective parenteral nutrition, gangrene of the midgut loop was incompatible with life. Now, massive resection of the small bowel can be compensated for, but a paradox still remains in that occlusion of the SMA is often fatal before the intestine has lost viability, and release of the occlusion leads to death more certainly and more quickly than if it is maintained.[11, 12, 13, 14] Total abolition of flow in the arterial side of the splanchnic

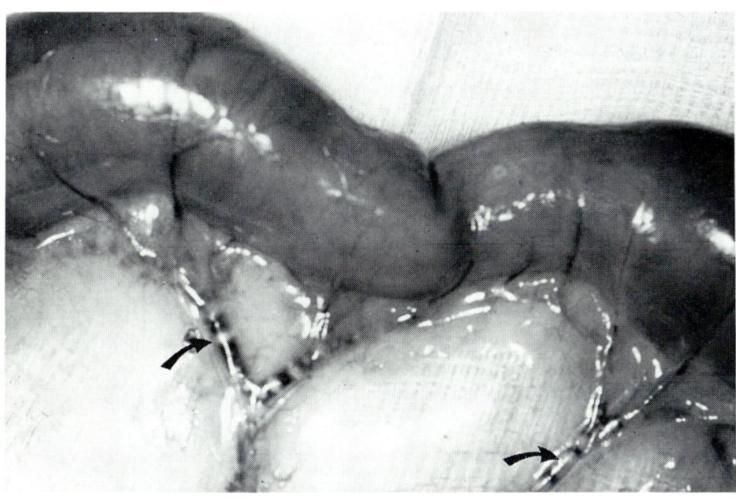

Fig. 3.4 Gas in the mesenteric veins.

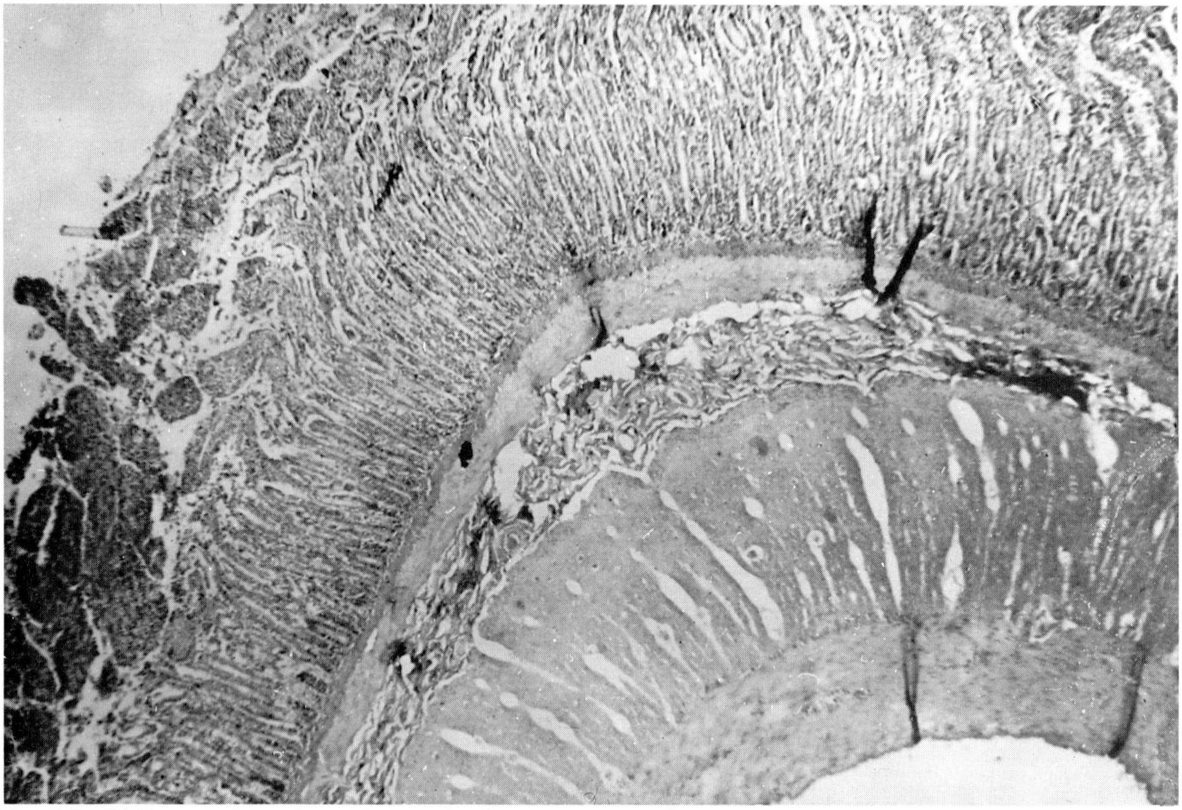

Fig. 3.5 SMA occlusion: photomicrograph of appearances at 3 hours.

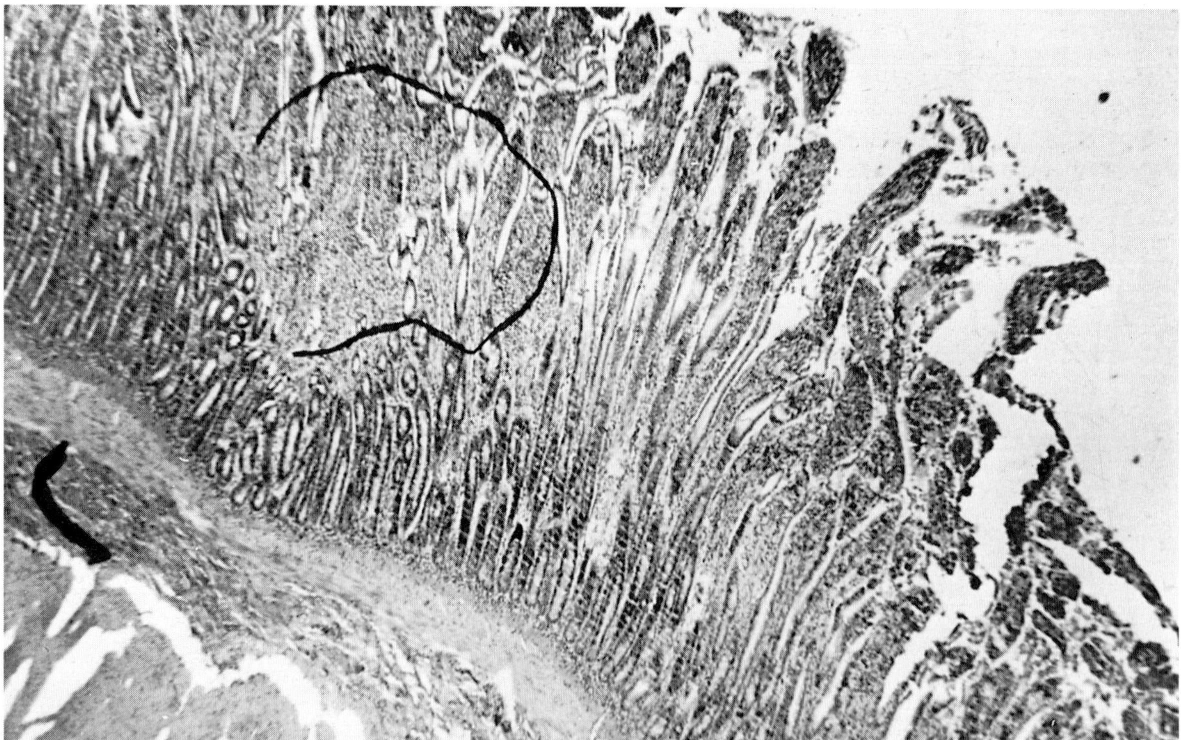

Fig. 3.6 SMA occlusion: photomicrograph of appearances at 6 hours.

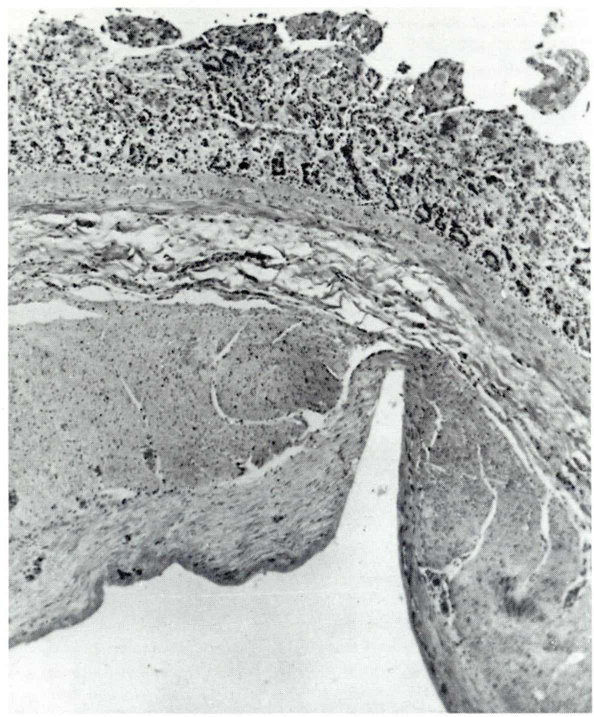

Fig. 3.7 SMA occlusion: photomicrograph of appearances at 9 hours.

circulation creates a complex physiological disturbance which can be analysed into several main components (Fig. 3.9).

Fluid loss

SMA occlusion is a variant of strangulation–obstruction. It is well established[15, 16] that between 15 and 65 per cent of the circulating volume can be lost in this condition, depending on the length of the strangulated loop. Whereas in short-loop strangulation the main cause of death is rupture and peritonitis, in long-loop strangulation it is loss of fluid. The classic experiments aimed to reproduce the type of intestinal obstruction which is seen clinically in a strangulated hernia, so the lesion in most cases involved a short loop of intestine, the veins, arteries and lumen of which were obstructed. This situation is rather different from total ischaemia of the midgut, where the veins remain patent. But an isolated arterial lesion does, in fact, lead to gross loss of extracellular fluid.

Our group[4, 17] demonstrated in 20 dogs a mean fall in blood volume of 34 per cent between the time of SMA occlusion and death. The red cell mass

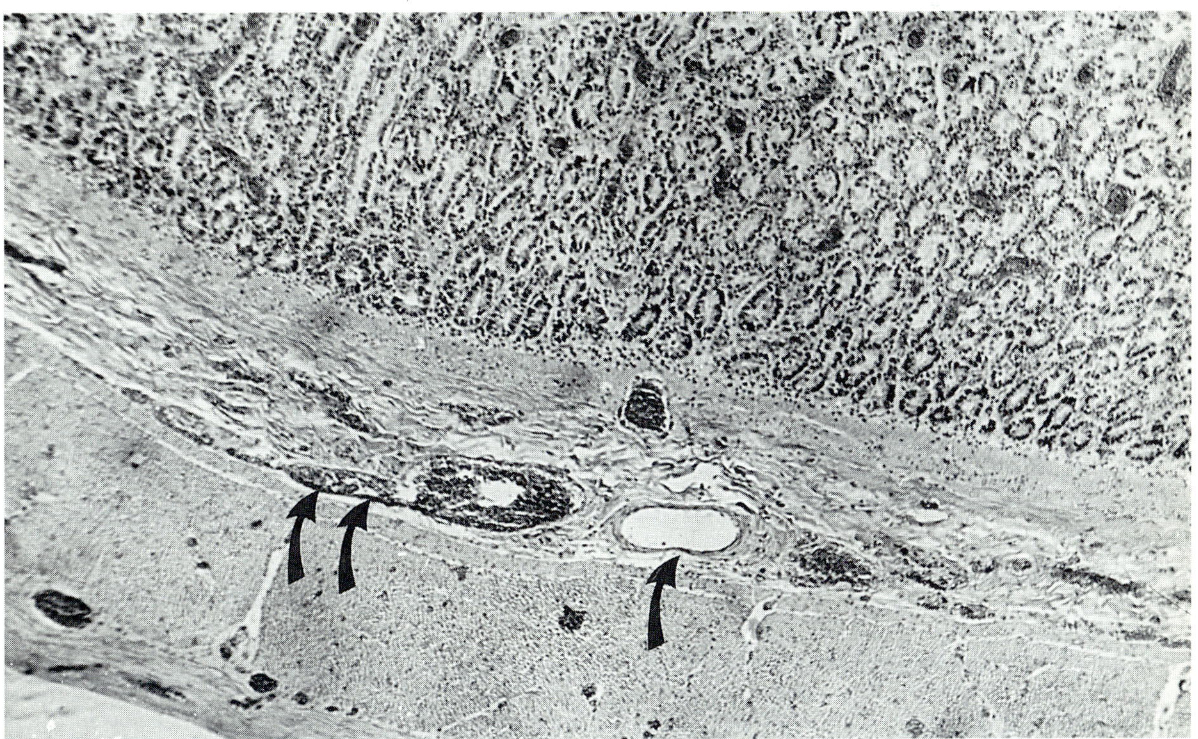

Fig. 3.8 SMA occlusion: photomicrograph showing collapsed arteries and thrombosed veins.

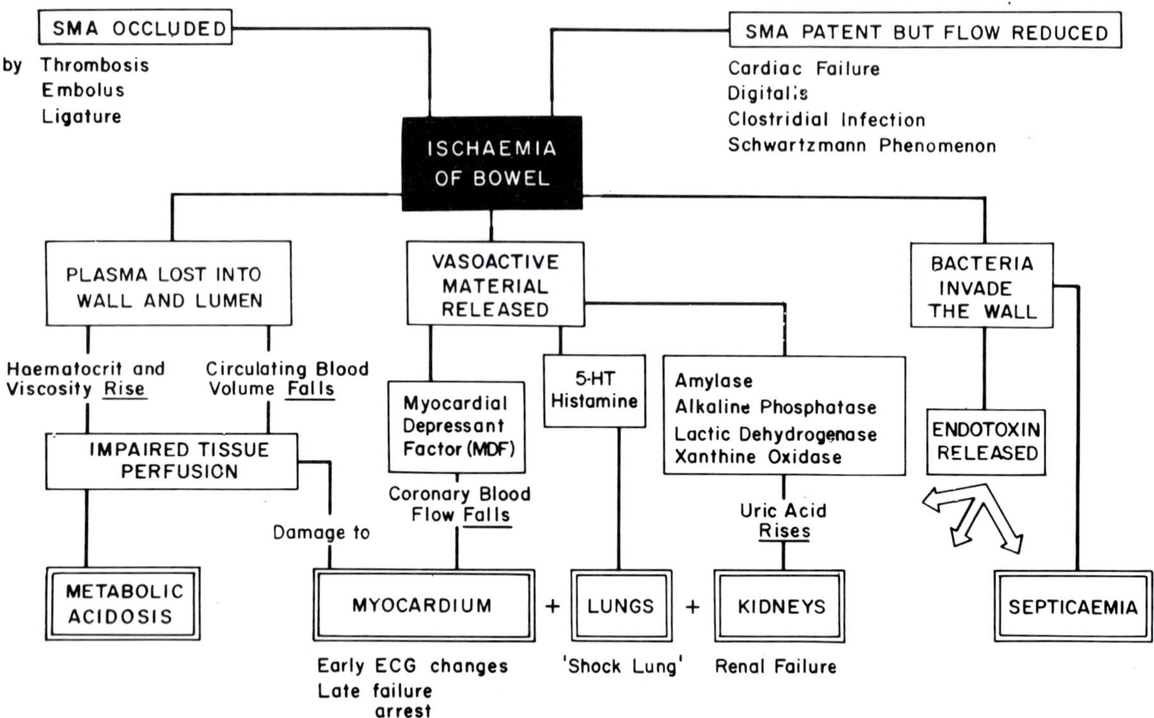

Fig. 3.9 Physiological consequences of massive small bowel ischaemia.

during this time fell by 10 per cent while the plasma volume fell on average by 54 per cent. The haematocrit frequently reached a level of 65–70 per cent immediately before death. This massive degree of haemoconcentration and fluid loss occurred in the absence of any significant portal hypertension, so the well-known syndrome of 'hepatic outflow obstruction' which tends to occur in dogs in response to stress was ruled out as a cause. The conclusion reached on the basis of these studies was that plasma leakage was occurring from the venous side of the circulation, into the wall and lumen of the bowel, via the damaged intestinal capillary.

These results were confirmed by Tjiong et al.,[18] who investigated the relative importance of fluid shift and metabolic change during and after occlusion of the SMA in 11 splenectomized dogs. Following measurements of blood volume and total body water, the SMA was clamped; the clamp was released 4 hours later, following which the spaces were measured at 0 and 2 hours. These authors were able to confirm the major shifts in body fluids observed by us, and at the same time demonstrated that blood cultures, in spite of changes characteristic of endotoxin absorption, were negative. While blood volume, total body water, serum potassium, pCO_2 and bicarbonate all declined, the arterial pO_2 remained constant.

Absorption of vasoactive material from the bowel

Vasocactive material is produced in the ischaemic bowel and absorbed via the peritoneum,[16] the veins[19] and the lymphatics.[6] Among the substances present are catecholamines,[20] histamine,[6] 5-hydroxytryptamine (5-HT),[21, 22] ferritin[22] and enzymes such as β-glucuronidase,[23] transaminases,[24] alkaline phosphatase,[25, 26] diamine oxidase[27] and β-*N*-acetylhexosaminidase.[28] Additionally, the portal blood is hyperkalaemic,[19, 29] hyperphosphatic[30] and rich in histamine[27] and bacterial endotoxin.[31]

Systemic effects can be demonstrated long before gangrene, or even much tissue damage, has occurred in the ischaemic intestine.[32] Williams and his group[33] have studied the early effects on the myocardium of short periods of small bowel ischaemia. Confirming and extending the earlier studies of Bounous et al.[7] and Dogru and Atasoy,[34] they demonstrated that within 1 hour of occlusion of the SMA in dogs there is a substantial decrease in cardiac output, accompanied by electrocardiographic change. Examination of the peripheral blood revealed the presence of a myocardial depressant factor (MDF), identified by its effect on the isolated rat myocardial strip.[35]

Similar results were obtained by Vyden, Nagasawa and Corday,[36] who studied the cardiovascular responses to acute occlusion of the SMA in dogs. They demonstrated initial transitory rises in arterial pressure and in coronary, renal and cerebral blood flow, which were followed by progressive increases in systemic vascular resistance with a concomitant fall-off in flow to all vital organs. The observed changes occurred early, before any great fall in plasma volume could have taken place, and were the opposite of what would have been expected from release of 5-HT from the damaged bowel. The authors lend their support to the view of Lefer and of Williams that a myocardial depressant factor is responsible, perhaps originating from the ischaemic pancreas.

Revascularization of the intestine

As has already been pointed out, once the SMA has been occluded for more than a few hours, release of the clamps leads to peripheral circulatory collapse and death of the animal.

The maximum tolerable period of midgut ischaemia in dogs was determined by Nelson and Kremen,[37] who found that the SMA could be safely occluded for 2 hours, but that release of the ligature after 3 hours' occlusion caused death in 60 per cent of dogs, and after 4 hours' occlusion in 80 per cent. The result of revascularizing the ischaemic intestine was haemorrhage into the bowel, accompanied by a fall in plasma volume and a rise in haematocrit.[12, 38] Revascularization of the ischaemic intestine is clearly unsafe, and this may help to explain the high mortality of mesenteric embolectomy in clinical practice.

Zuidema et al.[39] found that a 2-hour period of SMA occlusion in dogs produced leakage of ^{131}I-labelled polyvinylpyrrolidone (PVP) into the bowel, lowered serum albumin, decreased fat absorption, and a transient drop in blood urea nitrogen over a period of several days. Serum sodium and potassium levels were unaffected.

We[4] confirmed the abrupt fall in arterial blood pressure, peripheral resistance and blood volume which occurs following release of the occluded SMA, and demonstrated that whereas the fluid lost in the prerelease periods was largely plasma, revascularization led to massive haemorrhage into the intestinal wall and lumen, in itself quite enough to account for death of the animal.[4, 40]

It was further shown that when a normal donor dog was cross-circulated through the ischaemic bowel, it too died, but that this death could be prevented by blood replacement, suggesting that absorption of toxic material was a less important lethal factor than was haemorrhage under these circumstances.[40]

These early studies could be challenged in that they (1) took no account of the spleen's contribution to the blood volume, (2) measured total blood volume with the use of iodinated serum albumin which is now known to be misleading, and (3) drew conclusions from cross-circulation experiments involving unmatched blood. However, later work using a more refined approach has confirmed their findings. Thus Chiu, Scott and Gurd,[41] while admitting the importance of absorption of such toxic factors as histamine and β-glucuronidase, found that after 3 hours of SMA occlusion in the splenectomized dogs the mortality could be reduced from 89 to 36 per cent by adequate fluid therapy. Flushing of the mesenteric circulation following the same period of ischaemia did not produce circulatory failure. Kangwalklai et al.[42] carried out detailed space-studies during and after 3 hours' SMA occlusion. They confirmed our findings of progressive plasma loss (actually 3.9 per cent per hour as opposed to 5 per cent per hour, but this could be accounted for by differences in experimental detail) but found much less contraction in blood and plasma volumes after release of the clamp, although there was a contraction in total, and particularly in intracellular, body water. Later figures obtained by Tjiong et al.[18] of the same research team showed greater losses of whole blood.

However, this cannot be the whole story and it is well recognized that death from revascularization of the ischaemic bowel, long before the point of necrosis is reached, is often not preventable by maintenance of normal blood volume,[8] whereas preparation of the bowel by various measures designed to reduce endotoxin production and prevent vasoconstriction in the intestinal wall help to lower the mortality.[43]

Conclusions

The controversy as regards the relative importance of fluid depletion and toxic absorption as causes of death in mesenteric vascular occlusion is still not resolved, and perhaps never will be. Not surprisingly, there does seem to be a direct relation between the extent of the villous damage and the amount of cardiotoxic material released from the gut following induced periods of low perfusion. Haglund and Lundgren[44] have identified two heat-stable fractions from ischaemic cat intestine, one water soluble with a molecular mass of 500–1000 daltons and the other lipid soluble of unknown mass. However, provided the ischaemic damage is sufficiently slight to be wholly recoverable when the bowel is revascularized, the substances released into the systemic circulation following removal of the occlusion (potassium, histamine, 5-HT, cellular enzymes, endotoxin and other vasoactive materials) may not always reach concentrations high enough to cause death, provided that the circulatory volume is adequately maintained.

Factors which modify the effects of SMA ligation

These include the following.

Hypothermia
The tolerable period of SMA occlusion can be lengthened considerably by lowering the body temperature[38] to the extent that if the bowel is cooled to 5°C its entire circulation can be interrupted so that autotransplantation can be carried out.[12]

Antibiotics
Laufman[45] found that a 6-hour venous strangulation of the lower ileum in dogs was invariably fatal, whereas with massive penicillin therapy 8 out of 10 recovered, with varying degrees of stricturing and peritoneal adhesions. Cohn[46] was able to preserve normal mucosa in completely devascularized loops of intestine when tetracycline was given into the lumen. Benjamin et al.[47] extended these results to show that the mortality period following SMA ligation could be extended with systemic penicillin and streptomycin.

These laboratory findings have prompted clinicians to reduce the bowel flora with aminoglycoside drugs before undertaking reconstruction of the lower aorta and visceral arteries. Similar protection from endotoxin absorption in established ischaemia can be provided by peritoneal lavage.[48]

Anticoagulants
Martin, Laufman and Tuell[49] demonstrated that systemic heparin prevented sludging of blood and adherence of cells to the endothelial wall of the small gut vessels in major vascular occlusion; this work was confirmed by Nelson and Kremen,[37] who showed a substantial reduction of mortality in SMA occlusion and a prolongation of the safe occlusion period. The administration of low molecular weight dextran fractions[48, 50] has also been demonstrated as useful, although it may be that their beneficial effect is through plasma expansion. Heparin may also mitigate the damage caused by ischaemia by enhancing the effects of diamine oxidase,[27] whose protective antihistaminic effect in this situation is well established.[51]

α-Adrenergic blockade

Nahor, Milliken and Fine[13] studied the effect of coeliac blockage and of intravenous and intra-aortic phenoxybenzamine on standard SMA shock in dogs and rabbits, and showed that prerelease blockade significantly lowered the death rate. When this treatment was given following restoration of blood flow, results were less good although coeliac blockade still had some effect. The exact way in which these agents improve the intestinal circulation is not clear. Any remaining arterial spasm in the intestinal wall is presumably abolished and the collateral circulation dilated, but in the circumstances of extreme anoxia the minute vessels will already have been largely paralysed. At the same time, the sympathomimetic effect of the various vasoactive polypeptides, and of bacterial endotoxin, will be counteracted. Vasodilatation in the liver and spleen may also be of importance. There is, furthermore, some evidence that α-adrenergic blockade is capable of preventing the myocardial lesion which occurs in experimental endotoxin shock.[52]

The internal milieu
Gurd and his associates at McGill University have drawn attention to the importance of conditions within the intestinal lumen in the development of haemorrhagic lesions in the intestine in low-output states, or in experimentally induced ischaemia. An important cause of death in canine shock is intestinal autolysis associated with tryptic activity. Their work[7] has demonstrated that a 90-minute occlusion period of both SMA and IMA produces demonstrable lesions in the heart and kidney, which can be prevented by the preoperative feeding of an elemental diet. The diet consists of amino acids, sucrose, electrolytes and vitamins, and when the

standard ischaemic challenge is given the extra-intestinal lesions fail to appear. It appears that pancreatic proteolytic enzymes present in the lumen of the bowel are involved in the pathogenesis of the haemorrhagic intestinal necrosis, and that such enzymic activity can be abolished by altering the intraluminal content.

However, Manohar and Tyagi[53] found that ligation of the pancreatic duct, which abolished tryptic enteritis, does not in fact lessen the mortality from SMA shock, and that sterilization of the bowel has little effect. Survival time is prolonged by intravenous fluid therapy and cortisol.

Intraluminal oxygen

Haglund and Lundgren[44] found that small amounts of oxygen supplied to the mucosa via an intraluminal perfusion of oxygenated saline could prevent the development of haemorrhagic lesions in the tips of the villi, which occur during periods of reduced intestinal blood flow. This effect was not seen when nitrogenated saline was used.

This work was extended by Shute,[54] who found an 89 per cent mortality and gross histological damage to the bowel in rats subjected to SMA occlusion for 2 hours, which could be reduced to 29 per cent (with correspondingly reduced damage) by the use of gaseous oxygen introduced into the lumen. Not only were the mucosal changes much reduced by this treatment but also endotoxin absorption was significantly lowered[55] (Figs. 3.10 and 3.11).

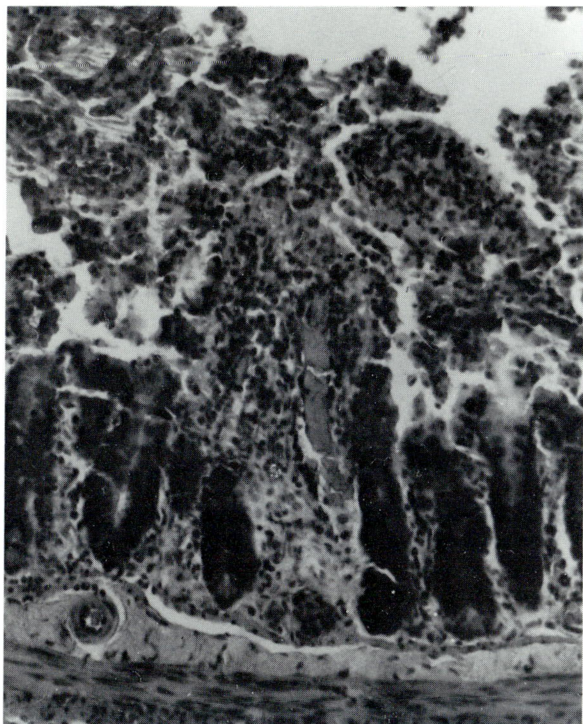

Fig. 3.10 Rat ileum following ligation of the SMA for 4 hours. (By courtesy of Mr Kenneth Shute.)

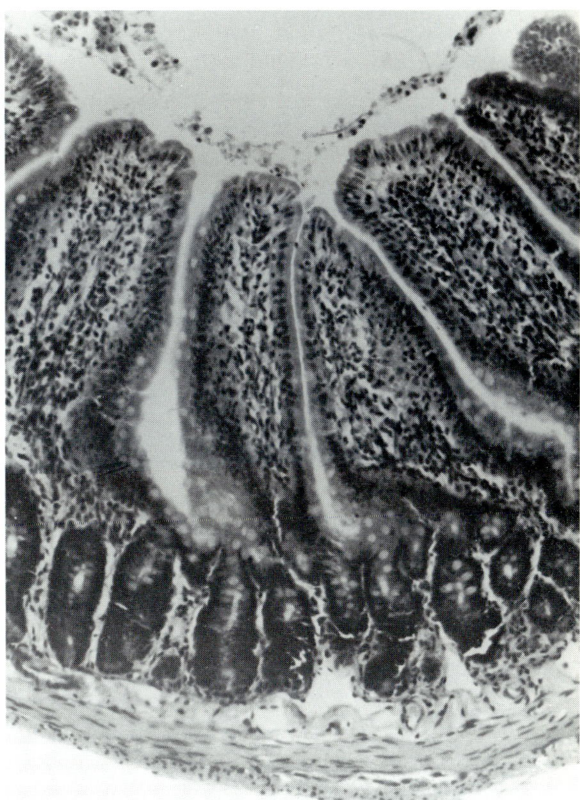

Fig. 3.11 The same as in Fig. 3.10, but with intraluminal instillation of oxygen. (By courtesy of Mr Kenneth Shute.)

Tests of viability

It is important, in the clinical context, to know whether a segment of bowel which has been damaged by ischaemia is capable of recovery. Estimation by eye of bowel colour, arterial pulsation and peristalsis is notoriously unreliable.[56]

Later, more refined methods have included the tetrazolium bromide (MTT) reduction test[57] and the use of labelled albumin microspheres,[58] but these essentially experimental methods have not been adopted clinically because they require complicated equipment which is unlikely to be at hand in an emergency. The two methods currently in use are Doppler ultrasound and intravenous fluorescein. Doppler techniques were first used in the laboratory by Wright and Hobson[59] and later in the operating theatre by Cooperman et al.[60] Cooperman et al. found that they were able to differentiate quite clearly between 4 patients who had viable bowel and good Doppler signals, 9 who had ischaemic bowel and no signal and who then underwent resection, and a third group of 10 patients who had clinically dubious bowel but in whom arterial signals were present. In this last group the bowel was retained and no problem resulted. Shah and Anderson[61] confirmed these findings in the laboratory, this time using venous rather than arterial interruption. However, other workers have not reproduced these results and in two experimental[62, 63] and one clinical[64] series where visual and Doppler assessment have been compared with fluorescein in injection the fluorescent technique was clearly more reliable. This method involves the intravenous injection of a bolus of fluorescein, followed by examination of the suspect loop of bowel under Wood's light. Fluorescence indicates vascularity, and, although this is not the same as viability, it is a good predictor; this is discussed in Chapter 4.

Chronic occlusion of the SMA and other main arteries

Gradual obliteration of the SMA is not lethal to man but may lead to disease. Recognition of this has led to many laboratory studies, the first of which was by Blalock and Levy[65] whose interest, in fact, was not in intestinal ischaemia *per se* but in the regulation of the arterial blood pressure. Following Goldblatt's demonstration that constriction of the renal artery gave rise to hypertension, they sought

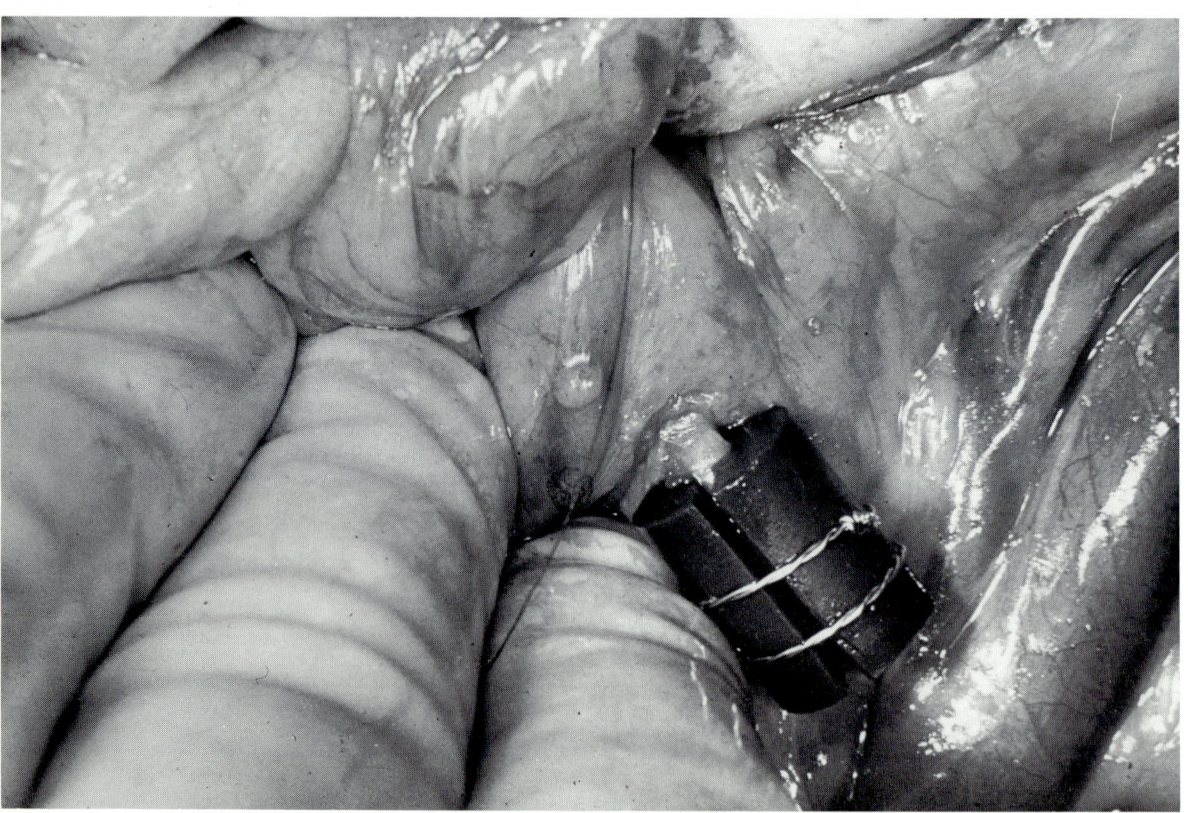

Fig. 3.12 The Ameroid cylinder.

this property in various other vessels, with negative results. By selective constriction of the coeliac axis, SMA and IMA with Goldblatt clamps, they were able to obtain 7 surviving dogs out of 29 whose intestinal arteries were completely closed. These animals appeared to be in good health, and no gross abnormality was found at autopsy.

Laufman[66] obtained complete occlusion of the SMA in 2 out of 5 dogs over a period of 4 months by wrapping cellophane tape around the origin of the vessel. These animals suffered a severe systemic upset, lost weight and became anaemic. Some pallor of the bowel and mucosal destruction were noted. Spencer and Derrick[67] reported a series of 7 dogs in which they narrowed the SMA to an estimated 66–91 per cent of its original diameter with a thread ligature. These animals again showed weight loss, diarrhoea and epilation over a 4-month period, at the end of which they were sacrificed. A control dog in whom the same dissection was performed but the ligature left loose remained in good health. Pallor of the bowel was noted *post mortem*.

In none of these three series of experiments were detailed biochemical, radiological or histological observations made. Chronic midgut ischaemia was not investigated fully in the laboratory until we re-studied the problem in 1963[40] using the Ameroid cylinder technique (Ameroid is a plastic which has the property of expanding at a constant rate when it is wet, so that, if outward expansion is prevented, any structure enclosed within it will be predictably compressed) (Fig. 3.12). Fourteen dogs were used in these experiments. Following a baseline estimation of weight, haematocrit, serum levels of vitamin B_{12} and folate, and a *d*-xylose absorption test, the collateral circulation above and below the superior mesenteric arterial territory was divided and an Ameroid cylinder positioned around the origin of the SMA. It was calculated that obliteration of the lumen of the vessel would be complete at about 3 weeks, and this was confirmed by aortography (Fig. 3.13) and a subsequent laparotomy at which the bowel was biopsied.

Apart from a transient disturbance some 4–7 days after insertion of the Ameroid, no obvious clinical abnormality was noticed in these dogs. At the final laparotomy, the bowel appeared pale but otherwise normal, and no pulsations could be detected in the arcades. A pressure gradient of 100 mm Hg was generally found across the occluded segment of artery. Vascular adhesions had formed around the Ameroid, the loops of bowel and the abdominal incisions. There appeared to be no hypertrophy of the coeliac axis, inferior mesenteric artery or lumbar and lower intercostal branches, and aortography (Fig. 3.13) showed that the bowel was nourished by a network of fine collaterals originating from extracoelomic vessels. No specific abnormalities were found in the serum folate and B_{12} levels although there was some drop in haematocrit. The xylose absorption studies were not conclusive and probably reflected the inaccuracy of the method (Fig. 3.14). Overall, absorption tended to decrease over the first 6 weeks and then gradually to revert to normal. There was little correlation between xylose excretion, haematocrit and body weight, which often tended to shift independently. Biopsies of the lower ileum obtained at intervals of from 3 to 13 weeks postoperatively were completely normal.

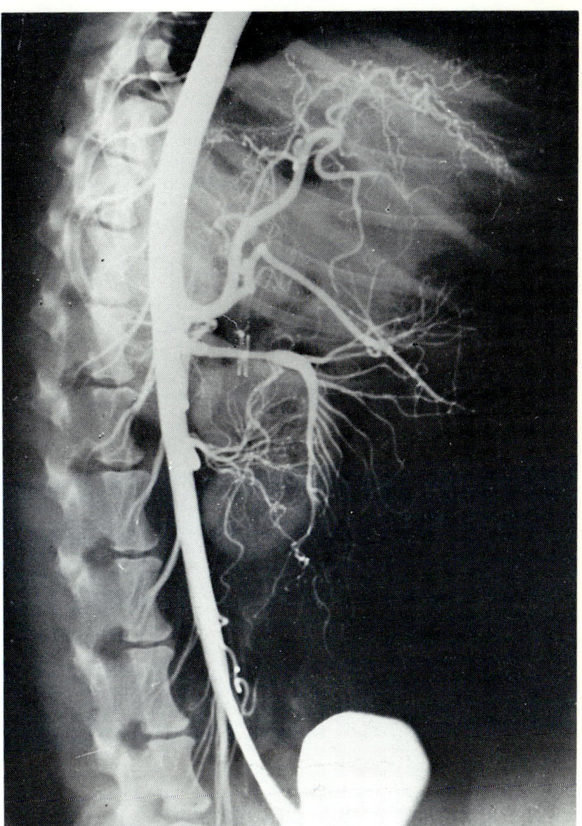

Fig. 3.13 Aortography showing poststenotic dilatation of SMA and enlargement of branches of CMA.

Similar studies using an Ameroid cylinder were

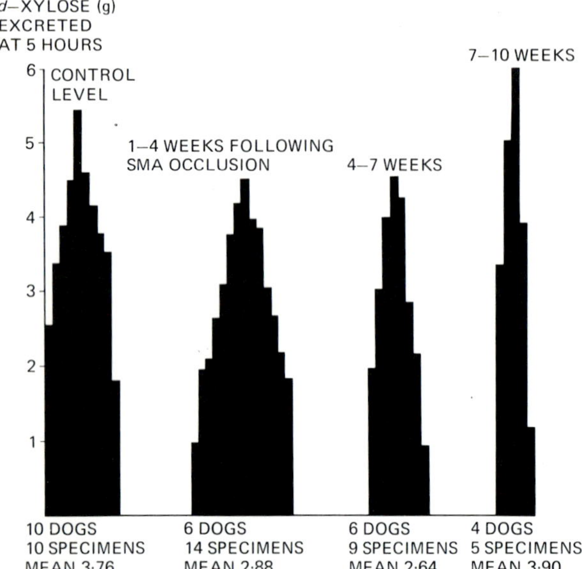

Fig. 3.14 *d*-Xylose absorption following chronic occlusion of SMA. (From Marston[17] by kind permission of the Hon. Editor, *Annals of the Royal College of Surgeons of England*.)

carried out by Popovsky.[68] These, too, had negative results.

In other words, the early results of Laufmann and of Spencer and Derrick could not be repeated, and although it is possible to produce chronic obliteration of the mesenteric arteries in the laboratory, it seems that the lesions do not correlate with intestinal structure or function.

Occlusion of segmental vessels

The small intestine

It is less easy than might be thought to produce consistent lesions in the small intestine by interference with the regional blood supply. Such attempts usually either kill the animal from intestinal rupture and peritonitis or else have no demonstrable effect on the bowel. Litten[1] ligated jejunal and ileal arteries in 19 dogs and found no intestinal damage. Maass[69] was able to demonstrate stenosis of the small intestine in rabbits after temporary interruption of the blood supply, but most later studies have not succeeded in causing parenchymal lesions unless both arteries and veins have been interrupted.[70, 71, 72]

Glotzer et al.[73] constructed an isolated jejunal loop in 17 dogs, and at a second operation produced mucosal ischaemia by constricting the pedicle of the loop for between 2 and 8 hours. Eight-hour periods of ischaemia resulted in gangrene of the loop and death of the animal. The depth of damage in the other groups was directly proportional to the duration of ischaemia, as was the period necessary for healing, which was between 1 and 100 days. The significance of this study was that it showed that complete repair, not only of the mucosa but also of the smooth muscle in the villi was possible after even a very deep ischaemic injury. Additionally, the regenerated villi were seen to be short, irregular, thick and branching, resembling the appearances found in coeliac disease or following radiation injury (see Chapter 9).

Our experience[40] was disappointing in that ligation of the arcade vessels produced neither gross nor histological abnormality. The same findings were obtained by Vest and Margulis,[72] who showed that interruption of these vessels resulted either in no change at all or in gangrene, perforation and death. There are, as already mentioned, significant differences in vascular architecture between different species, which may well account for the discrepancies between the results. Nevertheless, it is recognized that an ischaemic insult which is not sufficiently prolonged or severe to lead to gangrene, but at the same time prevents normal regeneration of the specialized layers of the bowel, can produce lasting damage, usually in the form of a fibrous stricture (see Chapters 8 and 9).

The 'potassium stricture'

A particular form of ischaemic damage in the small intestine is that caused by the application of high concentrations of potassium ion to the mucosa. This has particular relevance to the strictures encountered clinically in association with enteric-coated potassium chloride tablets. Stahlgren, Dapena and Roy[74] demonstrated that potassium chloride, alone or in combination with thiazide diuretics, could produce focal mucosal ulceration, which sometimes progressed to fibrosis and stricture formation. This was particularly prone to occur if the arterial arcades to the segment had been divided, which in itself, as already explained, is not a damaging situation in the small intestine. The fact that pre-existing intestinal ischaemia is likely to give rise to potassium stricture was underlined by the work of Mansfield et al.[75] who showed that animals with an experimentally constructed pressure gradient across the SMA were particularly vulnerable to insult by potassium. They pointed out that ulceration took place at the site of lymphoid follicles, which tallies with the clinical observation that most of these lesions occur in the ileum, where lymphoid tissue is concentrated. This is discussed further in Chapter 8.

The colon

The original experiments on acute segmental colonic ischaemia were carried out by Hukuhara, Kotani and Sato.[76] These authors were interested in the causation of congenital megacolon, and in 4 dogs produced a 4-hour period of ischaemia by isolating a segment of colon on a vascular pedicle perfused with Tyrode solution. They carried out barium studies at intervals in the postoperative period, and eventually sacrificed the animals for histological examination. They demonstrated contraction of the gut in a region corresponding to the perfused segment, but this area could be distended by increasing the head of pressure by barium and the authors concluded that the stricture was of a functional rather than a structural nature. Pathological appearances showed contracture and shortening of the bowel but no mucosal ulceration. Histological abnormalities were comparatively minor but no normal ganglion cells were found in the myoepithelial plexuses. It is interesting that later work by de Villiers,[77] using an almost identical technique, produced contrasting results in that there were marked changes in the mucosa and muscle layers of the ischaemic segments but ganglion cells were present in every specimen examined. De Villiers completely failed to reproduce the results of the Japanese workers, and could not concur in postulating ischaemia as a possible factor in the genesis of congenital aganglionosis.

Further studies in experimental devascularization of the colon were carried out by Boley et al.[78] These authors were interested in the clinical and radiological aspects of colonic ischaemia, and were able to reproduce in the laboratory their clinical experience by ligating the dog's intestinal arteries at or distal to the arcades. They followed up these studies[79] by a further series of experiments in which glass and ceramic microspheres of known diameter were injected into the caudal mesenteric artery via the aorta. They noted blanching and contraction of the involved segment during injection, which usually disappeared when the arterial clamps were released and blood flow was resumed. If the colour of the bowel did not return to normal, necrosis followed (although, conversely, return of colour did not preclude subsequent necrosis). According to the size and quantity of the microspheres injected, a varying degree of streaking, superficial ulceration, inflammation, perforation and eventual stricture formation was observed. Barium enemas were carried out under anaesthesia and showed 'thumb-printing', ulceration and late stenosis. No histological studies were reported by these authors.

Studies in our laboratory[26] confirmed and extended this work. In these experiments standard vascular interruptions were carried out as follows (Fig. 3.15):

1. Ligation of the caudal mesenteric artery.
2. Ligation of the caudal mesenteric artery and marginal artery.
3. Ligation of the caudal mesenteric and marginal arteries, plus the common colic artery.

Following operation, the animals were sacrificed at 1, 14 and 42 days. Observations made during the experimental period included routine clinical examination, sigmoidoscopy, barium enema, leucocyte count, and estimation of alkaline phosphatase, lactic dehydrogenase, aspartate transaminase and glutamate transaminase. In addition, all the lesions were examined both grossly and microscopically.

The aim of these studies was to reproduce as far as possible the effects of a mesenteric thrombosis affecting the colon. For this reason it was considered better simply to ligate the vessels rather than to introduce the added factors of intravascular foreign bodies or of the gross alterations in tissue electrolyte concentrations which are bound to occur following perfusion with saline or Tyrode solution. By varying the site of vascular interruption and by studying the lesions at successive degrees of maturity, it was hoped to obtain some information regarding the natural history of the condition. The main findings of this study were as follows.

Ligation of the caudal mesenteric artery (CMA) alone has little effect, but even quite severe degrees of colonic ischaemia are well tolerated by the healthy animal and do not usually cause a major systemic illness.

The most striking changes seen on sigmoidoscopy occurred the day following the operation, and consisted in a circumferential mucosal slough at the

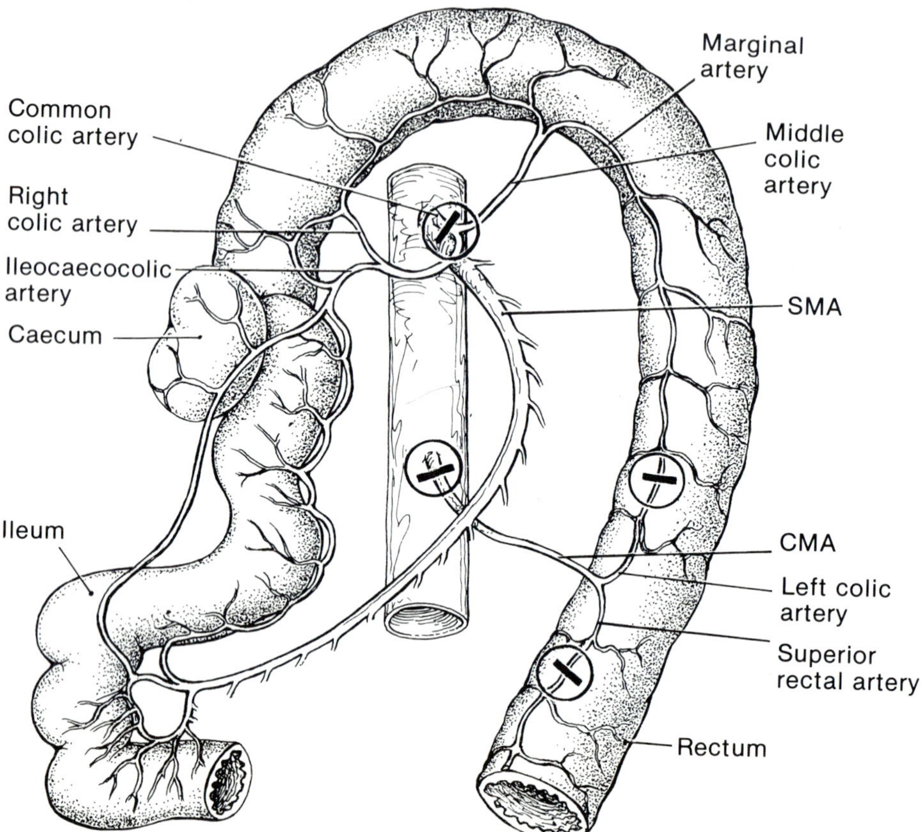

Fig. 3.15 The colonic circulation in the dog, showing sites of occlusion.

rectosigmoid junction with intense congestion above and below. At 14 days (Fig. 3.16) small discrete ulcers were seen, and at 6 weeks these were followed by stricture formation and contact bleeding. Less florid lesions, such as spasm, mucosal oedema and haemorrhage into the submucous lymphoid follicles, were frequent. Ligation of the caudal mesenteric artery alone produced minor abnormalities in 1 animal out of 6, the remaining 5 being unaffected.

The earliest radiological change was 'thumb-printing' of the affected segment, due to spasm, mucosal oedema and haemorrhage, which usually reverted to normal within a few weeks although occasionally a persistent stenosis resulted. The ulceration which was seen through the sigmoidoscope and on the pathological specimens proved difficult to demonstrate radiologically (Fig. 3.17).

Histopathological changes varied from surface inflammation to heavy deposition of fibrous tissue, depending on the extent and maturity of the lesion

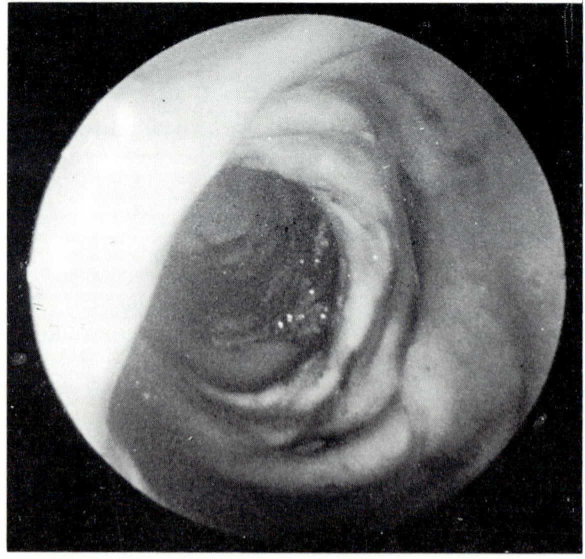

Fig. 3.16 Sigmoidoscopic appearances 2 weeks following ligation of CMA and IMA.

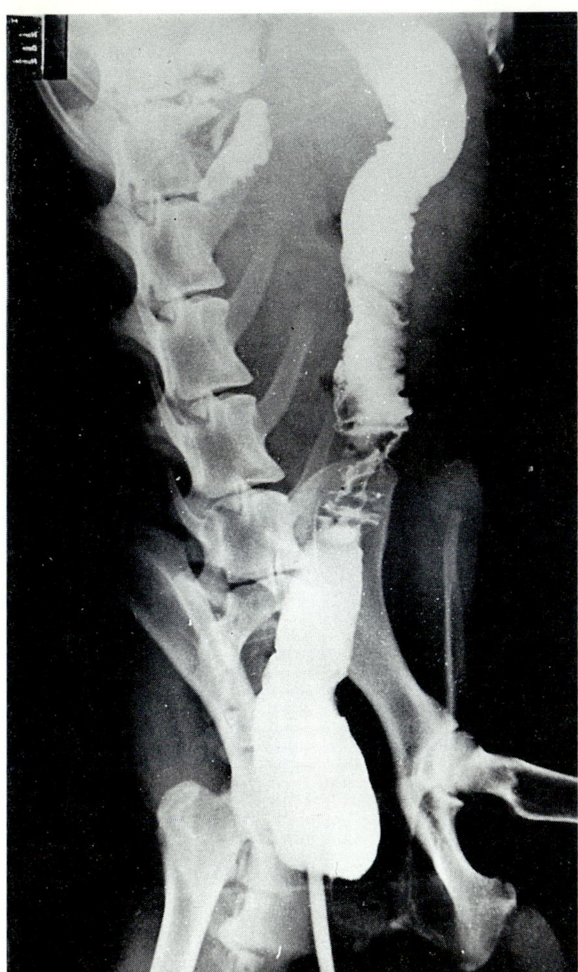

Fig. 3.17 Barium enema 42 days after ligation of CMA and IMA, showing (above) thumb-printing and (below) a stricture.

(Fig. 3.18). A conspicuous feature was the presence of haemosiderin-laden macrophages in the submucosa (see also Chapter 10).

There was a sharp rise in circulating leucoctyes following operation in all cases, which seemed unrelated to the degree of vascular injury.

Postoperative levels of lactic dehydrogenase and of aspartate and glutamate transaminases did not vary significantly from the preoperative baseline. However, the serum level of alkaline phosphatase rose abruptly in the immediate postoperative period, and this rise was directly related to the extent of devascularization and mucosal necrosis (Fig. 3.19). This finding prompted the question as to whether intestinal isoenzyme was being released into the circulation by the damaged bowel, which might form the basis of a potentially useful laboratory test for acute intestinal ischaemia.[26] However, when the isoenzymes were separated, no preponderance was found of the intestinal fraction, and the observed rise in alkaline phosphatase appeared to be coming from the liver. The differences noted between the groups of major colonic injury and the controls suggested, however, that the rise in enzyme level is not purely the result of handling of the liver during the operation because this happens to the same extent in both groups. A possible explanation is that the damaged colon leads to portal bacteraemia, which provokes an outpouring of hepatic enzyme. However, without bacteriological examination of the portal blood, this must remain a speculation. In fact, whatever the origin of the phosphatase, its peripheral effects — that is to say, liberation of inorganic phosphate into the systemic blood stream — are very gross. Jamieson and colleagues[30, 80] examined a large range of enzymes and inorganic substances in the laboratory and in patients, and showed that major rises in inorganic phosphate occur with gross arterial lesions, changes which are not seen in venous lesions or following interruption of small arteries. The clinical implications of this finding are obvious.

Further studies from our laboratory[81] were concerned with venous lesions of the colon. At first, attempts were made to produce thrombosis of the inferior mesenteric vein by simple application of ligatures, but those were unsuccessful. Subsequently, an isolated segment of vein was thrombosed by injecting thrombin according to the technique originally described by Polk.[82] In 13 dogs so treated, severe lesions were produced. The effects of arterial and venous occlusion were quite different. In the acute stages both showed congestion and oedema of the submucosa, but mucosal necrosis, which is so frequent in arterial lesions, was not found in those caused by interference with the veins. When it occurs, venous gangrene appears to affect mainly the submucosa and is usually associated with total necrosis of the muscle; the mucosa may be lost as a secondary process. The early histological picture shows congestion and dilatation of lymphatics and collateral veins. In the later stages, after resolution, there was evidence of erythrocyte sequestration, as seen by deposition of haemosiderin in the submucosa and also in the regional mesenteric lymph

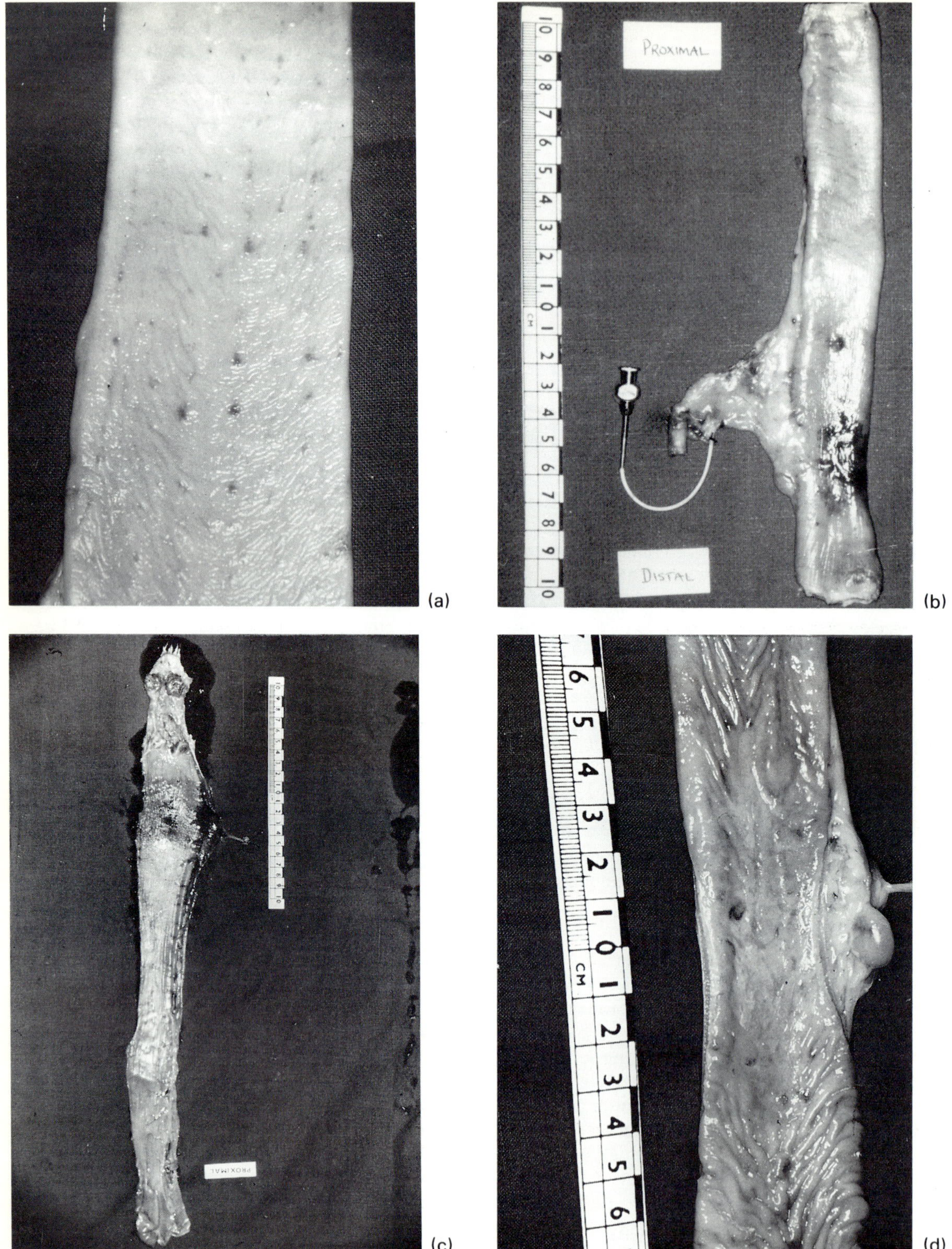

Fig. 3.18 Gross pathology of colonic ischaemia in the dog: (**a**) early minor vascular injury, (**b** and **c**) early major injury, (**d**) late changes.

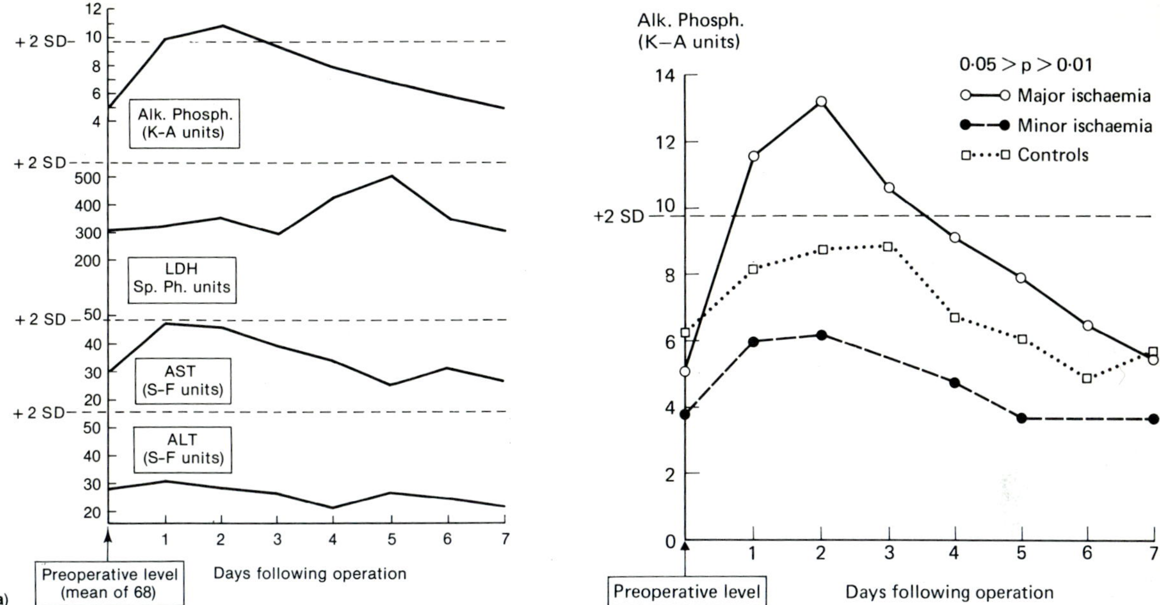

Fig. 3.19 Changes in (**a**) serum enzymes and (**b**) alkaline phosphatase levels following colonic ischaemia. (From Marston et al.[26] by kind permission of the Editor, *Gut*.)

nodes, the latter feature being highly characteristic. Sigmoidoscopy revealed widespread blue congestion of the mucosa, as distinct from the pale slough which appears following arterial interruption. The radiological and sigmoidoscopic features correlated well, particularly in the more severe cases, and 'thumb-printing' was more obvious after venous thrombosis. The changes in leucocyte count and serum enzyme levels following venous interruption were much the same as had been seen with arterial lesions.

The group of workers from Lausanne[83, 84] have for some years been interested in the functional as well as the morphological response of the colon to ischaemia. They have used a technique of total colonic ischaemia induced by clamping all afferent arteries for different periods of time, following which measurements of sodium flux, together with concentrations of Na/K/ATPase, across the mucosa are measured. The morphological changes produced were very much as have been described above. The authors drew attention to the comparatively slight effects of short periods of ischaemia on the colonic mucosa, contrasting with the autolytic destruction seen in the ileum after similar challenge. In this study two groups of dogs were used: an acute group in which the colons were removed for functional studies, and a recovery group in which the maturation of the lesion could be studied and its function estimated weeks later. It was found that active sodium transport disappeared after 2 hours of ischaemia, although ATPase activity persisted. Sodium flux was not a very convenient or reliable determinant of colonic function in the more severe lesions but Na/K/ATPase levels correlated well with recoverability, and the authors suggested that it may prove to be a useful clinical test. Matthews and Parks[85] have confirmed these results and have shown that, when SMA flow is reduced to below 20 per cent of normal, absorption of sodium ion is replaced by net secretion. They suggest that this may help to explain the diarrhoea observed in chronic intestinal ischaemia in that the diarrhoea may originate in the small bowel and that the ischaemic colon, being unable to absorb fluid bulk, acts as a passive tube for the transport of unaltered ileal contents.

Matthews and Parks[85] go on to observe that gradual occlusion of common colic and caudal mesenteric arteries in the dog does not bring about functional change in the colon but that, when SMA flow in such an animal is abruptly lowered by hypotensive drugs or venesection, then ischaemic changes in the colon are precipitated. This goes far to explain how ischaemic colitis can occur acutely in the clinical situation without there being an acute occlusion of a colonic blood vessel (see Chapter 10). This work is further borne out by the study of Gilmour et al.[86] which showed that minor degrees of hypovolaemia reduce colonic blood flow to dangerous levels and that retransfusion may not adequately compensate for this. Fiddian-Green and his group[87] have shown that it is possible to measure alterations in colonic vascularity, both in animals and clinically, by the introduction of a saline-filled probe and measuring the contained pCO_2 and arterial HCO_3, thus deriving the mucosal pH which is directly related to mucosal blood flow. The introduction of such methods into clinical practice may well improve our results in both colonic and aortic surgery.

Conclusions

In contrast to what obtains in the small intestine, experimental interference with the regional circulation to the colon is capable of producing predictable lesions, in both the short and the long term. Functional impairment may occur before there is any discernible anatomical change. Ischaemia produces transient superficial inflammation, linear ulceration progressing to loss of mucosa, fulminating inflammation and full-thickness necrosis, according to its degree and duration. Later lesions include chronic ulceration, and strictures of the colon due to the deposition of fibrous tissue in the submucosa. Broadly speaking, the morphological changes found following deliberate devascularization of the colon in the experimental animal are similar to those seen in human patients suffering from ischaemic colitis, bearing in mind that the very early changes created and studied in the experimental laboratory do not often come the way of the clinical pathologist, who is usually presented with a mature florid lesion. There are important early differences between arterial and venous lesions, although the later effects may be indistinguishable.

Summary

The effects of interruption of the blood supply to the gut of the experimental animal, whether involving large or small vessels, has been extensively studied for many years, and a vast literature has accumulated. While the reactions of the mammalian mesenteric circulation are probably similar in the broad sense, there are important species differences and it is difficult to know how much of this body of knowledge is applicable to clinical practice. Furthermore, it must be borne in mind that all laboratory work is concerned with healthy individuals, whereas human beings with mesenteric vascular disease have atherosclerotic lesions elsewhere.

References

1. Litten, M. Über die Folgen des Verschlüsses der Arteria Meseraica Superior, *Virchows Arch.* [Pathol. Anat.] (1875) **63**: 289–312.
2. Hertzler, A.E. *Surgical Pathology of the Peritoneum.* Philadelphia: J.N. Lippincott (1935).
3. Boyd, W. *Surgical Pathology*, 6th edn Philadelphia, Eastbourne: W.B. Saunders (1947) 565.
4. Marston, A. Causes of death in mesenteric arterial occlusion. *Ann. Surg.* (1963) **58**: 952–60.
5. Welch, W.H. Hemorrhagic infarction. *Collected Papers*, vol. 1, (1920) 66–109.
6. Khanna, S.D. An experimental study of mesenteric occlusion. *J. Path. Bact.* (1959) **77**: 575–81.
7. Bounous, G., Brown, R., Mulden, E.S., Hampson, L.G., Gurd, F.N. Abolition of tryptic enteritis in the shocked dog. *Arch. Surg.* (1965) **91**: 371–6.
8. Caridis, D.T., Cuevas, P., Fine, J. Treatment of acute ischemia of the intestine by peritoneal lavage in the rabbit. *Surg. Gynecol. Obstet.* (1973) **35**: 199–202.
9. Noonan, C.D., Rambo, O.N., Margulis, A.R. Effect of timed occlusion at various levels of mesenteric arteries and veins. *Radiology* (1968) **90**: 99–106.
10. Ahren, C., Haglund, U. Mucosal lesions in the small intestine of the cat during low flow. *Acta Physiol. Scand.* (1973) **88**: 1–9.
11. Chiu, C.J., McArdle, C. Intestinal mucosal lesion in low-flow states. *Arch. Surg.* (1970) **101**, 478–83.
12. Lillehei, R.C., Maclean, L.D. The intestinal factor in reversible endotoxin shock. *Ann. Surg.* (1958) **148**: 513–17.
13. Nahor, A., Milliken, J., Fine, J. Effect of celiac blockade and dibenzilene on traumatic shock following release of occluded superior mesenteric artery. *Ann. Surg.* (1966) **163**: 29–34.
14. Parkins, W.H., Ben, M., Vars, H.M. Tolerance of temporary occlusion of the thoracic aorta in normothermic and hypothermic dogs. *Surgery* (1955) **38**: 38–43.
15. Scott, H.G., Wangensteen, O.H. Blood losses in experimental intestinal strangulation. *Proc. Soc. Exp. Biol. Med.* (1932) **29**: 748–52.
16. Aird, I. Strangulation obstruction. *Ann. Surg.* (1941) **114**: 385–97.

17. Marston, A. Patterns of intestinal ischaemia. *Ann. R. Coll. Surg. Engl.* (1964) **35**: 151–81.
18. Tjiong, B., Bella, E., Weiner, M., Enquist, I.F. Fluid shifts and metabolic changes during and after occlusion of the SMA. *Surg. Gynecol. Obstet.* (1974) **139**: 217–21.
19. Mavor, G.E., Lyall, A.D., Chrystal, K.M.R., Proctor, D.M. Mesenteric infarction as a vascular emergency. *Br. J. Surg.* (1963) **50**: 536–9.
20. Kobold, E.E., Thal, A.P. Quantitification and identification of vasoactive substances liberated during various types of experimental intestinal ischemia. *Surg. Gynecol. Obstet.* (1963) **117**: 315–22.
21. Rosenberg, J.C. Circulating serotonin and catecholamines following occlusion of the superior mesenteric artery. *Ann. Surg.* (1964) **60**, 1062–5.
22. Hershey, S.G., Baez, S., Rovenstine, E.A. Intestinal ischemic shock in normal and dibenzyline protected dogs. *Am. J. Physiol.* (1960) **200**: 307–12.
23. Bounous, G., McArdle, A.H. Release of intestinal enzymes in acute ischemia. *J. Surg. Res.* (1969) **9**: 339–45.
24. Dagher, F.J., Panossian, A., Saab, S. The effect of experimental ligation of the superior mesenteric artery on serum xanthine oxidase activity and transaminase activity. *Surgery* (1967) **62**: 1044–50.
25. Rosato, F.E., Lazitin, L., Miller, L.D., Tsou, K.C. Changes in intestinal alkaline phosphatase in bowel ischemia. *Am. J. Surg.* (1971) **121**: 289–92.
26. Marston, A., Marcuson, R.W., Chapman, M., Arthur, J.F. Experimental study of devascularisation of the colon. *Gut* (1969) **10**: 121–30.
27. Kusche, J., Stahlknecht, C.D., Lorenz, W., Reichert, G., Richter, M. Diamine oxidase activity and histamine release in dogs following acute mesenteric artery occlusion. *Agents Actions* (1977) **7**: 81–4.
28. Polson, H., Mowat, C., Himal, H.S. Experimental and clinical studies of mesenteric infarction. *Surg. Gynecol. Obstet.* (1981) **153**: 360–2.
29. Bergan, J.J., Gilliland, V., Troop, C., Anderson, M.C. Hyperkalemia following intestinal revascularization. *J.A.M.A.* (1964) **187**: 17–19.
30. Jamieson, W.G., Marchuk, S., Rowsom, J., Durand, D. The early diagnosis of massive intestinal ischaemia. *Br. J. Surg.* (1982) **69**: S52–S53.
31. Einheber, A. Proceedings of a conference on recent progress and present problems in the field of shock. *Fed. Proc.* (1961) suppl. 9: 170.
32. Robertson, G., Lyall, A., Macrae, J.G.C. Acid base disturbances in mesenteric occlusion. *Surg. Gynecol. Obstet.* (1969) **128**: 15–20.
33. Williams, L.F., Goldberg, A.H., Polansky, B.J., Byrne, J.J. Myocardial effects of intestinal ischemia. *J. Surg. Res.* (1969) **9**: 319–22.
34. Dogru, M., Atasoy, H. La repercussion de l'ischémie gastrointestinale aigüe sur la coeur. *Bull. Soc. Int. Chir.* (1967) **26**: 536–45.
35. Lefer, A.M. Role of myocardial depressant factor in the pathogenesis of hemorrhagic shock. *Fed. Proc.* (1970) **29**: 1836–40.
36. Vyden, J.K., Nagasawa, K., Corday, E. Hemodynamic consequences of acute occlusion of the superior mesenteric artery *Am. J. Cardiol.* (1974) **34**: 687–90.
37. Nelson, L.E., Kremen, A.J. Experimental occlusion of the mesenteric vessels with special reference to the role of intravascular thrombosis and its prevention by heparin and sulphasuxidine. *Surgery* (1959) **28**: 819–24.
38. Medins, G., Laufman, H. Hypothermia in mesenteric arterial and venous occlusion. *Ann. Surg.* (1958) **148**: 740–51.
39. Zuidema, G.D., Turcote, J.G., Wolfman, E.G., Child, C.G. Metabolic studies in acute small bowel ischemia. *Arch. Surg.* (1962) **85**: 103–35.
40. Marston, A. Diagnosis and management of intestinal ischaemia. *Ann. R. Coll. Surg. Engl.* (1972) **50**: 29–44.
41. Chiu, C.J., Scott, H.J., Gurd. F.N. Volume deficit versus toxic absorption — a study of canine shock after mesenteric arterial occlusion. *Ann. Surg.* (1972) **175**: 479–88.
42. Kangwalklai, K., Saadat, S., Bella, E., Enquist, I.F. Space studies during occlusion of the superior mesenteric artery and upon its release. *Surg. Gynecol. Obstet.* (1973) **137**: 263–6.
43. Milliken, J., Nahor, A., Fine, J. A study of the factors involved in the development of peripheral vascular collapse following release of the occluded superior mesenteric artery. *Br. J. Surg.* (1965) **52**: 699–703.
44. Haglund, U., Lundgren, O. Intestinal ischemia and shock factors. *Fed. Proc.* (1978) **37**: 2729–33.
45. Laufman, H. Experimental evidence of factors concerned in the recovery of strangulated intestine. *Surgery* (1945) **28**: 509–13.
46. Cohn, I. Strangulative obstruction. *Surgery* (1956) **39**: 630–34.
47. Benjamin, H.B., Potos, W.B., Marnocha, J., Bartenbach, G.E. Correlation of clinical and experimental effects of antibiotic therapy for massive intestinal infarction. *J. Am. Ger. Soc.* (1960) **8**: 847–54.
48. Caridis, D.T., Cuevas, P., Fine, J. Treatment of acute ischemia of the intestine by peritoneal lavage in the rabbit. *Surg. Gynecol. Obstet.* (1972) **135**: 199–202.
49. Martin, W.B., Laufman, H., Tuell, S.W. Rat-

ionale of therapy in acute vascular occlusions based on micrometric observations. *Ann. Surg.* (1949) **129**: 476–81.

50. D'Angelo, G.J., Ameriso, L.M., Tredway, J.B. Survival after mesenteric vascular occlusion by treatment with low molecular weight dextran. *Circ. Res.* (1963) **27**: 662–3.
51. Kusche, J., Richter, H., Hesterberg, R., Lorenz, W. The role of hormonal factors and diamine oxidase activity in shock after intestinal ischaemia in rabbits. *Br. J. Surg.* (1973) **60**: 904–6.
52. Zwelfach, B.W., Nagler, A.L., Thomas, L. The role of epinephrine in the reactions produced by the endotoxins of Gram-negative bacteria. *J. Exp. Med.* (1956) **104**: 881–9.
53. Manohar, M., Tyagi, R. Experimental intestinal ischemia shock in dogs. *Am. J. Physiol.* (1973) **225**: 887–92.
54. Shute, K. Effect of intraluminal oxygen on experimental ischaemia of the intestine. *Gut* (1976) **17**: 1001–6.
55. Shute, K. Effect of intraluminal oxygen on endotoxin absorption in experimental occlusion of the superior mesenteric artery. *Gut* (1977) **18**: 567–70.
56. Bussemaker, J.B., Lindeman, J. Comparison of methods to determine viability of small intestine. *Ann. Surg.* (1972) **176**: 97–102.
57. Carter, K., Halle, M., Cherry, G., Myers, M.B. Determination of viability of ischemic intestine. *Arch. Surg.* (1970) **100**: 695–701.
58. Moossa, A.R., Skinner, D.B., Stark, W., Huffer, P. Assessment of bowel viability using Tc-labelled albumen microspheres. *J. Surg. Res.* (1974) **16**: 466–9.
59. Wright, C.B., Hobson, R.W. Prediction of intestinal viability using Doppler ultrasound techniques. *Am. J. Surg.* (1975) **129**: 643–5.
60. Cooperman, M., Martin, W.E., Carey, L.C. Evaluation of ischemic intestine by Doppler ultrasound. *Am. J. Surg.* (1980) **139**: 73–7.
61. Shah, S.D., Anderson, C.A. Prediction of small bowel viability using Doppler ultrasound. *Ann. Surg.* (1981) **194**: 97–9.
62. Gorey, T.F. The recovery of intestine after ischaemic injury. *Br. J. Surg.* (1980) **67**: 699–702.
63. Mann, A., Fazio, V.W., Lucas, F.V. A comparative study of the use of fluorescein and the Doppler device in the determination of intestinal viability. *Surg. Gynecol. Obstet.* (1982) **154**: 53–5.
64. Bulkley, G.R., Zuidema, G.D., Hamilton, S.R., O'Mara, C.S., Klacsman, P.G., Horn, S.D.Intraoperative determination of small intestinal viability following ischemic injury. *Ann. Surg.* (1981) **193**: 628–35.
65. Blalock, A., Levy, S.E. Gradual complete occlusion of the celiac axis and superior and inferior mesenteric arteries with survival. *Surgery* (1939) **5**: 175–80.
66. Laufman, H. Gradual occlusion of the mesenteric vessels — an experimental study. *Surgery* (1943) **13**: 406–11.
67. Spencer, D.C., Derrick, J.R. Acute and chronic effects of occluding the superior mesenteric artery in the experimental animal. *Am. Surgeon* (1962) **28**: 170–73.
68. Popovsky, J. Gradual occlusion of mesenteric vessels with ameroid cylinder. *Arch. Surg.* (1966) **92**: 202–5.
69. Maass, V. Über die Entstahung von Darmenstenose nach Brucheinklemmung. *Dtsch. Med. Wochenschr.* (1895) **21**: 365–7.
70. Boley, S.J., Krieger, H., Schultz, L., et al. Experimental aspects of peripheral vascular occlusion of the intestine. *Surg. Gynecol. Obstet.* (1965) **121**: 789–94.
71. Bonakdarpour, A., Ming, S., Lynch, P.R., et al. Superior mesenteric artery occlusion in dogs — a model to produce the spectrum of intestinal ischemia. *J. Surg. Res.* (1975) **19**: 251–7.
72. Vest, B., Margulis, A.R. Experimental infarction of the small bowel in dogs. *Am. J. Roentgenol.* (1964) **92**: 1080–87.
73. Glotzer, D.J., Villegas, A.H., Anekayama, S., Shaw, R.S. Healing of the intestine in experimental bowel infarction. *Ann. Surg.* (1962) **155**: 183–9.
74. Stahlgren, L.H., Dapena, A., Roy, R.L. Ulcerogenic properties of enteric-coated compounds in dogs. *Surg. Forum* (1965) **16**: 367–70.
75. Mansfield, J.B., Schoenfeld, F.B., Suwa, M., Geurkink, R.E., Anderson, M.C. The role of vascular insufficiency in drug-induced small bowel ulceration. *Am. J. Surg.* (1967) **113**: 608–14.
76. Hukuhara, T., Kotani, S., Sato, G. Effects of destruction of intramural ganglion cells on colon motility. *Jpn. J. Physiol.* (1961) **11**: 635–40.
77. de Villiers, D.R. Ischaemia of the colon — an experimental study. *Br. J. Surg.* (1966) **53**: 497–503.
78. Boley, S.J., Schwartz, S., Lash, J., Sternhill, V. Reversible vascular occlusion of the colon. *Surg. Gynecol. Obstet.* (1963) **116**: 53–60.
79. Boley, S.J., Krieger, H., Schultz, L., et al. Experimental aspects of peripheral vascular occlusion of the intestine. *Surg. Gynecol. Obstet.* (1965) **121**: 789–4.
80. Sawer, B.A., Jamieson, W.G., Durand, D. The significance of elevated peritoneal fluid phosphate levels in intestinal infarction. *Surg. Gynecol. Obstet.* (1978) **146**: 43–5.
81. Marcuson, R.W., Stewart, J.O., Marston, A. Experimental venous lesions of the colon. *Gut* (1972) **13**: 1–7.
82. Polk, H.C. Experimental mesenteric venous occlusion. *Ann. Surg.* (1966) **163**: 432–44.

83. Saegesser, F. Perspectives expérimentales et cliniques dans l'insuffisance vasculaire du gros intestin. *J. Chir.* (1972) **104**: 569–76.
84. Robinson, J.W.L., Rausis, C., Basset, P., Mirkovitch, V. Functional and morphological responses of the dog colon to ischemia. *Gut* (1972) **13**: 775–83.
85. Matthews, J.G.W., Parks, T.G. Ischaemic colitis in the experimental animal. *Gut* (1976) **17**: 671–7.
86. Gilmour, D.G., Aitkenhead, A.R., Hothersall, A.D., Ledingham, I.McA. The effect of hypovolaemia on colonic blood flow in the dog. *Br. J. Surg.* (1980) **67**: 82–4.
87. Wakefield, T.W., Whitehouse, W.M., Pittenger, G., Fiddian Green, R.G. Early diagnosis of colonic ischemia by hollow viscus tonometry. *Gastroenterology* (1983) **84**: 1344.

4

Tests of intestinal viability

Thomas F. Gorey

Introduction

Assessment of bowel viability after the release of strangulation, or after revascularization is a difficult clinical decision, which needs instrumental support. If non-viable bowel is not resected it may lead to sepsis with local perforation or, in the long term, to stricture formation. On the other hand unnecessarily to resect bowel which is capable of recovery may leave insufficient intestine for nutrition and survival. Classically, the surgeon waits for about 15 minutes after the release of strangulation and sometimes applies warm packs to stimulate local blood flow and then assesses viability on the criteria of colour, pulsation and peristalsis. Whilst a pink colour does provide evidence of restoration of the circulation it may not indicate actual cell viability. Another difficulty is that intramural haemorrhage, particularly in venous occlusions, may give a persistent dark colour. Return of arterial pulsation in the mesenteric vessels is a good indicator of viability but in cases of nonocclusive mesenteric infarction the pulsation here will not be lost initially. Peristalsis is a sign of returning muscle function but must not be confused with anoxic spasms, as describd by Laufman and Method.[1] The return of peristalsis may also be late and not apparent within the 15 minute observation period, even in loops destined to recover from ischaemic injury.[2] Many workers have found that clinical criteria alone were inaccurate in assessing bowel viability, particularly in borderline cases: Zarins et al.[3] found an accuracy in predicting viability of 42 per cent. Gorey[4] looked at the sensitivity of clinical criteria in a series of arterial, venous, and mixed arterial and venous occlusions. He found that in arterial and mixed occlusions that 40 per cent and 53 per cent of viable bowel segments respectively were missed although it was highly specific. In the case of venous occlusions, while clinical critera identified all non-viable bowel, there was a 17 per cent false positive rate which would have led to unnecessary resections. This experiment was designed to identify all non-viable bowel and therefore erred on the side of never missing necrotic intestine. The second area where clinical judgement of intestinal viability comes into play is the so called 'second look', exploration (see Chapter 5). The rational for this was outlined by Zuidema in 1961,[5] and 24 hours has been generally accepted as the period in which the bowel would have had adequate time in which either to recover or become obviously necrotic. However, Zuidema et al.[6] subsequently reported a case of small bowel resection with re-exploration at 18 hours when a further 17 cm of bowel was non-viable and required resection. Because of the unreliability of clinical criteria, and particularly in cases of massive small bowel ischaemia, other tests are necessary. In these cases salvage of an extra few centimetres of bowel may mean the difference between normal or long-term parenteral nutrition and indeed may mean the difference between life and death. In recent years many additional tests to assess bowel viability have been examined.

Dyes

Dye injection tests were among the first used, which depend on the dye reaching the intestine through a patent circulation and giving a characteristic visual pattern. Fluorescein is a vital dye actively taken up by living cells so that it may give an indication of cell viability as well as of reperfusion. Lange and Boyd,[7] were the first to use it to monitor re-establishment of blood flow after intestinal strangulation. They found uniform intestinal fluorescence in rabbits, after periods of ischaemia ranging up to three and three quarter hours, but with increased ischaemic time fluorescence was patchy. This was developed by Stolar and Randolph[8] to predict viability rather than reperfusion. They described three patterns of fluorescence only one of which was of predictive value in the immediate post-reperfusion period; the other two becoming apparent 24 hours later on reinjection of fluorescein. The Hopkins group further developed the fluorescent technique and described five patterns with an additional pattern specific to venous strangulation. These patterns all appeared immediately after reperfusion, and were of determinant value. Gorey[4] showed that the overall sensitivity of fluorescence in correctly identifying non-viable intestine was 96 per cent with a specificity of 95 per cent. It was slightly less specific in venous occlusions and had a 17 per cent false positive rate. In a series of experiments for the three types of vascular occlusion in rats it was significantly better in predicting viability than either Doppler ultrasonography or clinical criteria, whether applied immediately or at a 'second look' laparotomy. Wheaton et al.[9] produced similar fluorescence patterns in cats with an overall accuracy of 95 per cent. Fluorescein was used clinically in 28 patients by Bulkley et al.,[10] 71 ischaemic segments in all were evaluated and fluorescence compared with the Doppler test and clinical criteria, 15 minutes after release of strangulation. Patients were followed up clinically and resected specimens submitted to blind pathological analysis. Accurate histological criteria for bowel viability had been established in a previous large series of animals and if the bowel could not be labelled certainly as either non-viable or viable it was excluded; 17 equivocal segments were excluded on this basis. In the 54 ischaemic intestinal segments remaining for evaluation the overall accuracy of clinical critera was 89 per cent with no significant improvement from Doppler ultrasonography. However, the fluorescein test was correct in all 54 segments. The test was also found to be accurate by Marfuggi and Greenspan[11] in experiments of similar design. They also reported two clinical cases where fluorescence was correct in predicting gastric viability during resection for benign ulcer, and in delineating the resection margins in a volvulus.

Recent developments in fluorescence as an aid to assessment of viability have focused on quantitative fluorometric measurements, as well as the subjective patterns observed under ultraviolet light. Silverman et al.[12] reported an experiment in rats in which 5 cm segments were made ischaemic by an umbilical tape for periods ranging from 30 minutes to 8 hours. Fiberoptic fluorometry (which uses a branched fiberoptic light guide) transmits blue light to the fluorescein in the tissues being examined, the fluorescence being picked up by a photomultiplier tube which provides a measure of fluorescence in D F (Dye Fluorescence) units. The background fluorescence was first measured and, then later subtracted after injection of fluorescein, to eliminate the effects of autofluorescence.

This also has the advantage of allowing repeated measurements as previous fluorescence can be subtracted. The fluorometer can be linked to a computer to facilitate collection and analysis of data and computer-generated graphic patterns can be obtained which are consistent with viable and non-viable bowel. Alternately, readings can be taken at two time points and the fluorescein index calculated by dividing the reading in the experimental section by the reading in the reference section. The authors claimed that this method can increase the accuracy of prediction of viability from 53 per cent for qualitative fluorescence under Woods lamp, to 98 per cent. This method also takes into account the uptake and elimination of fluorescein. While visual fluorescence assessment has been proven to be accurate in practice and has the advantage of ease of application without the need for expensive equipment, a possible disadvantage is that repeat readings are difficult because dye may persist for up to 72 hours. This may be important when vaso-active drugs are used to improve the local circulation and a second fluorescent assessment is required. Perfusion fluorometry permits quantification of dye delivery and elimination, because if there is visible fluorescence from a previous injection it can be subtracted, making serial estimations possible. Silvermans group[12] found that a D F I (Dye Fluorescein Index) of over 35 was consistent with viability while under 15 was indicative of necrosis. However, intermediate values were unhelpful. Qualitative and quantitative fluorescence were also compared by Carter et al.[13]: this was a dynamic assessment of perfusion measuring both uptake and elimination. They also

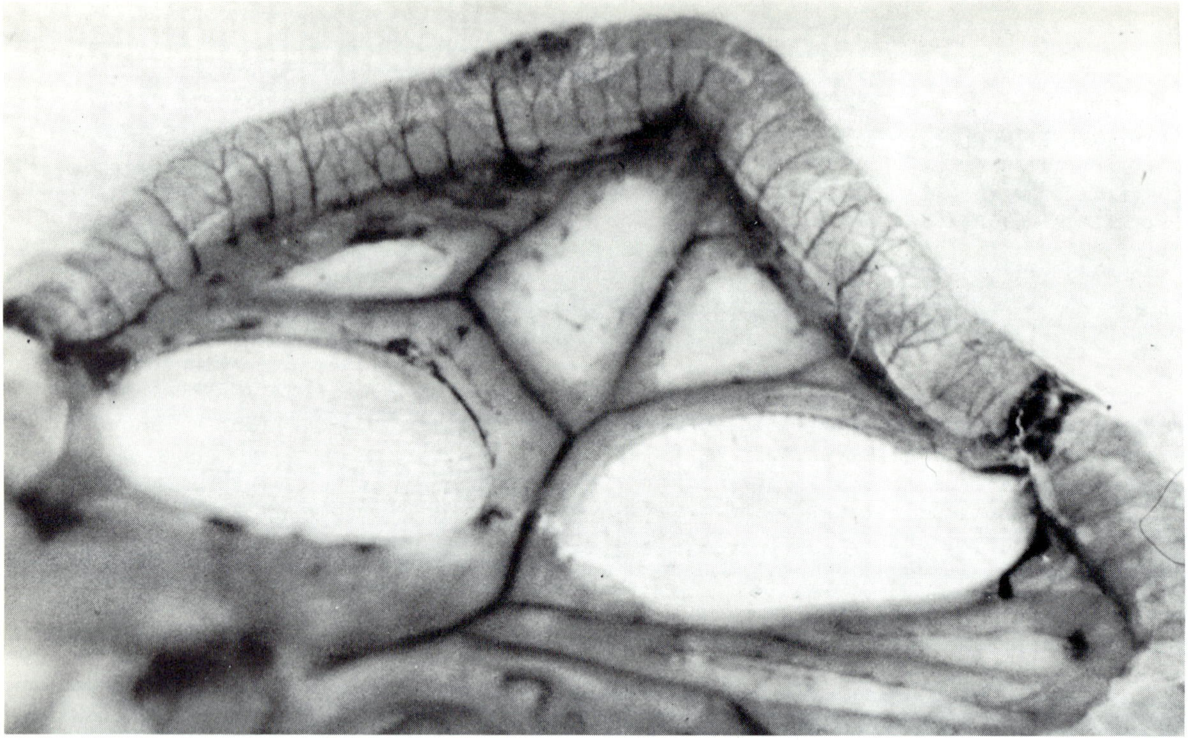

(a)

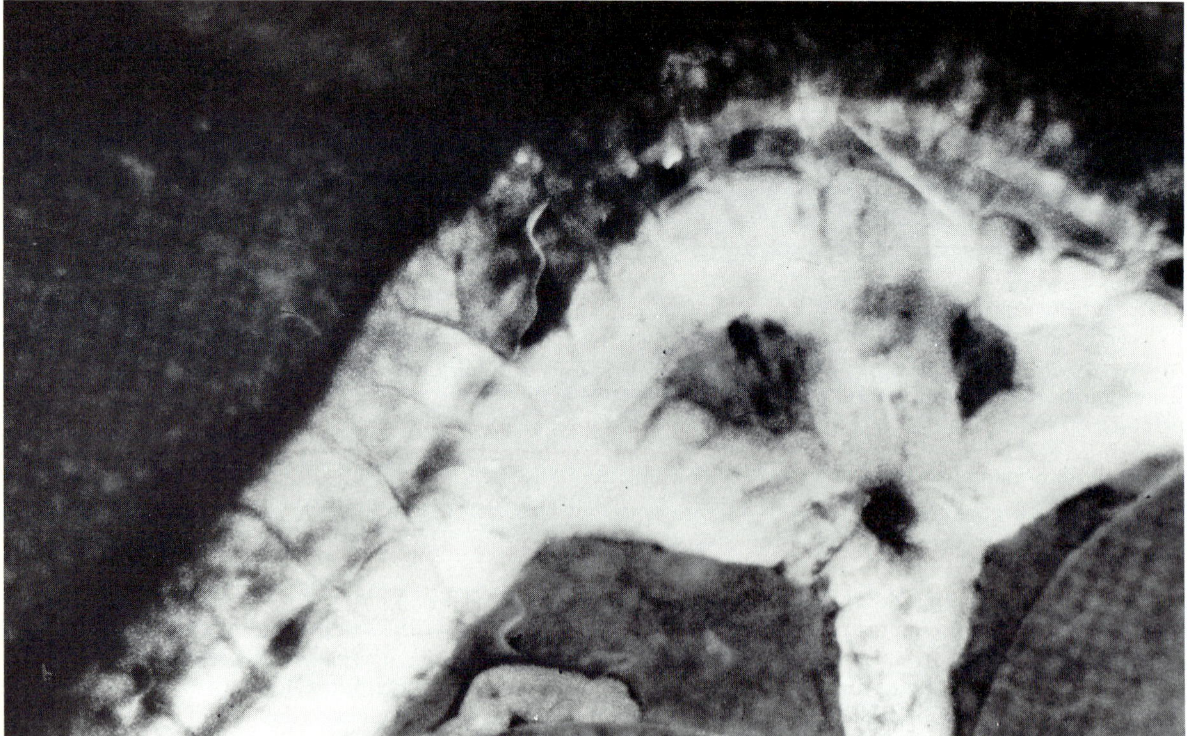

(b)

Fig. 4.1 (**a**) normal fluorescence; (**b**) patchy fluorescence; (**c**) non-fluorescence.

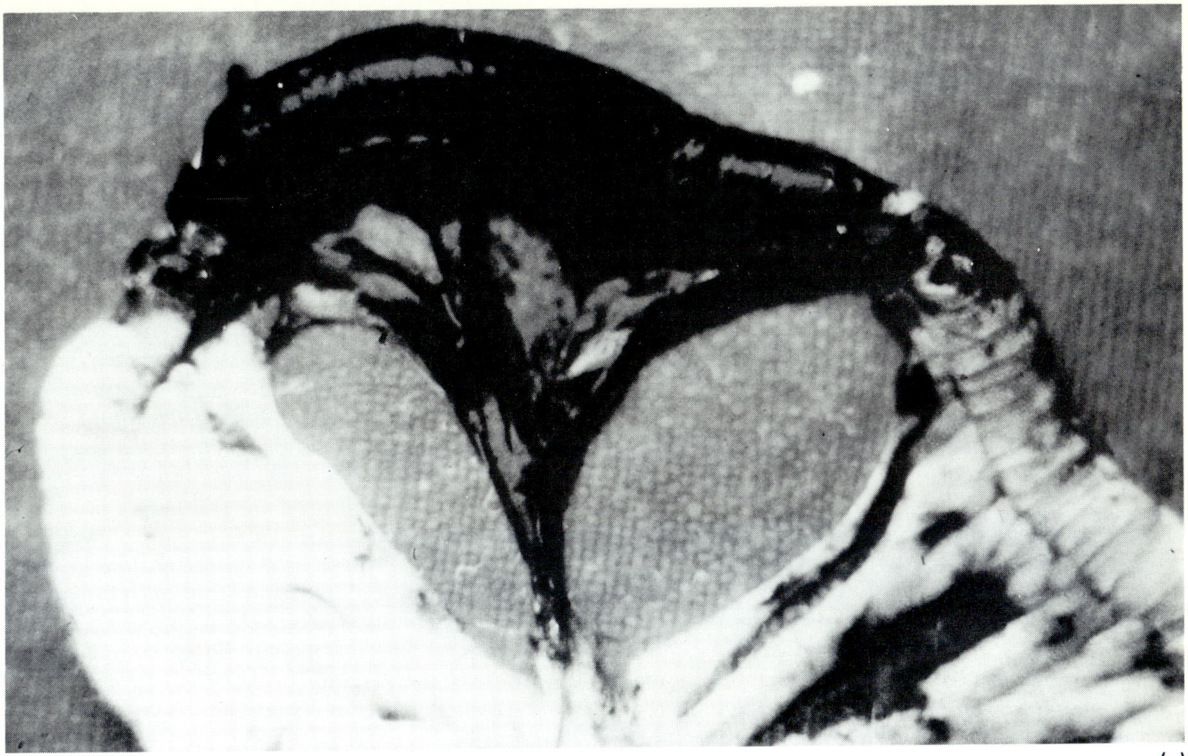

(c)

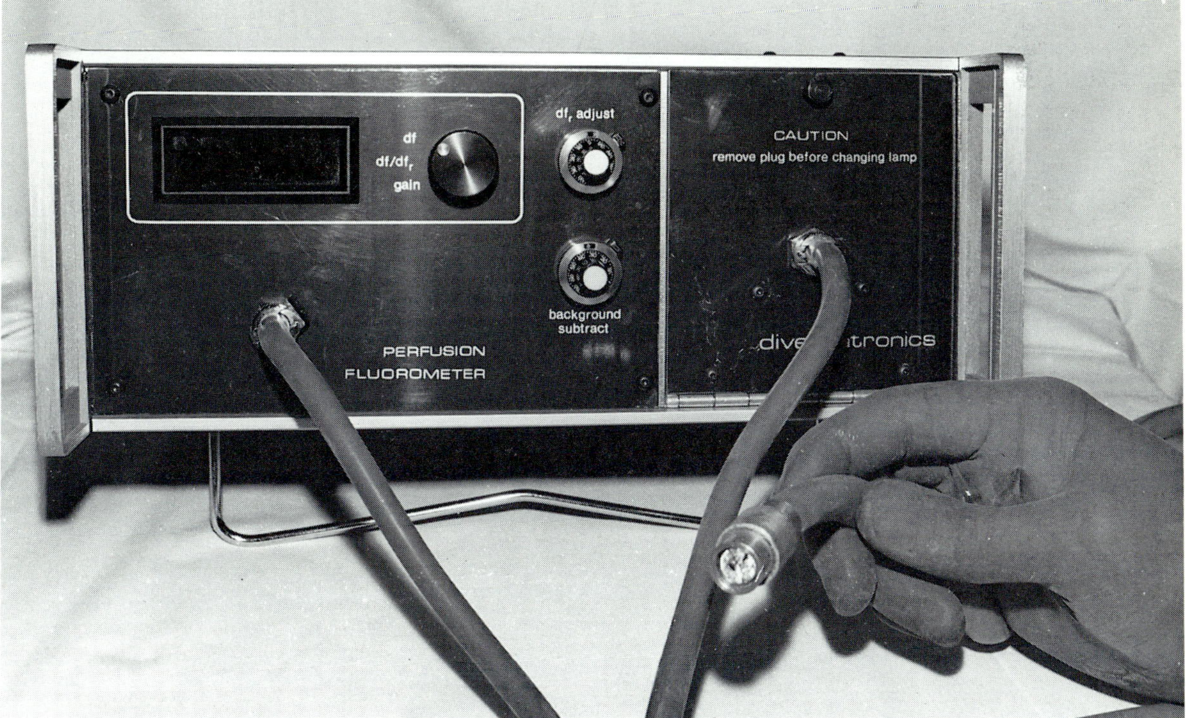

Fig. 4.2 A perfusion fluorometer with branched fiberoptic light and photomultiplier tube.

used a branched fibroptic light which had the advantage of being possible to use under normal lighting conditions when combined with a shield. They described two 'viable' uptake clearance curves; normal and hyperaemic with a peak and a rapid decline. There were three patterns consistent with non-viability; hyperfluorescence where the peak was again higher than normal but with delayed elimination, a low peak with a slow rise and impaired elimination, and a final pattern of complete non-fluorescence. These experiments were carried out in greyhounds using arterial occlusions and two doses of fluorescein were used: the lower 2 mg/Kg dose with the fluorometer and 5 mg/Kg using the Woods light.

The safety of fluorescence is well established: Herrlin, Glasser and Lange[14] used it to monitor the intestinal circulation, and referred to previous use in almost 500 patients without any adverse reactions. There are many reports of the safe use of fluorescein for different investigations in a great number of patients and Goodman and Gillman in the chapter on dyes[15] conclude that it is non-toxic apart from occasional nausea and vomiting. There are two reports of possible cardiovascular and allergic reaction: La Piana and Penner,[16] and four reports of possible myocardial problems associated with fluorescein administration in five patients (Cunningham and Balu,[17] Steinal,[18] Amaleric et al.,[19] and Deglin[20]).

Dyes other than fluorescein have been used to look at intestinal perfusion and prediction of viability. Papacristou and Fortner[21] injected trypan blue into the superior mesenteric artery in rats. They found the accuracy of clinical criteria to be 36 per cent compared to 69 per cent for reactive hyperaemia estimated with an electronic thermometer. The correlation between failure of dye uptake with subsequent necrosis and perforation had an accuracy of 84 per cent in this rat model. Myers and Cherry[22] used both fluorescein and patent blue V to delineate the vascularity of the colon. They found that while all fully stained intestine was viable, sometimes unstained intestine at the extremity of an ischaemic area also survived, which might have been unnecessarily resected. They found patent blue V was more easily visible than bromophenol blue which had been reported by Dineen et al.[23] Neither blue dyes are presently approved for use in patients. They also reported the use of fluorescein in

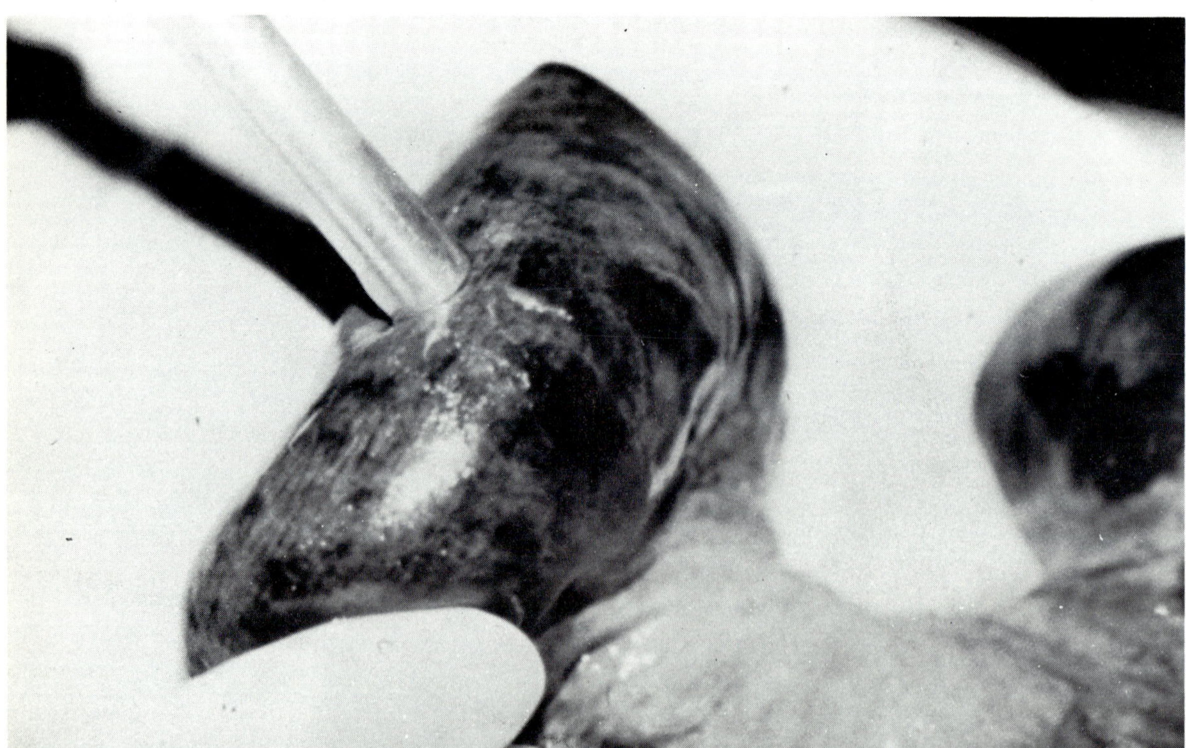

Fig. 4.3 A Doppler probe applied to the bowel surface.

10 patients and found that it was fully correct in determining colon viability. They pointed out that fluorescence is sometimes difficult to see in the red muscle of the rectum but that it can be examined in the mucosa after transection. It appears that the dye tests may be less reliable in the colon than in the small bowel.

Doppler tests

A Doppler probe was used to detect the presence of pulsitile blood flow in the small vessels in the bowel wall by Wright, Creighton and Hobson.[24] They developed a model of ischaemic intestine in dogs by clamping the vascular pedicle and found that the presence of intestinal blood flow correlated with ultimate viability on 'relook' 24 to 48 hours later. They measured blood flow at three locations; over the pedicle, at the junction of the mesentery and bowel wall and along the mesenteric border. Its value in predicting recovery of bowel was shown intraoperatively in 3 patients with intestinal ischaemia due to superior mesenteric artery thrombosis by O'Donnell and Hobson.[25]

Their findings were confirmed by 'second look' operation. There are many publications from Cooperman and his colleagues on the use of Doppler ultrasonography in predicting intestinal viability. Cooperman[26] found that the presence of a surface Doppler signal accurately predicted anastomotic viability after resection in experimental intestinal ischaemia in baboons. Subsequently, Cooperman, Martin, Evans et al.[27] carried out two layer anastomoses in 20 dogs with Doppler ultrasonography of the bowel ends prior to suture. They found that anastomoses carried out within one centimetre of the last audible Doppler signal were viable, but that if the length of bowel distal to the

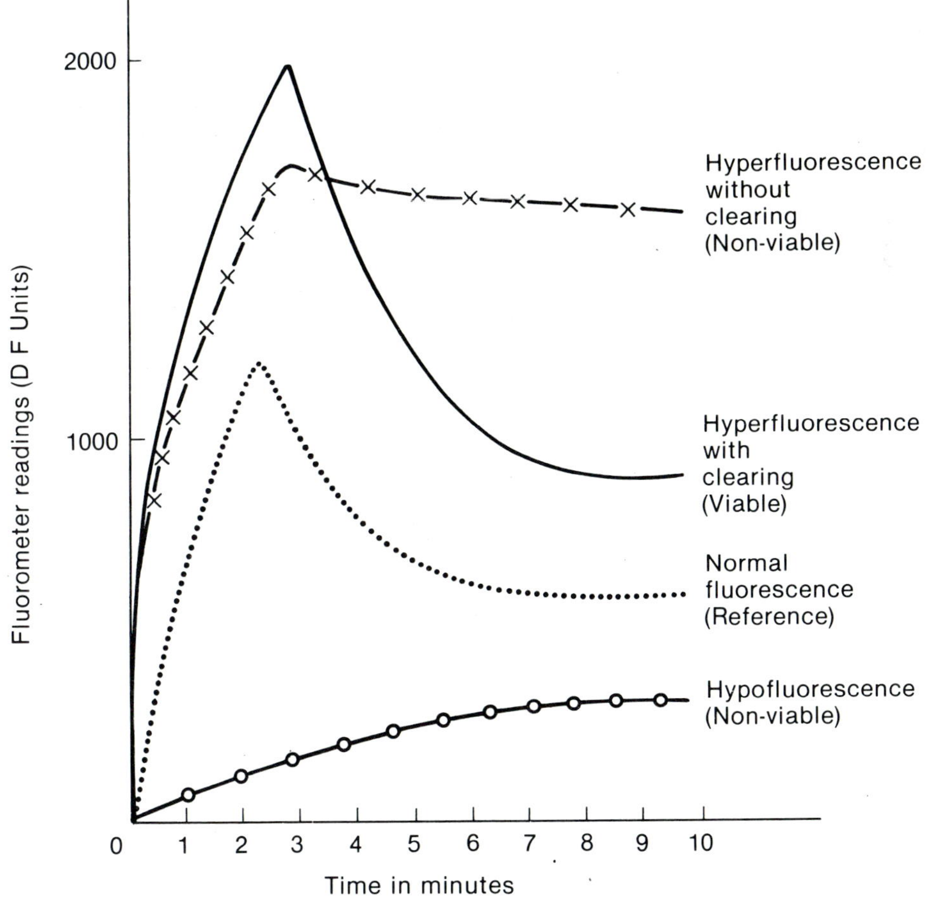

Fig. 4.4 Fluorescence uptake — clearance curves in perfusion fluorometry.

last signal was greater than this that there was a high incidence of disruption. Nevertheless, they had noted that all resection margins appeared viable grossly and bled when cut. Cooperman, Martin and Keith[28] reported 117 patients undergoing anastomosis or enterostomy. Clinical impression of viability coincided with Doppler result in 92 per cent of cases. In 6 cases the Doppler signal was absent; five of these had resection of additional intestine to within 1 centimetre of the nearest Doppler signal and all 5 healed. In the 1 patient not having additional resection there was subsequent anastomotic disruption. Shah and Anderson[29] evaluated Doppler ultrasonography in venous occlusion to 4–7 centimetre lengths of bowel in dogs. They found that almost half of the non-viable segments had signals at the junction of mesentery and bowel wall and that all of the non-viable segments had signals over the mesentery. They found, however, that there was a good correlation between loss of Doppler signal at the antimesenteric border and subsequent necrosis. In the segments in which the Doppler predicted viability intestinal function was also preserved, in that there was no malabsorbtion and no strictures after 6 months. Gorey[4] found that the overall sensitivity of Doppler ultrasonography in all types of vascular occlusion was 57 per cent, but that this was less accurate in venous occlusions. It had a high specificity in arterial and mixed vascular occlusions so that absence of a Doppler signal along the antimesenteric border would be consistent with subsequent necrosis. However, there were many inaccuracies in the technique, and in particular in the rat model used it was difficult to apply the large diameter probe to the bowel wall with consistency. Another difficulty involved the position of the bowel, so that undue manipulation of the bowel sometimes led to loss of signal, whilst if the bowel was left lying *in situ* false signals could be picked up due to transmission from underlying loops. A major difficulty with the Doppler technique is that it is not possible to screen large areas of bowel and to this end it may be complimentary to use it together with fluorescence. If the fluorescence technique draws attention to an under-perfused area the viability of this can then perhaps be confirmed with the Doppler probe.

Electromyography

The value of electromyography in assessing intestinal viability was reported by Schamaun.[30] The normal myoelectric rhythm consists of regular, slow, sinus-shaped potential variations present even in the absence of mechanical activity, while quick potential variations 'spikes' correspond to mechanical movements. Vascular occlusion was maintained from 4–11 hours in mongrel dogs, in three intestinal segments which either remained electrically active after occlusion or in which the amplitude and frequency returns to near the baseline within 15 minutes to one hour. All three segments were found to be intact after the dogs died. Two other segments were rendered ischaemic for 21 and 23 hours, and these demonstrated a total loss of electrical activity after occlusion, with no return of activity after reperfusion, and necrosis on follow-up. Katz et al.[31] reported further experience with electromyography. They created four 30 cm ischaemic loops of small bowel by applying a clamp to the segmental arteries supplying each loop after transecting collateral circulation. The normal slow-waves recorded before vascular occlusion had a frequency of 12–15 per minute and an amplitude of 2–6 millivolts. The period of ischaemia ranged from 2–6 hours. After vascular occlusion and throughout the period of occlusion all electrical activity was absent. After relief of occlusion in the 2 and 4 hour groups there was prompt resumption of electrical activity within 10 minutes. However, in the loop that was ischaemic for 6 hours there was no discernible electrical activity even after 30 minutes reperfusion. This loss of slow wave activity correlated with microscopic evidence of loss of muscle at three weeks and with fibrosis in both the muscularis externa and mucosae. Subsequently at 14 weeks the bowel was considerably shortened and stenosed. Shah and Anderson[29] compared Doppler ultrasonography and electromyography in assessing intestinal viability. For electromyographic measurement they used two subserosal electrodes placed 5 centimetres apart. They found return of electromyographic slow wave activity to be consistent with viable bowel. They also found that this correlated with Doppler signals at the antimesenteric border but that if the Doppler signal at this location was inconsistent or 'spotty' that electromyography was more sensitive in this equivocal group.

pH recordings

The value of intestinal pH readings in predicting viability was reported by Katz and colleagues.[31] They measured mucosal and serosal pH in isolated intestinal loops both before and after occlusion and again after restoration of blood flow. Initial serosal pH readings before occlusion were in the range of 7.90–8.10 and after vascular occlusion and manipulation of the bowel the readings dropped to the relatively acidotic range of 7.38–7.65. After three hours of vascular occlusion the serosal pH became alkalotic (7.90–8.40) which was associated with definite pre-gangrenous histological changes. As ischaemia progressed to frank gangrene the serosal pH readings returned to a neutral value of 7.50. They concluded that while mucosal pH merely reflected the act of revascularization, an alkalotic serosal pH of 7.95–8.40 indicated pre-gangrene. The transience of the shift however limited its clinical usefulness and isolated pH readings were of no predictive value. The relationship between surface pH and pCO_2 and the vascularity and viability of intestine was investigated by Myers, Cherry and Gesser.[32] The background to their work was that when a cell becomes ischaemic it suffers from both a lack of oxygen and inadequate removal of acid waste products. Then when anaerobic glycoloysis begins the pH falls and the pCO_2 rises. They carried out their experiments in rabbits by clamping the blood supply to a loop of ileum which they proved to be excluded from the circulation by injection of disulphine blue dye. They took control readings every 2 minutes for a 15-minute period, and then every minute after vascular occlusion, until equilibrium was obtained. The intestine was returned to the abdomen for periods of ischaemia ranging from 1–6 hours. After revascularization further pH and pCO_2 readings were taken for 15 minutes after which the animals were allowed to recover for seven days when they were killed for histopathological analysis of the bowel segments. The authors found that after occlusion of the blood supply there was an immediate drop in pH and rise in pCO_2 which levelled off after a maximum period of 45 minutes. Bowel segments which had suffered ischaemia for more than 4 hours became necrotic, but there was no direct correlation with pH or pCO_2. As in previous studies they concluded that while pH and pCO_2 could not reliably predict intestinal viability they might estimate the adequacy of perfusion and quantitate the effectiveness of splanchnic vasodilators, when these are used. They also pointed out that the electrodes could not be sterilized, thus preventing their intraoperative use.

Temperature

Several investigations tested the value of a rise in surface temperature after release of vascular occlusion as an indication of viability. The principle was established by Laufman and Method,[1] using a clinical mercury thermometer. They drew a series of temperature curves for both arterial and venous strangulations and found that a rise in temperature, measured at 3 minute intervals after release of strangulation, was consistent with viability of the segment as checked by post mortem examinations. The surface temperature between two electrodes was measured by a specially designed thermocouple by Bussemaker and Lindeman.[2] They found that 'reactive hyperaemia' could be detected 10 minutes after restoration of the circulation in intestinal segments ischaemic for 4 hours as the temperatures averaged 1.3 °C higher than in adjacent normal bowel. In contrast, segments ischaemic for longer periods and not destined to recover showed no hyperaemia. Similar findings were reported by Papachristou and Fortner[21] using a heat sensitive electronic probe on the antimesenteric border, to measure the temperature difference between ischaemic and control loops. Moss, Kressel and Brito[33] evaluated thermography in dogs with pure arterial occlusion in bowel segments ischaemic for periods of 2–8 hours. They measured surface temperature and studied thermograms at 5 minute intervals for 30 minutes after revascularisation. In the *short ischaemia* group (2–3 hours) there was uniform reactive hyperaemia and all 5 intestinal segments survived. In the *intermediate* group (3–7 hours) there was hyperaemia with some patchy areas and 4 of the 6 segments in this group survived, but all with some degree of transmural necrosis. In the *long term group* (8 hours ischaemia) there was no hyperaemic response and all 3 segments were necrotic with histological infarction. They concluded from this part of the study that a rise in temperature of 1°C after revascularisation was consistent with viability. A scanning telethermometer and thermistor probes were then used to measure bowel, rectal and room temperature and thermograms constructed with an AGA thermovision unit. These thermographic patterns were compared with histological appearances to determine if they could predict the degree and extent of viability of revascularised intestine after various periods of ischaemia. Autopsy was performed and histological analysis carried out when the animals died; otherwise they were killed electively at periods ranging between 17 and 90 days. The thermograms were blindly classified into 3 groups; uniform reactive hyperaemia, nonuniform and no reactive hyperaemia. Thermography was found to be more accurate than surface temperature measurement and this was thought to be due either to a sampling error or because the temperature probe was not applied uniformly in the intestinal surface.

The oxygen electrode

Piasecki[34] evaluated in dogs a surface polargraphic oxygen electrode as an indicator of intestinal viability. The principle was measurement of oxygen consumption, in that the oxygen used by the probe was replaced from the intestinal blood, so that the rate of oxygen uptake was proportional to the blood flow. The electrode was placed both on the serosa and mucosa to measure oxygen consumption while a graded constriction of the input artery allowed flow to be measured with a flowmeter. The experiment was designed so that graded constriction of the input artery could be used to demonstrate a relationship between readings from the instrument and varying blood flow. A good correlation was found between flow and muscle pO_2. There was a gradation of ischaemia from 40 mmHg to zero at 1 cm intervals along the bowel, passing from normal to ischaemic. The mucosal electrode was more difficult to place and there was no fall in oxygen until a critical level of 20 to 30% of flow was reached. With simultaneous mucosal and serosal electrodes, pO_2 decreased as flow decreased but when small collaterals were opened the pO_2 of the mucosa showed an increase about 2 minutes before that in the serosa demonstrating possible preferential distribution to the mucosa in a low-flow state. The oxygen probe was more sensitive at low flow and this is a situation that would be beneficial to a surgeon planning a partial resection.

Chemical tests

Katz[31] tested the value of tetrazolium analysis of the mucosa in the assessment of viability. Mucosal biopsies were taken for tetrazolium and histological analysis after various intervals of ischaemia. The homogenised tissue was incubated for 2 hours with tetrazolium which was reduced by the mucosal dehydrogenase enzyme system to produce diformazan. The diformazan was then extracted and assayed in a colorimeter to give a measure of dehydrogenase activity which reflects mucosal viability. This was found to be a reliable index of the mucosal damage but was of limited clinical application because of the time required for the analysis. Carter, Halle, Cherry and Myers,[35] performed quantitative analysis on a methyl tetrazolium bromide dye (MTT) and found that the time taken for tissue biopsies to change colour after reduction by the dehydrogenase enzymes was increased with prolonged periods of ischaemia. In experiments using ischaemic ileum in dogs they found that there was an apparent cut-off at 70 seconds, with MTT time less than this indicating viability and greater than this indicating necrosis. The estimation were performed on 1 c.c. biopsies of tissue which were excised and incubated at 37°C. The main difficulty with the test was the subjectiveness of the end point in determining the change from yellow to blue indicating reduction of the MTT. This together with a certain difficulty in determining the colour change in haemorrhagic bowel could probably be helped in the future by developing a photometric method of determining the end point colour change.

Radionuclides

Radioisotopes have been used in two major areas in monitoring intestinal viability, both by the use of injected radioactive microspheres and the external imaging of radiolabelled compounds. Zarins et al.[3] injected radioactive microspheres systemically to assess microcirculatory blood flow. It has been shown in two series of experiments that return of microcirculatory patency is directly related to intestinal viability after revascularisation, (Gorey,[36] Amano, Bulkley, Gorey et al.[37]). Zarins isolated 15 cm lengths of terminal ileum from the circulation in dogs using bulldog clamps on the pedicle and rubber bands to compress the intramural circulation. Ten minutes after revascularisation Tc 99M-albumin microspheres were injected into the aorta. The degree of revascularisation outlined by the scans was compared with viability predicted by return of colour and arterial pulsation 10 minutes after release of the occlusion. The ischaemic time was varied from 4–10 hours duration to produce 5 ischaemic scans, 4 normal scans and 5 hyperaemic scans. The 5 hyperaemic scans correlated well with visual prediction of viability and were all viable on final histological study. In the 4 normal scans the intestine was also evaluated as viable by visual criteria but on follow-up only 2 of the 4 segments were viable; one had perforated and one had formed a stricture. The technique proved most useful with the 5 ischaemic scans comprising the final group;

here 3 of the 5 segments were evaluated as viable by visual critera but all were necrotic on final histological diagnosis. The normal scintiscans were of indeterminate predictive value while the hyperaemic and ischaemic scans correlated well with histological evidence of viable and necrotic bowel respectively. To inject microspheres into the human aorta is not difficult but the technique requires a nuclear laboratory and expensive scanning equipment which are not readily available outside major centres, and are certainly cumbersome in the operating theatre. Skinner, Zarins and Moossa,[38], again demonstrated that the distribution of labelled microspheres was predictive of viability. Three to five microcuries were injected into the aorta and a hand held counting probe could determine the relative counts in normal and ischaemic tissue.

Haas et al.,[39] used external abdominal imaging after intravenous injection of Tc 99M-diphosphonate to demonstrate infarcted intestine in the intact animal. Tc 99M labelled phosphate complexes accumulate in necrotic tissue, and diffuse or focal abdominal activity of greater density than that of the chest was found to correlate well with transmural necrosis of intestine seen histologically. The fact that the scanning was carried out in the intact animal from 1–48 hours after the release of strangulation would make this technique less useful clinically as a predictor of viability. The authors considered that images obtained 2–3 hours after injection of the radioactive material gave the most accurate results. Similar studies using pyrophosphate have been performed by Beaujiz. This would be of little help to a surgeon trying to assess viability intraoperatively. Gharagozloo, Bulkley, Alderson et al.[40] evaluated intraperitoneal injection of Xe 133 in a dog model of nonocclusive mesenteric ischaemia created by transfemoral balloon occlusion of the superior mesenteric artery. The Xenon was rapidly absorbed from the peritoneal cavity by passive diffusion and in poorly perfused tissue it was selectively retained. This avoided the major problems of imaging ischaemic intestine where a paradoxical requirement for uptake of intravascular isotopes into hypoperfused tissue resulted in a low activity concentration ratio in ischaemic tissue. This meant that frank necrosis was required for positive images and also that isotope activity in adjacent organs obscured the area of no uptake. They found that external counts per minute at 30, 60 and 90 minutes after injection were higher in dogs with ischaemic intestine. Bulkley et al.[41] administered intra-peritoneal Xe 133 dissolved in saline to rats and dogs with strangulated bowel and found a delay in externally detected isotope washout from these animals, compared to those with simple obstruction or sham operations. There was an overall increased concentration of isotope in the ischaemic tissue and significant retention at 1 hour. The diminished clearance was due to a lower blood flow and was not dependent on isotope uptake in the necrotic tissue. Xenon is a lipid soluble inert gas that is 95% exhaled in a single passage through the lungs, so that the high concentration ratios in ischaemic tissue are based on differences in clearance and are unrelated to specificity of uptake.

Summary

Clinical judgement is not always accurate in deciding what bowel will recover after an ischaemic injury. If extensive lengths are involved, as in mesenteric vascular disease, preservation of all

Table 4.1

Test	Clinical (*C**) Laboratory (*L*)	Expense	Accuracy
Clinical judgement	C	–	+
'Second look'	C	+	+ +
Surface fluorescence	C	–	+ +
Perfusion fluorometry	C	+ +	+ + +
Doppler	C	+	+ +
Electro-myography	C	+ +	+ +
pH; pCO_2	L	+	+
Thermography	L	+ +	+
O_2 probe	L	+ +	+ +
Tetrazolium analysis	L	+	+ +
Isotope scans	L	+ +	+ +

*All clinical tests can also be used in the laboratory

potentially recoverable intestine is important for life and nutrition. A 'second-look' laparotomy is helpful but is a second operation in patients, often elderly and ill. There are many tests that increase accuracy; some of these require expensive equipment and specialized personnel. Others, already in clinical use, are helpful. Surface fluorescence increases the accuracy of identifying viable bowel. The equipment is inexpensive, it is somewhat observer-dependent and the dye is relatively safe. Perfusion fluorometry is more objective, allows repeat estimations with smaller doses of fluorescein and is more accurate. The equipment, however, is also more expensive. Doppler probes are widely available in hospitals, can be used intraoperatively and have a better accuracy than purely clinical judgement. They can, however, only access small lengths of bowel at a time and may be complementary to fluorescence which may pinpoint an area of particularly doubtful viability.

References

1. Laufman, H., Method, H. The role of vascular spasm in recovery of strangulated intestine. *Surg. Gynecol. Obstet.* (1947) **85**: 675–86.
2. Bussemaker, J.B., Lindeman, J. Comparison of methods to determine viability of small intestine. *Ann. Surg.* (1972) **176**: 97–101.
3. Zarins, C., Skinner, D., James, E. Prediction of the viability of revascularized intestine with radioactive microspheres. *Surg. Gynecol. Obstet.* (1974) **138**: 576–97.
4. Gorey, T.F. Prediction of intestinal recovery after ischaemic injury due to arterial, venous and mixed arterial and venous occlusions. *J. Roy. Soc. Med.* (1980) **73**: 631–4.
5. Zuidema, G.D. Surgical management of superior mesenteric arterial emboli. *Arch. Surg.* (1961) **82**: 267–74.
6. Zuidema, G.D., Reed, D., Turcotte, J.G., Fry, W.J. Superior mesenteric artery embolectomy. *Ann. Surg.* (1964) **159**: 548–53.
7. Lange, K., Boyd, L.J. The use of fluorescein to determine the adequacy of the circulation. *Med. Clin. N. Am.* (1942) **26**: 943–52.
8. Stolar, C.J., Randolph, J.G. Evaluation of ischemic bowel viability with a fluorescent technique. *J. Ped. Surg.* (1978) **13**: 221–5.
9. Wheaton, L.G., Strandberg, J., Hamilton, S., Bulkley, G.B. A comparision of three techniques for intraoperative prediction of small intestinal injury. *J. Am. Animal. Hosp. Assoc.* (1983) **19**: 897–902.
10. Bulkley, G., Zuidema, G., Hamilton, S., O'Mara, C., Klacsmann, P., Horn, S., Intraoperative determination of small intestinal viability following ischemic injury. *Ann. Surg.* (1981) **193**: 628–37.
11. Marfuggi, R., Greenspan, M. Reliable intraoperative predictions of intestinal viability using a fluorescent indicator. *Surg. Gynecol. Obstet.* (1981) **152**: 33–5.
12. Silverman, D.G., Hurford, W.E., Cooper, H.S., Robinson, M., Brousseau, D.A. Quantification of fluorescein distribution to strangulated rat ileum. *J. Surg. Res.* (1983) **34**: 179–86.
13. Carter, M., Fantini, G., Sammartano, R., Mitsudo, S., Silverman, D., Boley, S.G. Qualitative and quantative fluorescein fluorescence for determining intestinal viability. *Am. J. Surg.* (1984) **147**: 117–25.
14. Herrlin, J.O. (Jr), Glasser, S.T., Lange, K. New methods for determining the viability of the bowel. *Arch. Surg.* (1942) **45**: 785–90.
15. Harvey, S.C. Antiseptics and disinfectants; fungicides; ectoparasiticides. In: Goodman, L.S., Gilman, A., (Eds). *The Pharmacological Basis of Therapeutics*. New York: Macmillan (1975) 1004.
16. Lapiana, F.G., Penner, R. Anaphylactoid reaction to intravenously administered fluorescein. *Arch. Ophthal.* (1968) **79**: 161–2.
17. Cunningham, E., Balu, V. Cardiac arrest following fluorescein angiography. *J. Amer. Med. Ass.* (1979) **242**: 2431.
18. Stein, M.R., Parker, C.W. Reactions following intravenous fluorescein. *Am. J. Ophthal.* (1971) **72**: 861–8.
19. Amalric, P., Biau, C., Fenies, M.T. Incidents et Accidents Au Cours De L'Angiographie Fluoresceinique. *Bull. Ophthal. Soc.* (1968) **68**: 968.
20. Deglin, S.M., Deglin, E.A., Chung, E.K. Acute myocardial infarction following fluorescein angiography. *Heart Lung* (1977) **6**: 505–9.
21. Papachristou, D., Fortner, J.G. Prediction of intestinal viability by intra-arterial dye injection: A simple test. *Am. J. Surg.* (1976) **132**: 572–4.
22. Myers, M.B., Cherry, G. Use of vital dyes in the evaluation of the blood supply of the colon. *Surg. Gynecol. Obstet.* (1969) **149**: 97–102.
23. Dineen, P., Goulian, D., McSherry, C.K. A method of demonstrating intestinal viability. *Amer. J. Gastroent.* (1966) **45**: 335–7.
24. Wright, C.B., Hobson, R.W. Prediction of intestinal viability using Doppler ultrasound techniques. *Am. J. Surg.* (1975) **129**: 642–5.
25. O'Donnell, J.A., Hobson, E.Q. Operative confir-

mation of Doppler ultrasound in evaluation of intestinal ischemia. *Surgery* (1980) **87**: 109–12.

26. Cooperman, M., Pace, W.G., Martin, E.W., Pflug, B., Keith, L.M., Evans, W.E., Carey, L.C. Determination of viability of ischemic intestine by Doppler ultrasound. *Surgery* (1978) **83**: 6: 705–10.
27. Cooperman, M., Martin, E.W. (Jr), Evans, W.E., Carey, L.C. Assessment of anastomotic blood supply by Doppler ultrasound in operations upon the colon. *Surg. Gynecol. Obstet.* (1979) **149**: 15–17.
28. Cooperman, M., Martin, E.W., Keith, L.M., Carey, L.C. Use of Doppler ultrasound in intestinal surgery. *Am. J. Surg.* (1979) **138**: 856–9.
29. Shah, S., Anderson, C. Prediction of small bowel viability using Doppler ultrasound. Clinical and experimental evaluation. *Ann. Surg.* (1981) **194**: 97–9.
30. Schamaun, M. Electromyography to determine viability of injured small bowel segments: An experimental study with preliminary clinical observations. *Surgery* (1967) **62**: 899–909.
31. Katz, S., Wahab, A., Murray, W., Williams, L. New parameters of viability in ischemic bowel disease. *Am. J. Surg.* (1974) **127**: 136–41.
32. Myers, M.B., Cherry, G., Gesser, J. Relationship between surface pH and pCO_2 and the vascularity and viability of intestine *Surg. Gynecol. Obstet.* (1972) **134**: 787–9.
33. Moss, A.A., Kressel, H.K., Brito, A.C. Use of thermography to predict intestinal viability and survival after ischemic injury: A blind study. *Invest. Rad.* (1981) **16**: 24–9.
34. Piasecki, C. A new method for the assessment of gut viability. *Br. J. Surg.* (1981) **68**: 319–22.
35. Carter, K., Halle, M., Cherry, G., Myers, M.B. Determination of the viability of ischemic intestine. *Arch. Surg.* (1970) **100**: 695–701.
36. Gorey, T.F. The recovery of intestine after ischaemic injury. *Br. J. Surg.* (1980) **67**: 699–702.
37. Amano, H., Bulkley, G.B., Gorey, T.F., Hamilton, S.R., Horn, S.D., Zuidema, G.D. Role of microvascular patency in the recovery of small intestine from ischemic injury. *Surg. Forum.* (1980) **31**: 157–9.
38. Skinner, D.B., Zarins, C.K., Moossa, A.R. Mesenteric vascular disease. *Am. J. Surg.* (1974) **128**: 835–9.
39. Haase, G.M., Sfakianakis, G.N., Ortiz, V.N., Lobe, T.E., Boles, E.T. In vivo radionuclide imaging to detect intestinal necrosis. *Surg. Forum.* (1978) **29**: 486–9.
40. Gharagozloo, F., Bulkley, C., Alderson, P.H., Barth, K.H., White, R., Zuidema, G.D. Intraperitoneal Xenon 133 for the early detection of acute mesenteric ischemia. *Surg. Forum.* (1980) **31**: 144–6.
41. Bulkley, G. Gharagozloo, F., Alderson, P., Horn, S., Zuidema, G.D. Use of intraperitoneal Xenon-133 for imaging of intestinal strangulation in small bowel obstruction. *Am. J. Surg.* (1981) **141**: 128–35.

Acknowledgement

I wish to thank Gregory Bulkley of the Johns Hopkins Hospital, Baltimore, USA, with whom I collaborated as a research fellow. Drs Boley, Lanzafame, Copperman and Myers have shared their techniques with me. I am grateful to all my colleagues in Ireland who invited me to study their patients at operation. Finally, I wish to thank the editor Mr Marston whose work in this area has always been an inspiration.

5

Acute intestinal ischaemia

A.R. Moossa
Steven Shackford
Michael J. Sise

Introduction

Acute intestinal ischaemia produces an intra-abdominal catastrophe with a high mortality. Little improvement in survival has been achieved since the 1930s when a mortality rate of 70–100 per cent was observed.[1] The patient with acute intestinal ischaemia is usually at high risk due to advanced age (Fig. 5.1), underlying disease and the rapid progression to infarction. An aggressive diagnostic and therapeutic approach offers the only hope to reduce the morbidity and death rate of this syndrome. Selective angiography, intra-arterial vasodilators, embolectomy, thrombectomy, arterial reconstruction and bowel resection have been employed successfully when undertaken early in the course of the disease.[2, 3] In selected hands, these procedures have lowered deaths from acute intestinal ischaemia to between 20 and 30 per cent below the national average.

Clearly, prompt diagnosis is crucial. The early clinical features are vague and non-specific, and routine laboratory tests and plain x-ray are unhelpful. Recent preliminary data from Ontario, Canada, by Jamieson et al. appear highly promising. These workers have established that the gut wall of both dogs and humans contains high concentrations of both organic and inorganic phosphate. During ischaemia, phosphate is released from the bowel, which can easily be measured in blood, peritoneal fluid and urine.[4]

Canine gut can completely revert to normal after up to 6 hours of severe ischaemia. During these 6 hours, inorganic serum phosphate is elevated from hour 2 until hour 6. Thus, under hypoxic conditions, a time period of about 4–6 hours exists before irretrievable necrosis ensues (Fig. 5.2). During this crucial interval the serum phosphate is raised and prompt surgical intervention and revascularization may save the gut. Jamieson et al.[4] also report accurate clinical diagnosis in 20 consecutive patients with bowel ischaemia utilizing serum phosphate measurements. Three of their cases were diagnosed early, which led to revascularization without resection. If these observations are confirmed, this simple test will, by early diagnosis, lower the prohibitive mortality and morbidity associated with major mesenteric, arterial or venous occlusion.

Factors leading to acute intestinal ischaemia may be thought of as:

1. *Deficiencies in major blood flow*, as determined by the cardiac output or by local conditions in the mesenteric vessels. The four major causes of acute intestinal ischaemia are arterial embolus, arterial thrombosis, non-occlusive ischaemia and venous thrombosis. Iatrogenic occlusion of the mesenteric vessels following major abdominal operations or invasive radiology is also becoming more frequent. Each of these factors is reviewed with respect to presentation, diagnosis and management.
2. Factors operating *within the wall of the bowel*. These include radial muscular tension, and local tissue sensitivities leading to focal reactions such as the Arthus[5] and Schwartzmann phenomena. Among these may be included pharmacological agents such as digitalis, and pressor amines which act on the bowel wall and on its small vessels.
3. *Intraluminal factors*. These include:
   (a) the bacterial flora; and
   (b) tryptic activity and other influences which imperil the integrity of the mucosal barrier.

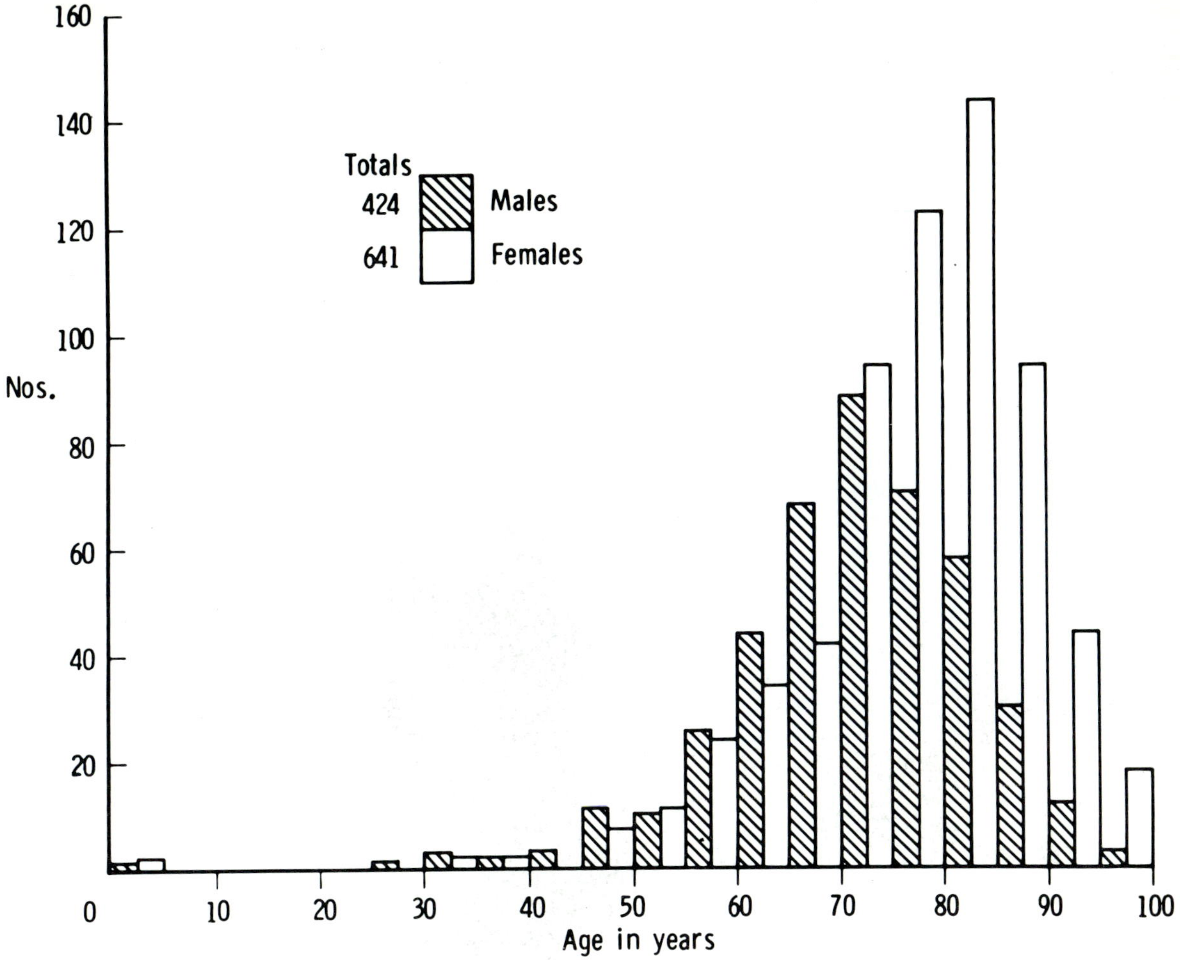

Fig. 5.1 Deaths from acute intestinal ischaemia related to age and sex (England and Wales, 1982).

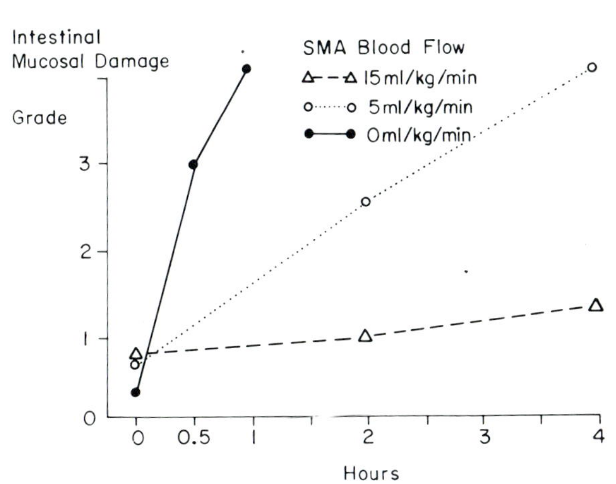

The bowel is unique in that it is normally populated by pathogenic bacteria which are capable of producing highly potent endotoxins and exotoxins. Any weakening of the mucosal defences will permit invasion to occur, resulting in local inflammation and generalized circulatory effects. Whether a sufficiently virulent strain of bacteria can invade a healthy gut with normal vasculature is a matter of dispute, but there is evidence that in certain circumstances this can occur. Ischaemia of the midgut induced by ligation of the superior mesenteric artery has been extensively studied in the laboratory and is discussed in Chapter 3.

Fig. 5.2 The relationship between SMA flow and the pace of mucosal damage. (From Chiu, C.J. *Archives of Surgery* (1976) **101**: 480, by kind permission of the author and Editor.)

Superior mesenteric arterial embolus

Causation

Embolic occlusion of the superior mesenteric artery (SMA) accounts for 25–30 per cent of acute intestinal ischaemia,[2, 6, 7] and 90–95 per cent of emboli arise from the heart, usually because of atrial fibrillation.[8] Other sources of embolism are mural thrombus in the left ventricle, vegetations or thrombi on diseased or prosthetic mitral or aortic valves, and dislodged debris from atheromatous plaques in the aorta. Paradoxical embolism from systemic veins can theoretically occur in the presence of an interatrial or interventricular septal defect, but is exceedingly rare.

The relative frequency of embolus and thrombosis is not easy to determine, but there appears to have been a steady decline in the incidence of emboli over the last two decades.

Johnson and Baggenstoss[9] outlined stringent criteria for the diagnosis of mesenteric embolism, namely:

1. There must be a source for an embolus.
2. There must be clinical symptoms of sudden onset.
3. A short section only of the SMA must be involved.
4. The microscopic appearance of the occlusion must suggest an embolus.
5. Embolic phenomena must have occurred elsewhere.

Applying these criteria, they found that an embolus accounted for 19 out of 45 cases seen at the Mayo Clinic between 1911 and 1949. If, however, the diagnosis of mesenteric embolus depended on findings which can only be verified *post mortem*, the reported incidence would be deceptively low. Although some authors have shown an equal or even preponderant number of emboli as against thromboses,[10, 11] it is now recognized that the relative frequency of embolus and thrombosis is an artificial statistic in that a mesenteric arterial block may bear little time relation to clinical events. The unique importance of the mesenteric embolus is that it is a condition which, if diagnosed early, is curable. This cannot be said of any other type of acute mesenteric vascular disease.

Clinical presentation

Mesenteric embolus presents most often with acute abdominal pain. The distribution of pain is peri-umbilical, but may be located in the right upper quadrant. Bowel wall ischaemia initiates intense peristaltic activity and gut emptying. Vomiting and loose stools frequently follow the onset. Bloody diarrhoea is usually not evident until several hours later in the course of the disease, when mucosal infarction has begun. The majority of patients with embolic occlusion are in the sixth or seventh decades and give a history of cardiac arrhythmia or recent myocardial infarction. A history of previous embolism to the brain, extremities or viscera can be elicited in 25–40 per cent of these patients.[8]

Physical findings are few in the early stages. Pain out of proportion to the objective signs is an important clue to the presence of ischaemia.

Peritoneal irritation heralds the onset of full-thickness bowel necrosis, and carries a grave prognosis.

Early in the course of the disease vital signs, including temperature, are normal. With progressive ischaemia, the intravascular volume contracts as fluid is lost into the intestinal lumen, the bowel wall and the peritoneal cavity. This will produce signs of hypovolaemia which, if untreated, can lead to profound shock. The temperature, if elevated, is usually below 38°C. Laboratory findings in acute ischaemia are initially unremarkable, with the exception of leucocytosis. Leucocyte counts in excess of 20 000 are common. Metabolic acidosis is a later finding and suggests bowel necrosis.

Plain radiographs of the abdomen are usually unhelpful.[12] However, the presence of air-filled loops of intestine with thickening of the wall, in this clinical setting, is suggestive of mesenteric ischaemia (Fig. 5.3).

Because of the lack of pathognomonic symptoms and signs, the differential diagnosis of patients with this presentation is wide, and includes acute pancreatitis, perforated ulcer (gastric or duodenal), small bowel obstruction, acute diverticulitis and aortic dissection.

Late in the course of embolic occlusion of the SMA, profound hypovolaemia, fever and refractory metabolic acidosis result.[13] At this point bowel infarction is clinically obvious, and circulatory collapse and death are inevitable unless the infarcted segment is resected.

Diagnosis

Mesenteric embolism occurs in an older population of patients with underlying cardiac disease who

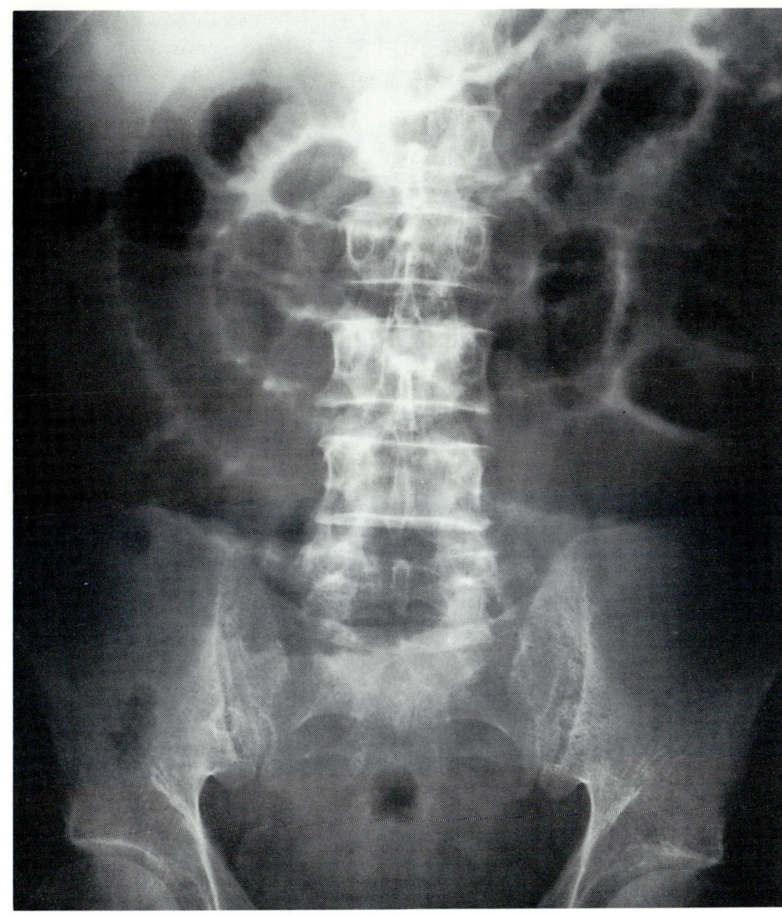

Fig. 5.3 Plain abdominal radiograph demonstrating dilated, air-filled small intestine with thickened wall in a patient with acute mesenteric ischaemia.

have little physiological reserve. An aggressive and timely diagnostic approach is the key to successful management.

If mesenteric ischaemia is suspected, the surgeon must decide whether to perform immediate exploratory laparatomy or to carry out a preliminary arteriogram. The decision to proceed directly to laparotomy depends upon the presence of signs of peritonitis or the presence of refractory hypovolaemia and metabolic acidosis, all of which suggest bowel infarction. Arteriography is the inital diagnostic step in those patients who have minimal or no signs of peritonitis and who appear to be haemodynamically stable. Percutaneous transfemoral retrograde arteriography can be performed safely in the majority of patients provided that they are not allergic to iodinated contrast material and have adequate renal function. It is important to keep these patients well hydrated before and during the angiogram because contrast material can be nephrotoxic and can also induce an osmotic diuresis which may further deplete the patient's fluid volume. Other than contrast reaction and renal failure, which occur infrequently, the morbidity from angiography is low. However, arteriography, even in the best centres, takes time and can delay definitive treatment.

Intra-aortic contrast injection at the level of the first lumbar vertebra is usually sufficient to visualize the SMA. Anteroposterior views will visualize the embolus which most commonly lodges just distal to the origin of the middle colic artery, 4–6 cm from the SMA origin[8] (Fig. 5.4).

The use of vasodilators infused through the catheter at the completion of the arteriogram has been advocated, since severe vasospasm accompanies all cases of acute mesenteric ischaemia, however caused. Papaverine can be used at an infusion rate of 30–90 mg per hour. Tolazoline has also been advocated. Glucagon, prostacyclin and methyl-

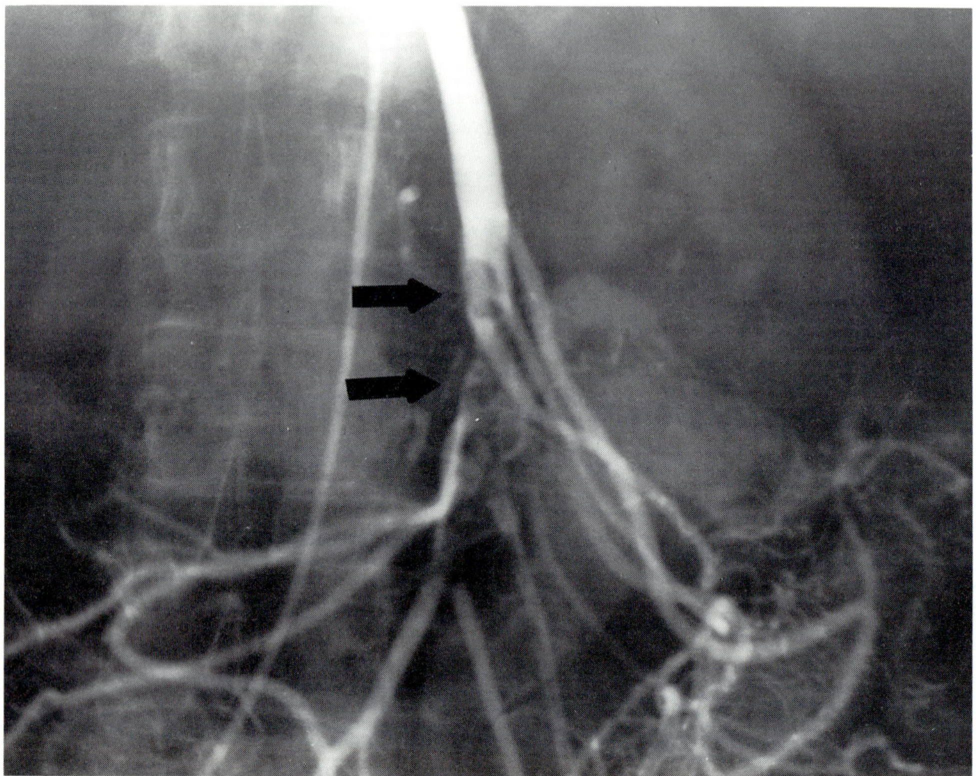

Fig. 5.4 Selective SMA angiogram revealing emboli (arrows) from a cardiac source.

prednisolone have been used experimentally with good results.[14]

The opponents of aortography argue as follows:

1. It is now widely recognized that varying degrees of occlusion of the visceral arteries are quite commonly encountered in normal people over the age of 45, often without any demonstrable effect upon their health. It therefore follows that the angiographic demonstration of a blocked mesenteric artery in a patient with indeterminate abdominal pain gives little guidance as to when the occlusion occurred or whether it is the cause of the symptoms.

2. Failure to show such a block is of no diagnostic help to the surgeon and, if signs of peritonitis are present, will not and should not deter him from exploring the abdomen. Some authors have claimed[15] that intestinal ischaemia, threatened or complete, can be diagnosed on the angiogram by the presence of a narrowed distal arterial tree with spasm of the intramural vessels. The situation can then be treated by epidural blockade or instillation of vasodilator substances (as mentioned above) into the SMA, and an unnecessary laparotomy avoided. Most experienced surgeons agree that the angiographic appearances may be far from specific, and that if doubt exists it is safer to operate.

When a new diagnostic facility is provided, it tends at first to be used without particular regard to its effectiveness. Now that angiography is readily available for emergency diagnosis of abdominal pain, a degree of abuse is inevitable.

Having said all this, it must in fairness be admitted that when embarking on an operation for suspected superior mesenteric vascular occlusion, most surgeons would be pleased to have an angiogram available.

Treatment

Once the diagnosis of embolic occlusion has been established by angiography, prompt operation with embolectomy and resection of any necrotic bowel should be undertaken.

Preoperatively, large-bore intravenous access is obtained to allow for volume replacement. A bladder catheter is inserted to monitor urine output. Invasive monitoring, by either a central venous or a pulmonary artery catheter, is mandatory to obtain optimum cardiac performance. An arterial line is placed to monitor blood pressure and to gain access for arterial blood gas determination. Blood samples are sent for typing and cross-matching.

Metabolic acidosis must be corrected. It arises through a combination of low tissue perfusion, haemoconcentration and absorption (via the peritoneal cavity and intestinal lymphatics) of the products of bacterial and gut necrosis. To this is added a respiratory component derived from impaired ventilation due to interference with respiratory movements and increased blood viscosity with intrapulmonary sludging. Measurements of base excess, pCO_2 and pH will determine the amount of bicarbonate therapy required. Given

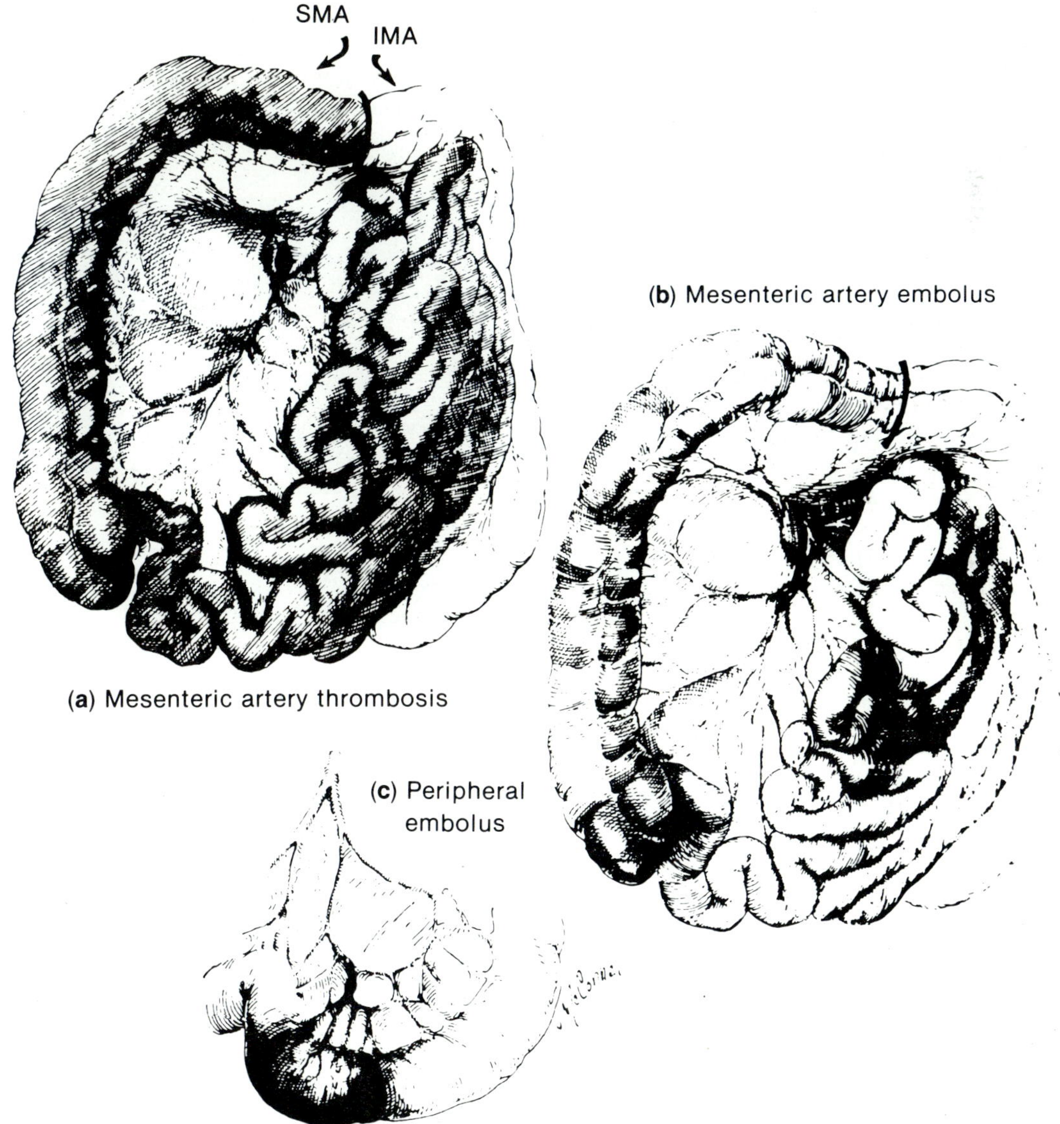

Fig. 5.5 (**a**) Distribution of ischaemia in thrombotic occlusion of the SMA. (**b**) Sparing of the proximal jejunum with embolism to the SMA resulting in acute ischaemia. (**c**) Segmental ischaemia from a small embolism in the peripheral arterial distribution. (From Bergan, J.J. Recognition and treatment of intestinal ischemia. *Surgical Clinics of North America* (1967) **47**: 109, by permission.)

reasonably normal pulmonary and renal function, however, restoration of the circulating blood volume will do much to restore correct acid–base equilibrium.

Systemic heparinization should be started as soon as the diagnosis is made so as to prevent distal propagation of thrombosis in the mesenteric vessels. Dextran may also be of benefit in this regard. Antibiotics with broad aerobic and anaerobic coverage should be administered intravenously early in the course of management.

Operative exploration is carried out through a generous midline incision to allow for thorough abdominal exploration and visualization of the entire length of intestines. Upon opening the abdomen, the small intestine may appear healthy. Closer inspection shows a loss of the normal glistening appearance of the serosa, and palpation of the mesenteric vascular arcades reveals loss of pulsation. Late in the course of mesenteric ischaemia, the bowel will appear grossly abnormal with a boggy bluish appearance.

At the time of exploration, the distribution of ischaemia is a useful indicator of the location of the arterial obstruction. Thrombosis of the SMA occurs at the origin and produces ischaemia throughout the midgut from the ligament of Treitz to the splenic flexure of the colon (Fig. 5.5). Emboli to the SMA usually lodge at, or distal to, the origin of the middle colic artery, thereby sparing the proximal jejunum.

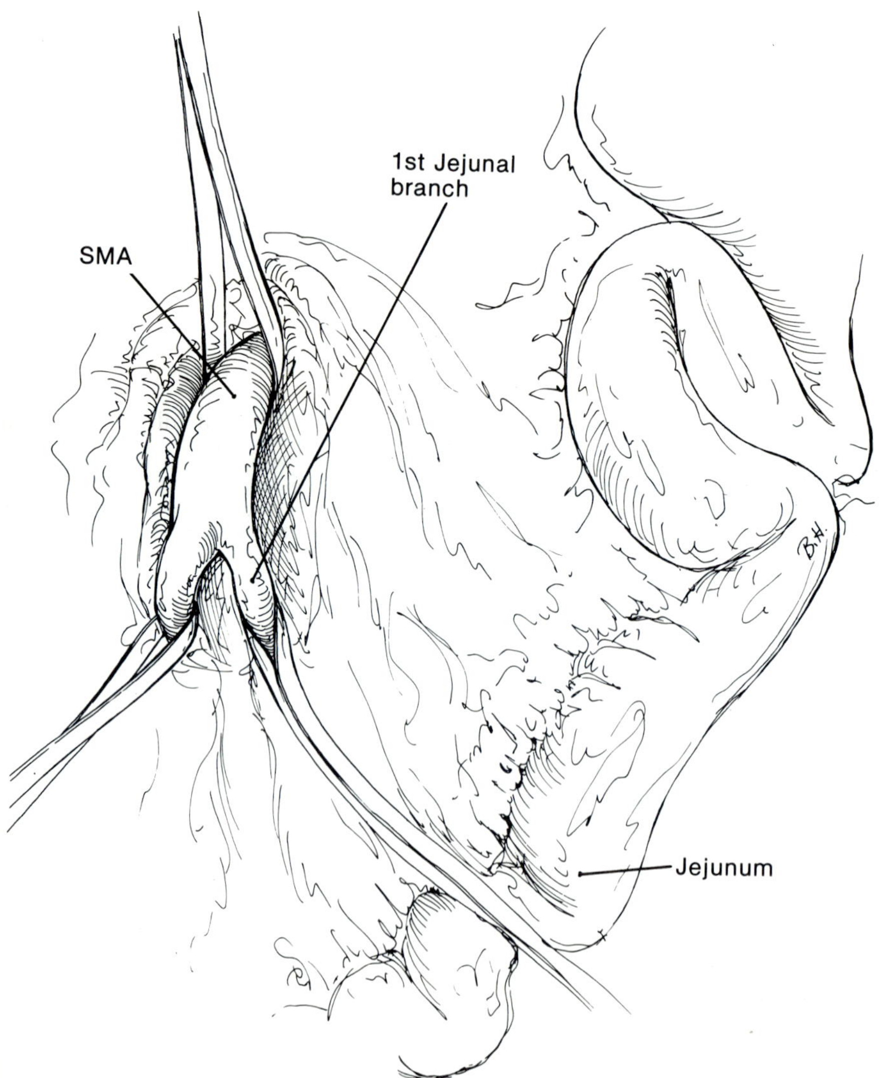

Fig. 5.6 Exposure of the proximal SMA.

Small emboli migrate peripherally and produce segmental ischaemia.

It must be emphasized that, once the peritoneal cavity is entered, it is a mistake to waste time in assessing bowel viability and planning the need or extent of resection. The entire small bowel must be quickly exteriorized and wrapped in moist warm packs, and immediate attention directed to the origin of the SMA.

The proximal SMA is exposed by retracting the transverse colon upwards and drawing down the small bowel mesentery (Fig. 5.6). The ligament of Treitz is incised and the fourth part of the duodenum and upper jejunum thoroughly mobilized. Palpation along the root of the mesentery anterior to the duodenum and at the inferior border of the pancreas will reveal a pulse in the artery proximal to the embolus. Proximal and distal control of the SMA is obtained by encircling the artery with silicone rubber (Silastic) and loops. Heparin 5000 units is given intravenously, the artery is occluded and a transverse arteriotomy made. The mesenteric arteries are thin walled and friable, and must be treated with the utmost care. Balloon catheter embolectomy is performed, taking care to avoid overinflating the balloon, which can result in arterial rupture or intimal injury (Fig. 5.7). After proximal and distal embolectomy is completed, the arterial bed is flushed with 30–40 ml of heparinized saline solution (10 units/ml) injected distally in the artery. The arteriotomy is closed with a fine vascular suture. Upon completion, an operative arteriogram is mandatory before closing the abdomen.[16, 17]

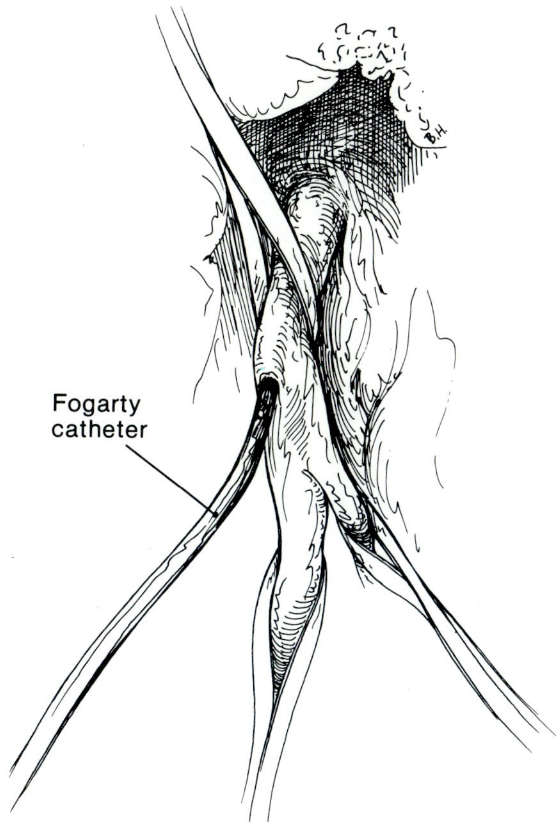

Fig. 5.7 Catheterization of the SMA.

Once adequate arterial flow has been established and documented with completion arteriography, the bowel must be carefully inspected in order to determine the need for resection. A 20–30 minute period of watchful waiting after revascularization will often reveal adequate perfusion of segments initially thought to be non-viable. Areas of obvious infarction should be resected at this time.

Intraoperative assessment of intestinal viability remains an unsolved clinical problem. Most surgeons rely on clinical judgement in deciding whether to resect non-viable bowel. The criteria usually employed for viability are the return of colour and pulsation and the resumption of peristalsis in the injured segment. The difficulty is often solved by resecting short bowel loops of doubtful viability if the patient's general condition is satisfactory. With seriously ill, unstable patients, especially in those with massive vascular occlusion, the decision becomes more difficult. It is often impossible to gauge the success of a revascularization procedure. When the surgeon is forced to perform a massive bowel resection to save the patient's life the length of remaining bowel and its adaptive capabilities become the critical factor for absorption and survival.

Several techniques designed to determine the presence of adequate perfusion of gut wall have been tried, advocated and abandoned (see Chapter 3). Probably the most useful current adjunct to clinical judgement is the use of the Doppler ultrasonic flow probe.[18]

At the end of the operation, the decision to re-explore in 24–48 hours must be made. The so-called 'second-look' operation is not mandatory. If all areas of revascularized bowel appear viable, re-operation is not required. If questionable areas of bowel are left in place, the re-exploration within 24–48 hours is required regardless of the patient's interval course. Most patients successfully treated with embolectomy will not require a second-look operation,[8] but if this is carried out primary anastomosis should *not* be performed. Rather, the divided ends of the bowel should be exteriorized and the stomas carefully watched.

Postoperatively, the cardiac status is continuously monitored because large amounts of fluid will be needed for the next 12–24 hours. If it has been decided to perform a second-look procedure, the patient is not extubated at the conclusion of the initial operation, but mechanical ventilatory support is continued through the second operation.[19]

If the embolus was of cardiac origin, the possibility of recurrent emboli should be remembered. Heparin is therefore continued, closely monitored by serial partial thromboplastin time determinations in order to prevent bleeding. Sodium warfarin is started when sufficient oral intake is resumed and should be maintained for the rest of the patient's life.

The period following SMA embolectomy may be complicated by a gastric hypersecretory response with high-volume intestinal fluid losses. This phenomenon is most likely the result of abnormal mucosal functions following ischaemia, and is usually limited to the 48–72 hours required for mucosal regeneration.[20, 21] It is imperative that all losses be measured and electrolyte concentrations determined in order to calculate accurate replacement. Early parental hyperalimentation should be considered in all patients.

Results

The mortality rate from embolic occlusion of the SMA remains 60–90 per cent.[1, 21, 22, 23] Rapid diagnosis and treatment will certainly improve the outcome, but the high-risk nature of this patient population is reflected by the heavy mortality in even the most successful series.[18, 23] Recurrent embolization is estimated to occur in 10–15 per cent of cases.[1, 18]

Mesenteric arterial thrombosis

Causation

Mesenteric arterial thrombosis results from occlusion of the principal arterial supply to the gut, in the setting of chronic atherosclerosis. Thrombotic occlusion accounts for 10–15 per cent of cases of acute mesenteric ischaemia.[3, 7, 8, 21] The site of the block is variable and depends upon the location and the degree of the underlying occlusive process. Both the SMA and the coeliac axis (CA) may be involved.

Atheromatous ulceration, with consequent platelet accretion, is commonly found at the origin of the SMA. Clearly, this will, on occasion, lead to acute occlusion of the lumen, with subsequent death of the bowel, in the same way that acute occlusion of a stenotic femoral artery can precipitate gangrene in the foot. The analogy, however, is not so simple. Not only can stenosis or occlusion of the SMA be present without causing any symptoms, but also the bowel can become infarcted in spite of there being a perfectly normal and patent vascular tree. It can be wrong, therefore, to conclude that a patient with an infarcted bowel and a blocked SMA has sustained a recent acute thrombosis. The block may have been there for months or even years and the acute intestinal ischaemia has occurred through a fall in cardiac output, a local Schwartzmann phenomenon or other unrelated cause. This is not to say that the occlusion should be ignored and no attempt made to restore patency. However, all reported evidence indicates that the results of operation for 'acute thrombosis' are much worse than when an embolus is present.

Clinical presentation

The syndrome of thrombotic occlusion of the SMA is more insidious in onset and its presentation is more subtle than embolic occlusion. Early signs are few, and the abdominal examination is rarely helpful. Mesenteric thrombosis frequently presents in the setting of major illnesses causing a low flow state, such as myocardial infarction or congestive heart failure, in a patient with pre-existing artherosclerotic narrowing of the origin of the SMA. In contrast to the intense pain seen with an embolus, the patient with thrombotic occlusion often presents with intermittent pain of moderate severity. However, once the point of infarction is approached, the symptoms and signs are similar to those of SMA embolism, and peritonitis and hypovolaemia ensue.

Symptoms of chronic intestinal ischaemia can be elicited in 30–50 per cent of patients presenting with SMA thrombosis, but it should be emphasized that partial occlusion of the SMA by an atheromatous plaque is a common finding in the elderly and does *not* necessarily mean that the chronic abdominal symptoms are of ischaemic origin.[23] In spite of these interpretative difficulties, one must remember Englebert Dunphy's advice — 'The clinical importance of vascular pain in the abdomen lies in the fact that it may be a precursor of fatal vascular occlusion' (see also Chapter 8).[24]

Diagnosis

Mesenteric thrombosis presents insidiously, and the diagnosis is often delayed.[23] A thorough history and physical examination, including palpation of the peripheral pulses will usually reveal manifestations of diffuse atherosclerosis. A high index of suspicion in these patients will expedite both diagnosis and treatment. A past history of claudication or cerebrovascular symptoms, in conjunction with diminshed pulses or bruits in the patient with persistent abdominal pain, should bring to mind the possibility of occlusion of the SMA.

Plain films of the abdomen are often non-specific, especially if they are obtained early in the patient's course (Fig. 5.8). Arteriography is essential to establish the diagnosis and to plan the operative approach (Fig. 5.9). Lateral views are required to visualize the origin of the coeliac and the superior mesenteric arteries (Fig. 5.10). The occlusion commonly occurs in the first segment of the SMA at the origin of the coeliac axis, and both arteries may be occluded. There may also be stenotic lesions at the origins of the renal arteries, the aorta itself may have ulcerated atherosclerotic plaques, the inferior mesenteric artery may be occluded and the iliac arteries severely diseased. Collateral vessels often arise through the lumbar and intercostal arteries, and to the midgut and foregut via the inferior

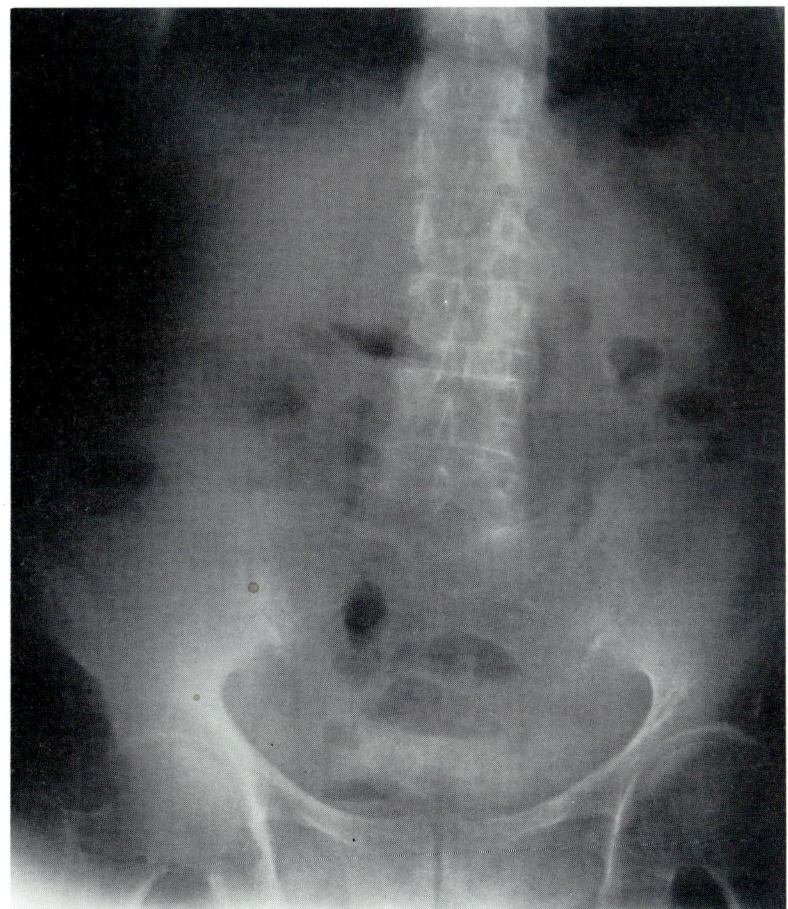

Fig. 5.8 Non-specific bowel gas pattern in a patient with thrombotic occlusion of the SMA.

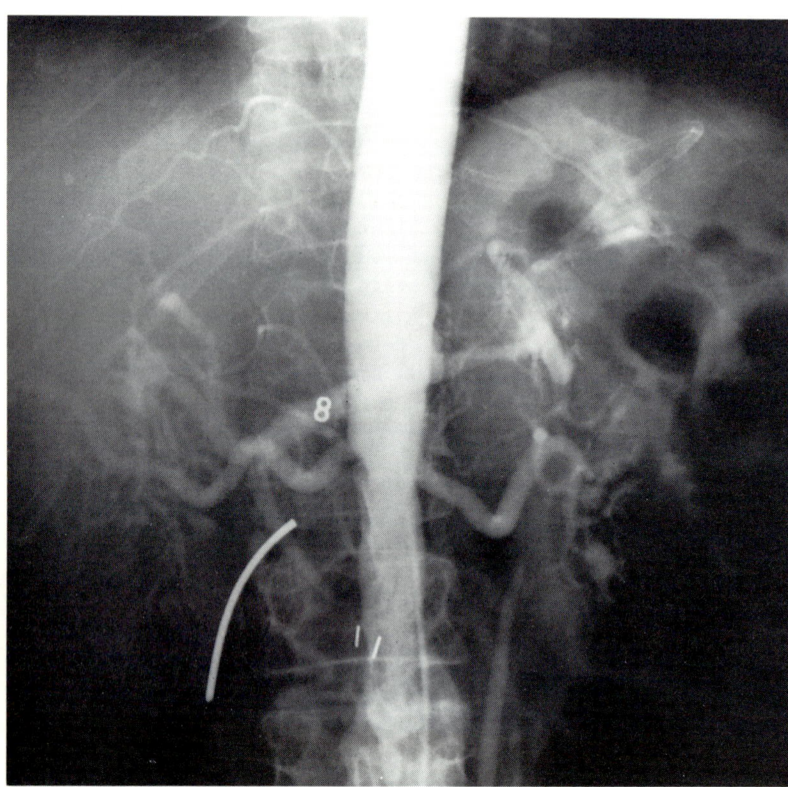

Fig. 5.9 Anteroposterior view of an aortogram obtained in a patient with thrombotic occlusion of the SMA, demonstrating lack of visualization of artery.

mesenteric artery (IMA), which can be two to three times its normal size.

Treatment

Selective catheterization of the mesenteric vessels may not be possible, and therefore vasodilator infusion cannot always be instituted. However, it should be attempted, since vasospasm may worsen gut ischaemia. The agents and doses used are similar to those described for embolic occlusion.

Infusion of a fibrinolytic agent (streptokinase, urokinase) through the arterial catheter might succeed in unmasking a stenosis which could then conceivably be dilated by the Grüntzig technique, thus obviating the need for operation. However, fibrinolysis and balloon dilation are not without risks (haemorrhage, distal embolization) and, therefore, should be undertaken only in centres with experience in the technique. Moreover, this form of treatment should only be attempted early in the course of the disease, before the onset of advanced ischaemia. In the presence of peritonitis, time must not be wasted on non-operative management; rapid resuscitation followed by laparotomy are mandatory.

The preoperative care of patients with SMA thrombosis is similar to that used in the management of patients with embolic occlusion, and includes invasive monitoring, aggressive fluid resuscitation, broad spectrum antibiotics and systemic heparinization.

Upon opening the abdomen through a long midline incision, the bowel will appear ischaemic for a varying length depending upon the underlying occlusive disease. If two of the three mesenteric vessels were previously occluded due to chronic atherosclerotic changes, acute thrombosis of the remaining vessel may result in ischaemia from the oesophagogastric junction to the rectum. The vessel most commonly involved is the SMA, resulting in ischaemia from the proximal jejunum to the splenic flexure. The effects are less if the IMA is patent and adequate collateral flow occurs through the marginal artery of Drummond.

Thrombosis of the SMA requires a reconstructive

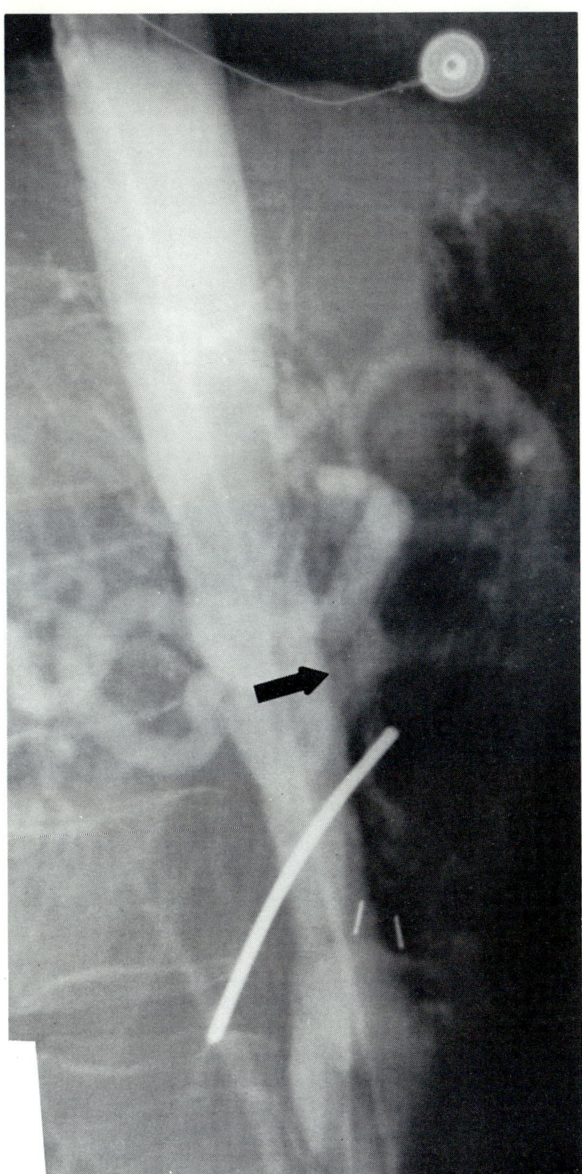

Fig. 5.10 Lateral aortogram of the patient in Fig. 4.9. The arrow indicates the appropriate location for origin of the SMA.

vascular procedure.[25] The mesenteric vessels are approached by exposing the aorta at the level of the renal arteries and origin of the SMA (Fig. 5.11a, b). Extensive thromboendarterectomy of the mid-aortic region, including the origins of the visceral vessels, has been advocated.[2, 26] However, bypass grafting from the infrarenal aorta to the mesenteric vessels just distal to their origin is more commonly performed.[8] In the presence of advanced bowel ischaemia or bowel infarction, autologous saphenous vein is the preferred graft material. Careful alignment of the graft from the aorta to the superior mesenteric or coeliac arteries is required to prevent occlusion of the graft from kinking (Fig. 4.11c, d). Just before completing the bypass, a balloon catheter is passed to ensure patency of the distal arterial tree.

Such a direct attack on the origin of the SMA for emergency revascularization of the gut involves a dissection which is often difficult and prolonged, especially in an obese patient. Access is hampered by the portal vein, the neck of the pancreas with its many vascular connections and the thick lymphatic tissues in the root of the mesentery. However, success can occasionally be achieved by this means, and in a thin patient it may be worth attempting a direct attack.

An alternative approach[23] is illustrated in Fig. 5.12. It consists in exposing the ileocolic artery by reflecting the caecum medially and dissecting in its mesentery, and using this route for the revascularization procedure.

The common iliac arteries are cleared and controlled with snares and atraumatic clamps in order to prevent dislodgement of thrombus into the legs. The ileocolic artery is then dissected proximally until a reasonable diameter (3–4 mm) has been attained, and is controlled with tapes. The vessel is easily found in the caecal mesentery, and is usually of quite adequate calibre. A 1 cm arteriotomy is then made in this vessel, and a size 4F Fogarty embolectomy catheter is passed up into the origin of the SMA. The catheter is gently but persistently worked into the aorta, using three or four passages if necessary, and repeatedly drawn back so as to retrieve as much occlusive material as possible. As the occlusion is extracted the ileocolic artery progressively dilates. When all possible thrombus has been withdrawn, the mesentery is milked back to clear the distal vessels, the SMA is flushed from the aorta and the catheter is passed again. The iliac arteries are checked, and if any debris is felt to have accumulated within them this is removed through short longitudinal incisions.

If at this point the SMA picks up pulsation and the bowel becomes pink and is obviously revascularized, the incision in the ileocolic artery is closed, or (if the pattern of collateral appears to make this safe) the vessel is simply ligated. If, however, there is still some doubt regarding restoration of blood

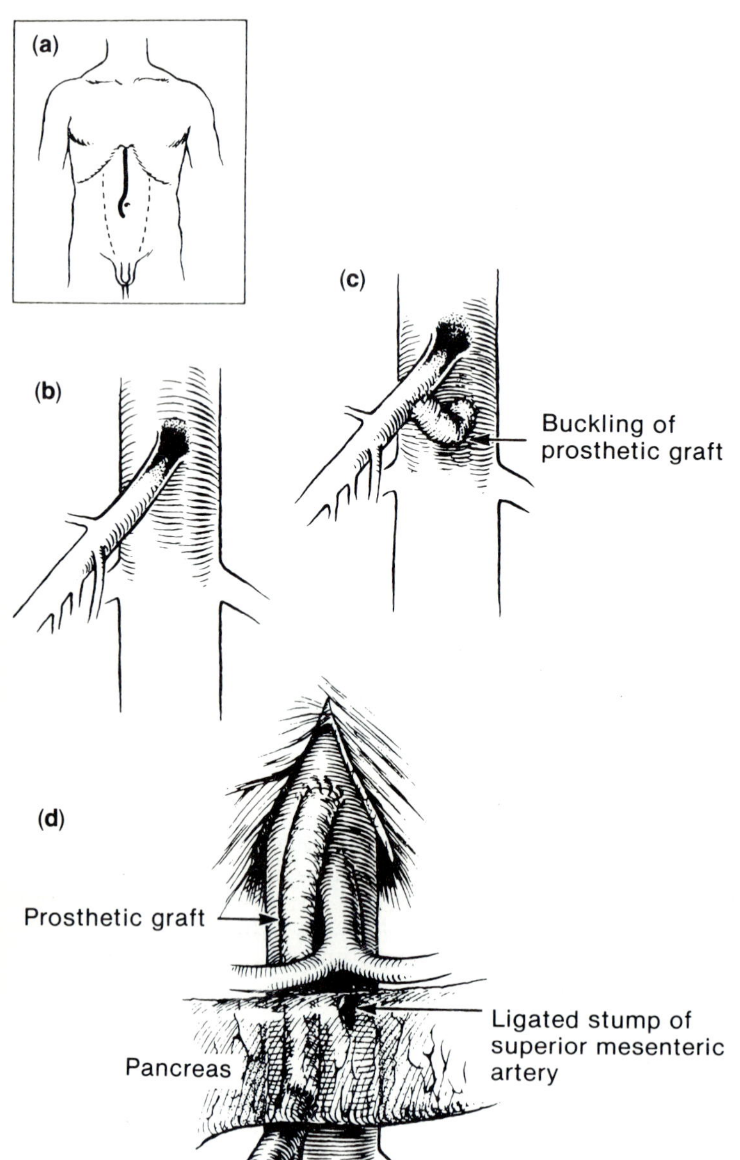

Fig. 5.11 (**a**) Incision for approach to the visceral arteries. (**b**) Thrombotic occlusion of the SMA. (**c**) Buckling of bypass graft not properly aligned. (**d**) Alternate route of graft from supracoeliac aorta. (From *Vascular Surgery Principles and Techniques*, Haimovici, H., ed. New York: McGraw-Hill (1976) p. 676, by permission.)

supply and it is felt that the occlusion at the origin has not been completely relieved, the bowel must be revascularized in another way. It is quite a simple matter to make a short (1.5 cm) arteriotomy in the common iliac artery and to carry out a side-to-side anastomosis between this vessel and the already opened ileocolic, using two running sutures of 4/0 or 5/0 material. When clamps are finally removed, the bowel is revascularized in a retrograde fashion, the blood passing up the ileocolic artery into the SMA and hence to the arcades.

Following revascularization of the gut, the principles of bowel resection discussed earlier concerning mesenteric embolism apply in these patients as well. If bowel resection is required, anastomotic leak, peritonitis and fistula formation are major postoperative risks. Serious consideration should again be given to exteriorizing the bowel

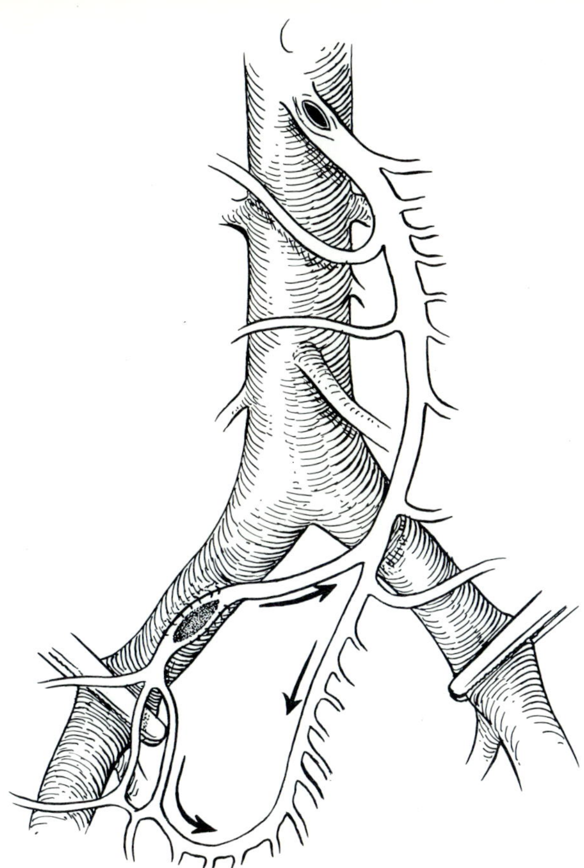

Fig. 5.12 Alternative techniques in mesenteric embolectomy.

ends instead of performing a primary anastomosis under less than optimum conditions.

Postoperative care of the patient with mesenteric thrombosis is similar to that of the patient with embolism. However, systemic heparinization need not be continued into the postoperative period if good technical vascular reconstruction is achieved and the patient will not require oral anticoagulants.

Results

Survival following mesenteric arterial thrombosis depends upon the speed and adequacy of revascularization. Successful revascularization has been shown to have good long-term results; however autogenous vein grafts have not produced adequate long term patency rates sufficient to prefer their use to Dacron or autogenous artery[3, 8] except in the presence of bowel necrosis or perforation.

The overall prognosis in this group of patients remains very poor. Mortality rates from 50 to 100 per cent have been reported,[1, 22, 23] Early vascularization, and resection if needed, continue to be the only effective method of treatment.

Non-occlusive mesenteric ischaemia

Causation

Cases of intestinal ischaemia which are not due to mechanical blockage of the major arteries have, as already explained, been classified under a variety of different names, the most inclusive of which is the term 'non-occlusive ischaemia'.[27, 28, 29, 30, 31, 32, 33] The great majority of these patients have in common some central factor leading to diminished cardiac output and mesenteric flow. The more important of these factors which have been described are as follows.

Congestive cardiac failure is a common and important predisposing cause of intestinal ischaemia.[34, 35, 36] Kligerman and Vidone's[37] series reported that 75 of 109 patients with intestinal ischaemia were also in heart failure. Renton[38] reviewed the literature up to 1972 and showed that 220 patients out of the 284 (77 per cent) reported had severe heart disease, including acute or chronic congestive failure and a history of myocardial infarction and angina. About half the patients were in atrial fibrillation or other arrhythmia; the importance of arrhythmia in reducing cardiac output and precipitating intestinal damage has been underlined by Britt and Cheek,[15] who were able, in the experimental laboratory, to demonstrate an abrupt fall in mesenteric flow following induction of atrial fibrillation. Other authors[39] have demonstrated a drop in mesenteric blood flow during paroxysmal atrial tachycardia, and have described areas of ischaemia and necrosis of the bowel in such cases.

The role which *digitalis* has to play in this situation is uncertain. Cardiac glycosides have a selective vasoconstrictive action on the mesenteric circulation, and many of the clinical series reported contain a high proportion of patients suffering from digitalis overdosage.[40, 41] However, the local effect of digitalis on the bowel is often counterbalanced by the control which the drug exercises on left ventricular failure, with a corresponding rise in cardiac output. Certainly, intestinal ischaemia is not confined to patients who are on digitalis, and it has been reported in those who have stopped taking the drug.[40] Another factor which frequently operates in these patients is the *haemoconcentration* which follows administration of rapidly acting diuretic agents.[42]

The true incidence of non-occlusive ischaemia remains unknown, due largely to the reversible nature of the process and the underlying major illnesses which are associated with it. Infarction without occlusion of the mesenteric vessels has become a phenomenon of increasing frequency.[23] This is related to the emergence of intensive care units in which patients with major cardiovascular disease are sustained through crises such as myocardial infarction, severe aortic insufficiency and congestive heart failure, only to present later with complications of the low flow state. Non-occlusive ischaemia may now account for up to 50 per cent of cases of bowel infarction.[1, 2, 8]

Clinical presentation

The presentation of non-occlusive mesenteric ischaemia is variable and depends upon the underlying disease process. Most patients have been severely hypovolaemic or suffered a low flow state secondary to cardiac failure. Drugs, such as digitalis, vasopressin and ergot alkaloids, which cause decreased splanchnic blood flow, have been implicated in many of these cases. Similarly, the use of pressor drugs to sustain blood pressure during periods of decreased cardiac output may further diminish mesenteric blood flow.

Once ischaemia is present, the symptoms of non-occlusive mesenteric insufficiency resemble those of embolism or thrombosis. However, abdominal pain may not be readily apparent in patients who are critically ill. Gut emptying and, later, rectal bleeding may be the first indications of ischaemia and infarction. Increased fluid volume requirement and unexplained metabolic acidosis are other clues which should raise the suspicion of non-occlusive ischaemia in the critically ill patient in an intensive care unit.

Diagnosis

The arteriogram reveals patent vessels with normal anatomy. Late phase films are necessary to rule out the presence of mesenteric venous thrombosis. At the completion of diagnostic arteriography, the SMA is catheterized and the catheter is left in place to allow for the infusion of vasodilators. As occurs in thrombotic and embolic occlusion, vasospasm plays a prominent role in the pathophysiology of non-occlusive mesenteric ischaemia, and vasodilators may improve mesenteric flow.[43]

Treatment

Pharmacological treatment is the mainstay of the successful management of non-occlusive mesenteric ischaemia. If vasodilator infusion can be maintained successfully for 24 hours without the appearance of peritonitis, repeat arteriography should be performed to rule out segmental occlusion of the mesenteric vessels. If peritoneal signs persist or develop during the infusion, the patient must be presumed to have bowel infarction and operation is mandatory. The onset of increasing fluid requirement or unexplained metabolic acidosis is also an indication for exploratory laparotomy, as these signs are highly suggestive of bowel infarction.

The place of splanchnic block

Orr, Lorhan and Kaul[44] treated 2 patients — 1 with total and 1 with partial small bowel ischaemia — by infiltration of the coeliac and mesenteric plexuses with lignocaine, which in each case was followed by recovery. Some experimental confirmation of this was provided by Liavåg[45] in dogs. More recently, there have been one or two threads of clinical evidence[46] that this procedure may be useful in human beings. Having completed the resection of infarcted bowel and/or the arterial reconstruction, it is reasonable to infiltrate widely the origin of the coeliac axis, the root of the mesentery and the pre-aortic region around the inferior mesenteric artery with a long-acting local anaesthetic such as bupivacaine.

Results

The prognosis for non-occlusive mesenteric ischaemia remains poor. Its frequent association with serious underlying cardiac disease leads to an overall mortality rate of 80–85 per cent.[1, 2, 46] However, increasing awareness of the condition has prompted a more aggressive and timely application of visceral angiography and pharmacological intervention. Survival can approach 100 per cent in those patients who have not developed peritoneal signs prior to the initiation of vasodilator infusion,[46] but, as outlined above, this group of seriously ill patients is not easy to identify.

Trauma and 'shock'

The ischaemic intestinal lesion of shock is very much a fact in the dog, and haemorrhagic necrosis of the alimentary tract is frequent following the challenge of oligaemia, trauma or endotoxaemia. It has been known since the classic work of Wiggers[47] and of Fine[48] that experimentally induced shock in the exsanguinated dog becomes irreversible due to the development of intestinal necrosis.

There are, however, considerable species differences in the intestinal response to shock. The rabbit, cat and monkey behave quite differently from the dog, which is the experimental animal most accessible to researchers. The clinical counterpart to the experimental canine lesion, if it exists, does not appear to be of fundamental importance.[49, 50] Clinical experience accumulated from two world wars and from the Korean and Vietnam conflicts have produced no convincing evidence that intestinal necrosis is an important cause of death in fit human beings who have lost blood because of wounding.

There is a small body of clinical evidence which suggests that intestinal ischaemia can, on occasion, follow trauma. Renton[38] described the case of a fit 18-year-old male who developed necrosis of the entire bowel from the upper jejunum to the pelvic colon 24 hours after a traffic accident involving multiple fractures. There was no intra-abdominal injury and no occlusion of any intestinal vessel. More recently, Haglund and his associates[51] in Göteborg have described haemorrhagic mucosal lesions with epithelial lifting, entirely charcteristic of mucosal ischaemia, in a series of 7 patients suffering from varying degrees of circulatory depletion. Three of their patients had occlusive infarction of the gut in areas distant from the mucosal lesion, and should probably be excluded on these grounds. The other 4 patients, however, had no such problem, and may be considered to be pure examples of the 'intestinal shock' lesion. This is the first time that this lesion has been described in man.

Haemoconcentration and intravascular coagulation

Fogarty and Fletcher[40] emphasized the importance of the haematocrit in the genesis of intestinal ischaemia. They pointed out that values are substantially higher in patients who develop necrosis in the absence of arterial occlusion, and emphasized that a lowered cardiac output coupled with rising blood viscosity will inevitably lead to a fall in mesenteric flow. This point has been further emphasized by Sharefkin and Silen[42] with regard to diuretic agents.

Whitehead[52] showed that intestinal ischaemia is frequently associated with the presence of microthrombi in other organs such as the lungs and kidneys, and has many of the features now known to be characteristic of disseminated intravascular coagulation (DIC).[27] The factors which precipitate this syndrome in man are not fully understood, but include multiple trauma (as may have been the case in Renton's patient), severe burns, septicaemia and anaphylaxis. The Schwartzmann reaction, which is a manifestation of sensitivity to Gram-negative endotoxin, is another potent cause of DIC, and a generalized Schwartzmann reaction could well be an important factor in the causation of intestinal ischaemia. Indeed, a similar lesion can be produced in rabbits by injecting a small sensitizing dose of endotoxin into the colonic wall and following this up with a larger does intravenously.[53] Bearing in mind the constant high level of endotoxin in the intestinal lumen, it is easy to see how this situation could occur clinically.

Perhaps arising from a similar mechanism, intestinal necrosis has been reported[54] as occurring as a complication of renal transplantation. It usually affects patients who have had a difficult post-transplantation course, with high doses of immunosuppressive agents and repeated episodes of rejection. Whether the intestinal lesion is a result of tissue sensitization following the transplant, or whether the immunosuppressive therapy lowers mucosal resistance to bacterial invasion, remains undecided.

Abnormalities of the bowel

Dilation of the lumen of the bowel due to a distal obstruction will cause a corresponding decline in mucosal flow and, if sufficiently severe and prolonged, may precipitate necrosis. An example of this is the ischaemic colitis which occurs above an obstructing carcinoma.[55] However, the damage is usually focal and the cause obvious. Similar acute and massive necrosis has been described in association with rheumatoid arthritis, polyarteritis and diabetes. Although it is difficult to be certain that these are not in fact examples of mechanical infarction due to small vessel involvement, it does seem that on occasion massive necrosis, out of all proportion to the local vascular lesion and apparently normal parts of the bowel, may occur.

Anthony and Drury[56] have described sudden unexpected intestinal necrosis as a complication of functioning carcinoid tumour, and speculated that this is due to bradykinin and 5-hydroxytryptamine (5-HT) secreted by the tumour and conveyed in the intestinal lymphatics (see Chapter 8).

Contents of the bowel

Bacterial activity

Under normal circumstances (given a normal blood supply) the intestinal mucosa is well able to resist bacterial challenge, and when organisms such as clostridia are found within the wall of the gut they are there as secondary invaders. Nevertheless, these organisms produce powerfully constrictive exotoxins, and the question arises as to whether the balance between bacterial aggression and mucosal defence can ever be shifted the other way: that is, whether an organism of unusual virulence can invade a mucosa which has a normal vascularity. There is evidence that this can occur. The problem is fully discussed in Chapter 6.

Tryptic activity

As well as the bacterial content, the chemical content of the bowel exerts a strong influence on its behaviour following any type of ischaemic challenge. The first, and perhaps most important, line of defence is the mucous barrier which coats the epithelium. There is evidence that haemorrhagic necrosis of the gut as seen in the experimentally shocked animal occurs from tryptic digestion of this mucus. Thus, proteolytic enzymes can penetrate through the mucosa, in which the lysosomes have been damaged by ischaemia, and lay it open to bacterial invasion. Prior use of an elemental diet which reduces or abolishes this tryptic activity has been shown[57] to confer some protection against standard ischaemic injury. While at present there is no information on the clinical relevance of these findings, it would seem likely that the mucosal barrier provides the same protection in man as it does in the experimental animal.

The aortoiliac steal syndrome

By a 'steal' is meant redistribution of flow from one vascular bed into another, due to a pressure gradient created by a stenosis between the two respective arteries of supply. The first such syndrome to be described was the 'subclavian steal', in which a block in the subclavian artery creates a head of pressure between the circulations to the brain and the arm, so that blood flows out the circle of Willis, retrogradely down the vertebral artery and so into the subclavian beyond the block. The existence of a similar state of affairs in the mesenteric circulation has been postulated,[58] and the term 'aortoiliac steal' has been used to describe two different sets of circumstances.

With occlusive disease of the aortoiliac segment, ischaemia of the legs may occur in the post-absorption period. This is discussed in Chapter 8.

Of greater interest is the situation whereby the iliofemoral circulation appears to 'steal' blood from the bowel. Kountz, Lamb and Connolly[59] reported a series of patients who died from intestinal infarction following sympathectomy and/or reconstructive aortoiliac surgery. This was particularly likely to occur in patients with occlusive disease of the mesenteric arteries and the authors' view was that it was the result of reflex vasoconstriction in the gut vessels rather than simple mechanical redistribution of blood following the surgery. Experiments on dogs demonstrated that lumbar sympathectomy increased flow and lowered resistance in the legs, but had the opposite effect on the gut. Subsequent authors[60, 61] have suggested that it is the opening up of the vessels in the legs which causes a direct steal of blood.

It is clearly important to know whether restoration of blood supply to the legs by sympathectomy or arterial surgery is likely to infarct the bowel. It may be said that, for a number of reasons, this seems not to be the case. In the first place, small bowel (as opposed to colonic) ischaemia following aortic surgery is very rare, amounting to less than 1 per cent.[62] Secondly, it is well recognized that acute intestinal ischaemia can follow any sort of operation, even haemorrhoidectomy[60] or no operation at all, and many patients undergoing arterial surgery will have the sort of cardiac history which is the normal background to this event. Finally, study of the haemodynamics of steal syndromes in general, and of subclavian steal in particular, has cast considerable doubt on their validity except as angiographic curiosities.[60] Theoretical analysis of the likely consequences of increasing flow in the distal aorta suggests that, given a normal cardiac output, even very large increases would not affect SMA perfusion pressure (and hence mesenteric flow) unless there were gross aortic obstruction above the origins of the mesenteric vessels, as in a coarctation. It has been calculated[63] that quadrupling the flow to the legs would 'steal' about 8 ml per minute from the mesenteric circulation; most arterial operations do little more than double the flow, and then only transiently. However, where cardiac reserve is diminished so that output cannot rise if the peripheral resistance is lowered, and particularly if there is a coexistent stenosis of the SMA, then this may not apply and shutdown may occur.

On the whole, the consensus of evidence suggests that the iliofemoral circulation does not divert blood from the bowel, either during exercise or following operation, unless there is a combination of diminished cardiac output and local abnormality in the mesenteric circulation. It is questionable whether this is fairly described as a 'steal' syndrome.

Mesenteric venous thrombosis

Causation

Mesenteric venous thrombosis accounts for less than 10 per cent of cases of intestinal ischaemia. Current thinking attributes the majority of cases to one of a variety of different pathological states, which includes:[2, 64, 65, 66]

1. *Trauma*: penetrating injuries due to stab or gunshot wounds to the abdomen are being seen with increasing frequency. Operative injuries may result from inexpert attempts at pancreatoduodenal resections or 'radical' right hemicolectomy for cancer of the ascending colon.
2. *Hypercoagulable states*: e.g. antithrombin III deficiency, polycythaemia vera, thrombocytosis, cryofibrinogenaemia.
3. *Portal vein thrombosis* due to any cause.
4. *Low flow states*.
5. *Vasoconstrictor usage*: e.g. vasopressin, pressor agents.
6. *Intra-abdominal sepsis*.
7. *Neoplasms*, especially those involving the mesenteric lymph nodes, or blood dyscrasias.
8. *Mechanical bowel obstruction* by bands, volvulus or adhesions.

Clinical presentation

Mesenteric venous thrombosis tends to be insidious in onset. The duration of symptoms prior to presentation or diagnosis is much longer with venous thrombosis than with arterial occlusion. Vague abdominal pains, distension, change in bowel habit (usually diarrhoea), nausea and mild fever are common. Mild abdominal tenderness, hypoactive bowel sounds and leucocytosis are often present. The features of an acute abdomen appear late. The most common acute presentation is that of cramping epigastric or periumbilical pain with nausea, vomiting and diarrhoea. Physical examination usually reveals generalized tenderness and abdominal distension. Evidence of hypovolaemia may also be present. Signs of peritoneal irritation and shock suggest bowel infarction and carry a very poor prognosis. Leucocytosis and hyperamylasaemia are common.

Diagnosis

Plain x-ray of the abdomen usually shows features of small bowel obstruction with dilated loops and air–fluid levels. Pneumatosis intestinalis is a late finding. The role of angiography is now clearly established in the diagnosis of mesenteric venous thrombosis. Preliminary arteriography excludes mesenteric arterial occlusion which is often suspected because of its more frequent occurrence. The angiographic features of mesenteric venous thrombosis are well described, and include:

1. Reflux of contrast into the aorta.
2. Spasm of the SMA and its branches.
3. Opacification of only a few distal arterial branches.
4. Prolongation of the arterial phase beyond 40 seconds.
5. Non-opacification of the SMV within 40 seconds.

6. Intense opacification of the thickened bowel walls.
7. Visible contrast within the bowel lumen.

While angiography may be of great diagnostic value, it is often time consuming if subtle changes in the mesenteric venous circulation are to be demonstrated, and may delay treatment. It is therefore essential to individualize the need for angiography based on the patient's general condition and on the availability of expert personnel and equipment. The diagnosis is made at laparotomy in many instances.

Treatment

Mesenteric venous thrombosis is a surgical emergency and the need for early operation must be stressed. Intravenous fluids, antibiotics and heparin are given before operation. Patients operated upon within 12 hours of acute presentation have a mortality rate of 25 per cent. If laparotomy is carried out between 25 and 48 hours of acute onset the mortality rate rises to 72 per cent. Withholding surgery is 100 per cent fatal.

The first step in the operation is quickly to exclude arterial occlusion. In patients with mesenteric venous thrombosis, the bowel infarction is often limited and segmental. Thus, short bowel syndrome is less likely to occur than after treatment of arterial occlusion. All infarcted bowel must be resected. Venous thrombectomy of the superior mesenteric vein is essential. The SMV can be approached in three ways from the right side of the root to the mesentery of the small bowel:

1. The right colon is mobilized extensively from right to left until all the right lumbar gutter structures are visualized and the SMV is visualized as it crosses the third part of the duodenum.
2. The lesser peritoneal sac is opened by detaching the greater omentum from the transverse colon and following the middle colic vessels until the middle colic vein dips underneath the neck of the pancreas to join the SMV.
3. Using a very extensive Kocher manoeuvre, the supraduodenal portion of the portal vein can be exposed behind the hepatic artery and the common bile duct, and thrombectomy can be performed through the portal vein using balloon Fogarty catheters.

All these approaches may be necessary in order to ensure adequate venous thrombectomy.

After resection of infarcted bowel, primary anastomosis must not be attempted. Postoperative anticoagulant therapy is essential. Judicious planning of the second-look laparotomy and the timing for the restoration of bowel continuity are also essential for optimum results.

Results

No large series of patients with mesenteric venous thrombosis has been reported. The three causes of high morbidity and mortality are:

1. Failure to remove all non-viable bowel.
2. Anastomotic leak and sepsis.
3. Recurrent thrombosis and infarction.

Unless a correctable hypercoagulable state is identified, it is advisable to keep all patients on long-term anticoagulation.

Acute ischaemia of the colon

Causation

Hindgut ischaemia is a less common clinical problem but is easier to diagnose. The clinical syndromes produced are well delineated and often simulate those of more common non-vascular lesions of the colon, with clear evidence of the site of the lesion and the need for surgical intervention. Acute hindgut ischaemia differs from small bowel ischaemia in that it can most often be treated successfully using well-established general surgical principles without having to resort to a reconstructive arterial procedure.

The commonest cause of IMA occlusion is arteriosclerosis.[67, 68] Some cases follow ligation of the IMA during operations on the distal aorta. There is also a reported association with rheumatoid arthritis, the contraceptive pill and phaeochromocytoma.[68, 69, 70, 71]

The most frequent sites for acute colon ischaemia are at the splenic flexure and the rectosigmoid junction.[68] Anatomical defects in the marginal artery have been described angiographically. Whether these defects are the result of congenital maldevelopment or of occlusion by the arteriosclerotic process is debatable.

The clinical patterns of acute hindgut ischaemia are discussed in Chapter 10. In this chapter we will be concerned exclusively with infarction.

Infarction of the hindgut is about one-tenth as common as small bowel gangrene and presents with severe peripheral circulatory failure, sepsis and obvious clinical features of generalized peritonitis and rectal bleeding. The exact cause of the abdominal catastrophe is often only recognized at laparotomy or at autopsy. It may follow aortic thrombosis, aortic surgery or even aortography. The syndrome has also been reported from the fourth to the fourteenth day following many unrelated non-vascular operations, including haemorrhoidectomy, vagotomy and pyloroplasty, ureteric transplantation and above-knee amputations. It is postulated that an episode of low cardiac output from heart failure is the underlying aetiology even though the main IMA may still be patent. Thus, the equivalent of the non-occlusive bowel ischaemia may be much more common in the colon than is generally recognized. Evidence in support of this is that colon necrosis occurs only in about 1 per cent of cases following ligation of the IMA during resection of abdominal aortic aneurysms. Much, of course, depends on the state of the collateral pathway from the SMA, the internal iliac and the middle colic arteries. In the presence of advanced disease of the SMA and coeliac axis, the IMA becomes the main visceral artery and its ligation may cause ischaemia which extends beyond the distal colon.

Acute necrotizing colitis is now recognized as a complication of colonic obstruction.[55] The increased intraluminal pressure diminishes blood flow through the colon wall even in the absence of major vessel occlusion. Ischaemia confined initially to the mucosa may begin a train of events which allows resident bacteria, especially clostridia, to become lethally invasive. The changes observed at laparotomy have ranged from mucosal necrosis to frank gangrene of the colon proximal to the obstructing lesion. Gram stains of resected colon have demonstrated Gram-positive bacilli invading the mucosa and submucosa[55] (see also Chapter 6).

Treatment

The initial management of colonic gangrene consists of fluid resuscitation, intravenous antibiotics and nasogastric suction. Other supportive measures for any underlying cardiac condition are usually needed. Vasoconstrictor drugs are contraindicated and heparin should not be given because it will increase the risk of haemorrhage. Some authorities advocate the use of low molecular weight dextran to promote small vessel flow in marginally ischaemic areas.

Arterial reconstruction has nothing to offer in the management of colonic ischaemia. In the emergency situation, resection of all the gangrenous colon is essential with construction of an end-colostomy and a mucous fistula or a Hartmann's procedure. Resection must be wide of the involved area, and adequate bleeding from the cut bowel ends must be confirmed. Primary anastomosis is mentioned to be condemned. A temporary proximal colostomy leaving the ischaemic colon behind is also contraindicated.

Course and prognosis

The severe cases of colon necrosis have a high mortality, and usually die from circulatory failure and sepsis. The ultimate survival depends on the status of the patient's underlying cardiovascular disease.

References

1. Ottinger, L.W. Nonocclusive mesenteric infarction. *Surg. Clin. North Am.* (1974) **54**: 689–98.
2. Boley, S.J., Lawrence, L.J., Veith, F.J. Ischemic disorders of the intestine. *Curr. Probl. Surg.* (1978) **15**: 6–80.
3. Stoney, R.J., Olcott, C. Visercal artery syndromes. *Surg. Clin. North Am.* (1979) **59**: 637–47.
4. Jamieson, W.G., Marchuk, S., Rowson, J., Durand, J. The early diagnosis of massive acute intestinal ischaemia. *Br. J. Surg.* (1982) **69**: Suppl. S52–S53.
5. Goldgraber, M.B., Kirsner,B. The Arthus phenomenon in the colon of rabbits. *Arch. Path.* (1959) **67**: 566–71.
6. Baue, A.E., Austen, G.W. Superior mesenteric artery embolism. *Surg. Gynecol. Obst.* (1963) **116**: 474–7.
7. Kairalvoma, M.I., Karkola, P., Heikinnen, E., et al. Mesenteric infarction. *Am. J. Surg.* (1977) **133**: 188–93.
8. Bergan, J.J., Yao, J.S. Acute intestinal ischemia. In: Rutherford, P., ed. *Vascular Surgery* 2nd ed. Philadelphia: W.B. Saunders (1981) 948–63.
9. Johnson, C.C., Baggenstoss, A.H. Mesenteric

vascular occlusion. *Proc. Mayo Clin.* (1949) **24**: 649–53.

10. Bigot, J.M., Monnier, J.P., Chermet, J., Kieny, R., Cinqualbre, J., Tongio, J. Les ischémies mesenteriques aigues. *Ann. Radiol.* (1976) **19**: 377–85.
11. Mackenzie, R.L., Provan, J.L. Recognition and management of embolism to the superior mesenteric artery. *Can. Med. Ass. J.* (1974) **111**: 1207–10.
12. Frimann-Dahl, J. *Roentgen Examinations in Acute Abdominal Disease*, 2nd edn. Oxford: Blackwell (1960) 324–8.
13. Vyden, J.K. The systemic effects of acute superior mesenteric vascular insufficiency. In: Boley, S.J., ed. *Vascular Diseases of the Intestine.* New York, London: Appleton-Century-Crofts (1972) 279–94.
14. Kazmers, A. Zwolak, R., Azselman, H.D., et al. Pharmacologic interventions in acute ischemia: improved survival with intravenous glucagon, methylprednisolone and prostacyclin. *J. Vasc. Surg.* (1984) **1**: 472.
15. Britt, L.G., Cheek, R.C. Nonocclusive mesenteric vascular disease. *Ann. Surg.* (1969) **169**: 704–11.
16. Sasser, C., Farringer, J.L., Pickens, D.R. Successful mesenteric arterial embolectomy. *Am. Surg.* (1971) **37**: 86–92.
17. Schoofs, E., Vereecken, L., Derom, F. Acute occlusive van der arteria mesenterica superior. *Acta Chir. Belg.* (1975) **74**: 86–92.
18. O'Donnell, J.A., Hobson, R.W. Operative confirmation of Doppler ultrasound evaluation of intestinal ischemia. *Surgery* (1980) **87**: 109–12.
19. Editorial. Ketone body ratio — an index of multiple organ failure? *Lancet* (1984) **1**: 25.
20. Joske, R.A., Shamma'a, M.H., Drummey, G.D. Intestinal malabsorption following temporary occlusion of the superior mesenteric artery. *Am. J. Med.* (1958) **25**: 449–57.
21. Bergan, J.J., Dean, R.H., Conn, J., et al. Revascularization in the treatment of mesenteric infarction. *Ann. Surg.* (1975) **182**: 430–4.
22. Krauz, M.M., Many, J. Acute superior mesenteric arterial occlusion — a plea for early diagnosis. *Surgery* (1978) **83**: 482.
23. Marston, A., Szilagyi, D.E., Kieny, R., Taylor, G.W. Intestinal ischemia. *Arch. Surg.* (1976) **111**: 107–12.
24. Dunphy, J.E. Abdominal pain of vascular origin. *Am. J. Med. Sci.* (1936) **192**: 109–12.
25. Kieny, R., Cinqualbre, J., Pinke, R., Jeanblanc, B. *Chirurgie des Lesions Atheromateuses des Artères Digestifs.* Paris: Expansion Scientifique (1974) 141–8.
26. Brittain, R.S., Early, T.K. Emergency thromboendarterectomy of the superior mesenteric artery. *Ann. Surg.* (1963) **158**: 138–43.
27. Bhagwat, A.G., Hawk, W.A. Terminal hemorrhagic necrosis enteropathy (THNE). *Am. J. Gastroenterol.* (1966) **45**: 163–88.
28. Brawley, R.K., Roberts, W.G., Morrow, A.G. Intestinal infarction resulting from nonobstructive mesenteric arterial insufficiency. *Arch. Surg.* (1966) **92**: 375–8.
29. Drucker, W.R, Davis, J.H., Holden, W.D., Regan, J.R. Hemorrhagic necrosis of the intestine. *Arch. Surg.* (1964) **89**: 42–53.
30. Frengley, J.D., Reid, J.D. Nonspecific enteritis resulting from mesenteric vascular insufficiency. *N.Z. Med. J.* (1964) **63**: 212–18.
31. Heer, F.W., Silen, W., French, S.W. Intestinal gangrene without apparent vascular occlusion. *Am. J. Surg.* (1963) **110**: 231–8.
32. McGovern, V.J., Goulstone, S.G.M. Ischaemic enterocolotis. *Gut* (1965) **6**: 213–20.
33. Prandi, D., Degott, C., Molas, G., Lortat-Jacob, I.-L. Entérites et colites ischémiques aigües postopératoires. *Arch. Franc. Mal. App. Dig.* (1975) **64**: 209–14.
34. Berger, R.L., Byrne, J.J. Intestinal gangrene associated with heart disease. *Surg. Gynecol. Obst.* (1961) **112**: 529–35.
35. Ende, N.P. Infarction of the bowel in cardiac failure. *New Engl. J. Med.* (1959) **260**: 258–61.
36. Grosh, J.L., Mann, R.H., O'Donnell, W.M. Nonthrombotic intestinal infarction in heart disease. *Am. J. Med. Sci.* (1965) **250**: 613–20.
37. Kligerman, M.J., Vidone, R.A. Intestinal infarction in the absence of occlusive mesenteric vascular disease. *Am. J. Cardiol.* (1965) **16**: 562–70.
38. Renton, C.J.C. Non-occlusive intestinal infarction. *Clin. Gastroenterol.* (1972) **1**: 655–71.
39. Irving, D.W., Corday, E. Effects of cardiac arrhythmias on the renal and mesenteric circulation. *Am. J. Cardiol.* (1961) **8**: 32.
40. Fogarty, T.J., Fletcher, W.S. Genesis of nonocclusive mesenteric ischemia. *Am. J. Surg.* (1966) **111**: 130–37.
41. Polansky, B.J., Berger, R.L., Byrne, J.J. Massive nonocclusive intestinal infarction associated with digitalis toxicity. *Circulation* (1964) **30**: suppl. 141–5.
42. Sharefkin, J.B., Silen ,W. Diuretic agents inciting factors in nonocclusive mesenteric infarction? *J.A.M.A.* (1974) **229**: 1451–3.
43. MacGregor, A.M.C., Abney, H.T., Morris, L. Pharmacodynamic response in nonocclusive mesenteric ischemia. *Am. Surg.* (1974) **40**: 381–3.
44. Orr, T.G., Lorhan, P.H., Kaul, P.G. Mesenteric vascular occlusion. *J.A.M.A.* (1954) **155**: 648–51.

45. Liavåg, I. Acute mesenteric vascular insufficiency. *Acta Chir. Scand.* (1967) **133**: 631–9.

46. Boley, S.J., Sprayregan, S., Siegelman, S.S. et al. Initial results from an aggressive rontgenologic and surgical approach to acute mesenteric ischemia. *Surgery* (1977) **82**: 848–55.

47. Wiggers, C.J. Splanchnic pooling in hemorrhagic shock. *J. Exp. Med. Surg.* (1943) **1**: 2–10.

48. Fine, J. The role of the intestine in traumatic shock. *Am. J. Gastroenterol.* (1958) **29**: 596–7.

49. Marston, A. The bowel in shock. *Lancet* (1962) **2**: 365–70.

50. Carey, C.S., Okada, F., Monson, D.O., Yao, S.T., Shoemaker, W.C. Intestinal infarction in shock with survival after resection. *J.A.M.A.* (1967) **199**: 422–5.

51. Haglund, U., Hulten, L., Asken, C., Lundgren, O. Mucosal lesions in the human small intestine in shock. *Gut* (1976) **16**: 979–84.

52. Whitehead, R. Ischaemic enterocolitis, an expression of the intravascular coagulation syndrome. *Gut* (1971) **12**: 912–17.

53. Berry, C.L., Frazer, G.C. The experimental production of colitis in the rabbit with particular reference to Hirschsprung's disease. *J. Pediatr. Surg.* (1968) **3**: 36–42.

54. Perloff, L.J., Chou, H., Petrella, E.J., Grossman, R.A., Barker, C.F. Acute colitis in the renal allograft recipient. *Ann. Surg.* (1976) **183**: 77–83.

55. Teasdale, C., Mortensen, N.J. McC. Acute necrotizing colitis and obstruction. *Br. J. Surg.* (1983) **70**: 44–7.

56. Anthony, P.P., Drury, R.A.B. Elastic vascular sclerosis of mesenteric blood vessels in argentaffin carcinoma. *J. Clin. Pathol.* (1970) **23**: 110–18.

57. Bounous, G. Tryptic enteritis, its role in the pathogenesis of stress ulcer and shock. *Can. J. Surg.* (1969) **12**: 397–402.

58. Harris, P.L., Charlesworth, D. Chronic intestinal ischaemia due to aorto-iliac steal. *J. Cardiovasc. Surg.* (1974) **15**: 122–4.

59. Kountz, S.L., Lamb, D.R., Connolly, J.E. Aorto-iliac steal syndrome. *Arch. Surg.* (1966) **92**: 490–94.

60. Connolly, J.E., Stemmer, E.A. Intestinal gangrene as the result of mesenteric arterial steal. *Am. J. Surg.* (1973) **126**: 197–204.

61. Williams, L.F., Kim, R.M., Tompkins, W., Byrne, J.J. Aorto-iliac steal — a cause of intestinal ischemia. *N. Engl. J. Med.* (1968) **278**: 777–8.

62. Johnson, W.C., Nabseth, D.C. Visceral infarction following aortic surgery. *Ann. Surg.* (1974) **180**: 312–18.

63. Strandness, D.E., Sumner, D.S. (editors) Aorto-iliac steal. In: *Hemodynamics for Surgeons*. New York: Grune and Stratton (1975) 376–80.

64. Berry, F.B., Bougas, J.A. Agnogenic venous infarction. *Ann. Surg.* (1950) **132**: 450–54.

65. Cuschieri, A., Brearley, R., Bradley, J., Moossa, A.R. Recurrent venous thrombosis and portal hypertension. *N. Engl. J. Med.* (1972) **287**: 1083–5.

66. Vanway, C.W., Brockman, S.K., Rosenfeld, L. Spontaneous thrombosis of the mesenteric veins. *Ann. Surg.* (1971) **173**: 561.

67. Demos, N.J., Bahuth, J.J., Urnes, P.D. Comparative study of arteriosclerosis in the inferior and superior mesenteric arteries. *Ann. Surg.* (1962) **155**: 599–605.

68. Marston, A., Pheils, M.T., Thomas, M.L., Morson, B.C. Ischaemic colitis. *Gut* (1966) **7**: 1–11.

69. Cotton, P.B., Thomas, M.L. Ischaemic colitis and the contraceptive pill. *Br. Med. J.* (1971) **3**: 27–9.

70. Marcuson, R.W., Farman, J.A. Ischaemic disease of the colon. *Proc. R. Soc. Med.* (1971) **64**: 1080–83.

71. Rosati, L.A., Augur, N.A. Ischaemic enterocolitis in pheochromocytoma. *Gastroenterology* (1971) **60**: 581–3.

6

Pseudomembranous colitis

M. R. B. Keighley
D. W. Burdon

Pseudomembranous colitis (PMC) is a disease of the colon and rectum characterized by the formation of elevated yellowish-white mucosal plaques. The dominant clinical feature of the disease is diarrhoea ranging in severity from occasional soft stools to frequent and incapacitating watery motions. Nearly all cases are related to antibiotic therapy, especially with lincomycin, clindamycin, ampicillin and the cephalosporins. There is now substantial evidence that PMC is caused by toxin elaborated by *Clostridium difficile.* The condition may be spread by patients who are excreting the organism, particularly if they are nursed on an open ward. Diagnosis is usually by detection of faecal toxin or by biopsy of a plaque during sigmoidoscopy. Death is now uncommon in diagnosed patients who receive appropriate therapy, but the disorder is still identified in unsuspected cases at post-mortem examination. Treatment with oral vancomycin or metronidazole is effective but metronidazole may also be given by intravenous infusion in patients who cannot take oral therapy. Relapse is seen in 10–20 per cent of patients despite a favourable clinical response to initial therapy.

Definitions

Originally PMC was regarded as a histopathological diagnosis and few cases were recognized before death. Many early cases were recorded after surgical procedures, particularly following operation for obstructing carcinoma.[1] The disorder was reported before antibiotics came into use, and the principal predisposing factors were thought to be obstruction and ischaemia.[2] These may still play a part, although their importance is now less certain. The toxin of *C. difficile* is occasionally recovered in patients with diarrhoea who have not received an antibiotic.[3]

Improved diagnostic methods based on detection of *C. difficile* toxin have revealed a wider spectrum of pathology than PMC. Illness caused by *C. difficile* now appears to include diarrhoea in patients who do not have pseudomembranes and in whom non-specific inflammatory change may or may not be found in the colonic and rectal mucosa. In a prospective colonoscopy study, absence of rectal disease was documented in 23 per cent of patients with *C. difficile* colitis.[4] Suitable nomenclature for the disease in such patients might be antibiotic-associated *C. difficile* colitis or diarrhoea, respectively. However, it is impossible to distinguish between these two manifestations with confidence without a complete colonoscopic examination. Consequently, it is difficult to arrive at an appropriate diagnostic label which covers all patients with diarrhoea and *C. difficile* toxin in their faeces. The distinction is of little importance if one allows that a natural progression and regression between diarrhoea, colitis and pseudomembrane formation may occur. It is, however, essential to assess the degree of involvement before deciding whether specific therapy should be started. For convenience, the full spectrum of disease associated with *C. difficile* toxin is considered here under the single but possibly misleading heading of PMC.

Aetiology

An animal model of PMC

The occurrence of colitis as a complication of antibiotic administration has long been recognized in several animal species. When a single dose of lincomycin or of clindamycin is given to hamsters, a caecitis with watery diarrhoea is induced followed by death in 3–5 days. The affected caecum is distended, and shows haemorrhages on the mucosal and serosal surfaces. The terminal ileum and ascending colon may also be involved. Vancomycin protects hamsters against clindamycin-induced caecitis but the caecitis recurs once the vancomycin is stopped.[5] Similar results were obtained by Bartlett, Onderdonk and Cisneros[6] with vancomycin and bacitracin, but they found that if vancomycin was given for 3 days before the clindamycin challenge, all animals survived. It was subsequently observed that the disease could be transferred to healthy hamsters by the intracaecal injection of either caecal fluid or bacteria-free filtrates of such fluid from clindamycin-treated hamsters.[7] Similarly, caecitis could be induced by intracaecal injection of a certain clostridicum or by germ-free filtrates from the organism, which had been isolated from the caeca of clindamycin-treated hamsters and which was later identified as *C. difficile*. These data established that clindamycin induced caecitis in hamsters was caused by a clostridial toxin. It was then shown that although the organism producing the toxin was *C. difficile* it could be neutralized by *C. sordellii* antitoxin.[8] The neutralization of *C. difficile* toxin by *C. sordellii* antitoxin is the result of an antigenic similarity between the toxins of the two clostridia, and has prompted enquiries into the pathogenicity of *C. sordellii*. Although it has been isolated from hamsters with caecitis, *C. difficile* was also present in these animals[9] and pure isolates of *C. sordellii* did not cause caecitis when injected into hamsters. Allo[10] has, however, recovered four isolates of *C. sordellii* from experimentally obstructed intestinal loops in dogs and shown that three of these cause diarrhoea and two cause caecitis in hamsters.

Role of *C. difficile* in human disease

The discovery of a cytotoxin in the faeces of patients with PMC provided the first clue that human colitis had a bacterial cause.[11] Shortly afterwards, it was reported that this cytotoxin could be neutralized by *C. sordelli* antitoxin,[12, 13] thus supporting the validity of the hamster model of PMC. Finally, *C. difficile* was isolated from the faeces of patients with PMC and it was demonstrated that the isolates produced a toxin *in vitro* which had the same cytotoxic characteristics as faeces, including neutralization by *C. sordellii* antitoxin.[14, 15] In patients treated with vancomycin or metronidazole, disappearance of clostridia and faecal cytotoxin coincided with clinical improvement,[16, 17] strengthening the association between disease and the presence of *C. difficile*.

Pathogenesis

Relationship to antibiotic therapy

PMC was first described in the nineteenth century, and a number of factors such as gastrointestinal operations, intestinal ischaemia, heavy metal poisoning, salmonella infection, leukaemia and uraemia have been associated with its pathogenesis. Involvement of the small bowel, stomach and even the oesophagus is recorded in some cases. This widespread form of the disease was attributed to staphylococcal enterotoxin. Staphylococcal enterocolitis was frequent in the 1950s and 1960s, and was commonly associated with gastrointestinal surgery and with treatment by antibiotics, particularly tetracycline. PMC caused by *C. difficile* differs from many of these earlier cases, being confined to the colon and rectum. It is almost invariably associated with antibiotic therapy[18] although a few cases have been reported in which antibiotics have not been used.[3, 19, 20] PMC occasionally occurs in patients receiving cytotoxic drugs.[21] The antibiotics most often linked with PMC are lincomycin and clindamycin[22, 23] but ampicillin and the cephalosporins are also implicated. Most other antibiotics have been incriminated, the only important factor being a concentration of antibiotic within the gut which is high enough to alter the bacterial flora. It is likely that oral therapy carries a greater risk than does parenteral administration of antibiotics, and this is certainly true for the combination of an aminoglycoside with metronidazole used in prophylaxis for colorectal surgery.[24] However, there is growing evidence that even a single dose of systemic antimicrobial therapy may be associated with the emergence of *C. difficile*.

Changes in intestinal flora associated with PMC

The mechanism by which antibiotics precipitate colitis is not established but it is thought to involve reduction in the number of certain components of the intestinal flora which normally suppress the growth of *C. difficile*. An alternative hypothesis is that *C. difficile* can only be detected in faeces when the normal flora is suppressed. Whatever the mechanism may be, it remains operative for long periods, since colitis may develop as much as 3 weeks after the predisposing antibiotics have been withdrawn. The changes in intestinal flora which permit overgrowth of *C. difficile* have not been identified. In clindamycin-treated hamsters, the total aerobic count was unchanged, any increase in *Escherichia coli* and enterococci being compensated by a decrease in corynebacteria. The anaerobic flora showed a marked decrease in streptococci, a moderate decrease in *Bacteroides* species, and no change in the number of clostridia.[9] Although similar changes are seen in some patients with PMC, there is no uniform pattern of altered bowel flora.[25]

Influence of a single dose of antibiotic on emergence of *C. difficile*

There is now increasing evidence that even short-term antimicrobial exposure, as used for prophylaxis in intestinal surgery, can be followed by *C. difficile* colitis. Studies in our hospital brought to light 5 cases which occurred after 24-hour cover with lincomycin[26] and 6 patients who developed PMC after only two doses of prophylactic cefoxitin.[27] Morris et al.[28] have reported 3 more cases in 109 patients receiving a single 2 g dose of latamoxef. Such clinical observations prompted a study of the influence of single-dose systemic antimicrobials on the changes in faecal flora and the emergence of *C. difficile* (Table 6.1). We were unable to demonstrate any specific changes in faecal flora except in one group receiving cefotetan where there was a dramatic reduction in both the aerobic and anaerobic bacterial counts.[29] The most marked changes in bacterial flora were amongst patients receiving broad-spectrum third-generation cephalosporins, particularly those which were excreted in high concentrations in the bile. *C. difficile* was not recovered after cephaloridine or any of the penicillins, but was observed with all other cephalosporins, and was particularly common with those agents which had the greatest influence on faecal flora, such as cefoxitin, cefotaxime, cefotetan and latamoxef. Furthermore, at least half of the subjects who developed *C. difficile* had associated diarrhoea, indicating that this was more than a laboratory finding and represented a potentially important clinical observation.

Source of *C. difficile* and cross-infection

C. difficile is known to be present in the faeces of about 40 per cent of newborn infants,[30, 31, 32] which

Table 6.1 Influence of single-dose systemic antibiotic administration on emergence of *C. difficile*

Number studied	Antibiotic	Number who excreted *C. difficile*	Number with toxin
6	No antibiotic	0	0
6	Benzylpenicillin	0	0
6	Ampicillin	0	0
6	Piperacillin	0	0
6	Mezlocillin	0	0
6	Ticarcillin	0	0
6	Cephaloridine	0	0
6	Cephazolin	1	0
6	Cefuroxime	1	0
6	Cefotaxime	2	1
6	Cefoxitin	2	1
6	Latamoxef	3	1
6	Ceftriaxone	2	0
6	Cefotetan	4	2

suggests that it is acquired from the mother and is a part of the normal adult flora. However, culture of adult faeces is generally negative and *C. difficile* was found in only 4 of 137 patients whose faecal flora was studied in detail.[33] It seems, therefore, that if *C. difficile* is a normal inhabitant, it must be present in very low numbers.

An alternative view to the concept of overgrowth by a normal intestinal commensal is that PMC is the result of an acquired exogenous infection. Experimental support for this idea has been obtained in a study of hamsters which remained well unless they were exposed to *C. difficile* when given clindamycin in protected environments.[34] Cross-infection is implicated by the observation that PMC occurs in clusters, often in circumstances where there have been no previously recorded cases and in which the usage of antibiotics has not changed.

Patients may continue to excrete *C. difficile* for some weeks after exposure to antimicrobials and after the clinical symptoms of PMC have disappeared. These asymptomatic carriers of *C. difficile* may therefore be a threat to a hospital community. We have observed an outbreak of PMC following the readmission of an unsuspected carrier requiring closure of colostomy 6–8 weeks after a bowel resection which was originally complicated by *C. difficile* colitis.

The possibility that *C. difficile* colitis could be a transmissible infection was investigated in our unit by examining stool cultures from ward staff and patients. No evidence of *C. difficile* carriage was found in the staff but 3 of 53 asymptomatic patients had *C. difficile*. While our own unit was closed for cleaning, 5 new cases of colitis were recorded elsewhere in the hospital within 1 month, but typing of the clostridia revealed that these were different from strains previously isolated. Within a few weeks of reopening the unit there were new cases of colitis caused by the same strain which had previously been associated with that unit. No known carriers had been readmitted, and it seems clear that the organism had survived in the ward environment and had reinfected the patients. This would be consistent with other observations regarding contamination of the environment,[35] and the ability of clostridial spores to remain viable for long periods. As a result of sterilizing the sigmoidoscopes and treating all asymptomatic carriers by elimination of *C. difficile* from the stool, the frequency of *C. difficile* colitis was greatly reduced in our unit and the epidemic strain eventually disappeared (Fig. 6.1).

As well as the evidence of case clustering in our own unit and that described by Greenfield,[36] Rogers et al.[37] reported an outbreak of *C. difficile* from a paediatric unit where children who received oral antimicrobials were found to excrete the organism. Cross-infection occurred from contamination of the bedpan washing machine, from which *C. difficile* was isolated.

On account of the evidence for cross-infection, many physicians now advise that patients with *C. difficile* colitis should be barrier nursed. Environmental contamination occurs rapidly,[38] especially if there is faecal incontinence or a stoma, and *C. difficile* has also been isolated from the hands.

C. difficile Toxins

C. difficile produces several soluble extracellular antigenic substances, of which two are known to be

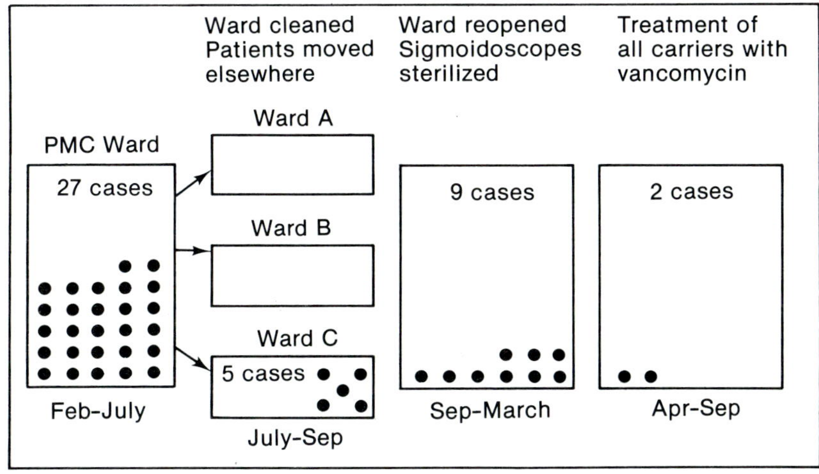

Fig. 6.1 Epidemiological study at the General Hospital, Birmingham.

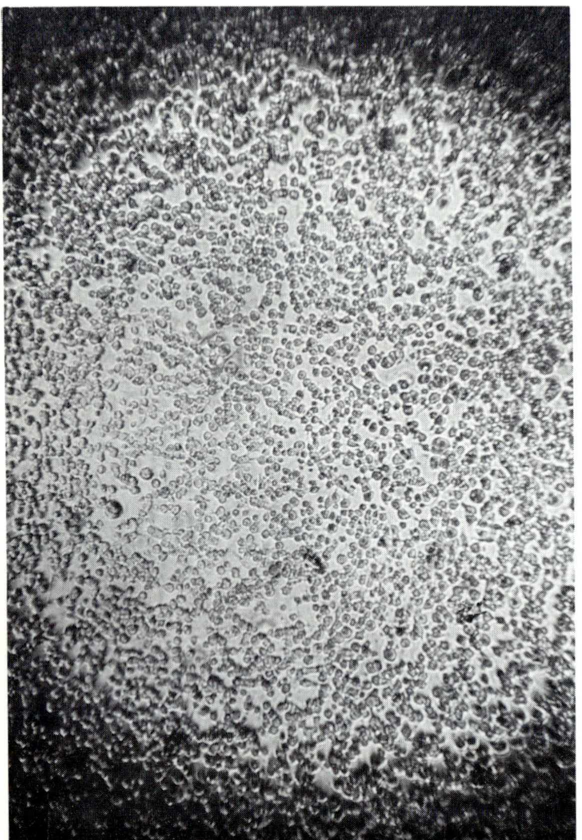

Fig. 6.2 Cytopathic effect of *C. difficile* cytotoxin on HeLa cells. The monolayer of confluent irregularly shaped cells has separated to form discrete rounded cells.

toxins. The cytotoxin now renamed toxin B was discovered in the faeces of patients with PMC by Larson et al.[11] Toxin B is recognized by the cytopathic effect which it produces on tissue culture cell lines such as HeLa and human embryonic lung fibroblast cells, the individual cells becoming rounded and separated from one another (Fig. 6.2).

Toxin B is present in the bacterial cytoplasm and is released upon cell lysis.[39] Activity is destroyed by proteolytic enzymes and by heating at 56°C for 30 minutes.[13] Estimates of the molecular weight of toxin B range from 240 000 to 600 000.[39, 40, 41] Partial purification of crude toxin preparations resulted in the separation of a protein fraction with enterotoxic properties distinct from the cytotoxin.[42, 43] This toxin, named toxin A, produces a pronounced haemorrhagic dilation in the rabbit ileal loop test and, in comparison with toxin B, is only weakly cytotoxic. Toxin B gives a negative response in the ileal loop test, and when injected into the hamster caecum causes only minor inflammatory changes. Immunization against both toxins is necessary to protect hamsters against fatal caecitis, and immunization against either toxin A or toxin B alone does not protect them.[44]

Relationship to underlying disorders

No clear relationship has emerged between the occurrence of PMC and any underlying disease. It has been suggested that the disease is more common after operations for carcinoma of the colon than after other gastrointestinal operations,[1] but this report did not take into account the different antibiotics used. Table 6.2 shows our data[18] in which the incidence of PMC is related to the use of antibiotics. The difference between the operative groups is not significant when only patients given antibiotic are compared. In a review of 66 cases of PMC of which 85 per cent were in surgical patients there was a predominance of patients with disease of the large bowel (Table 6.3), a third of the patients having a carcinoma.[45] This association is probably coincidental and reflects the surgical interest of our unit, in which an outbreak of PMC was occurring amongst patients, most of whom received antibiotic prophylaxis.

Table 6.2 Postoperative pseudomembranous colitis and antibiotic therapy (General Hospital, Birmingham)

Operations		Patients given antibiotic	Patients with PMC	Percentage incidence of PMC in patients given antibiotics
Biliary	72	12 (17%)	1 (1.4%)	8.3
Gastric	70	24 (34%)	1 (1.4%)	4.2
Colorectal	81	74 (91%)	9 (11%)	12.2
Others	18	9 (50%)	0	
Total	241	119 (49.4%)	11 (4%)	9.2

Table 6.3 Underlying gastrointestinal disease in a group of 66 patients with PMC (General Hospital Birmingham)

Large bowel:	
Carcinoma of colon	10
Carcinoma of rectum	12
Diverticular disease	5
Other large bowel disorders	10
Small bowel:	
Acute small bowel obstruction	5
Crohn's disease	1
Gastric	4
Biliary	5
Miscellaneous (non-gastrointestinal)	14

PMC was also seen in a group of compromised non-surgical cases. The underlying disorders included leukaemia, drug addiction, chronic respiratory disease and collagen disorders.

Incidence

It is difficult to provide an accurate assessment of the incidence of PMC, since this depends upon the diligence with which it is sought. Many cases of diarrhoea are not thoroughly investigated by sigmoidoscopy, colonoscopy or faecal cultures. Not only is observer awareness an important factor, but also there are probably local factors which influence the frequency of diagnosis. Moreover, there is marked fluctuation in the frequency of cases, even within a single institution (Fig. 6.3). A high population of patients at risk will undoubtedly bias the reported incidence. In our own unit, we have a large number of patients with colorectal cancer and other disorders of the large bowel, many of whom are elderly and have received therapeutic or prophylactic antibiotics. There has also been some evidence of cross-infection in the past. The incidence is also high within orthopaedic units, particularly in elderly patients requiring emergency admissions for fractures who receive prolonged antimicrobial therapy.

In order to try to determine the incidence of *C. difficile* colitis in our own unit a prospective survey was undertaken on all patients admitted from 1 September 1977 to 28 April 1978. Every patient with diarrhoea, defined as more than three stools a day, or a colostomy output greater than 1 litre per 24 hours, was studied for evidence of *C. difficile* colitis. Of the 241 patients admitted for major intestinal operations, 119 (49.4 per cent) had received antibiotics and 58 (24 per cent) had diarrhoea. Of the group with diarrhoea, 9 had *C. difficile* toxins. This represents a 3.7 per cent incidence of PMC in patients undergoing gastrointestinal operations. These data were, however, collected during an outbreak caused by a single epidemic strain of *C. difficile*. Following eradication of this strain from our hospital the incidence and severity of *C. difficile*-associated illness were substantially reduced for a period of 4 years. Recently the severe form of colitis reappeared in an outbreak lasting 2 months. There were 15 cases of colitis, of which 7 occurred on orthopaedic wards and 4 elderly patients died.

Relationship to inflammatory bowel disease

It has been suggested that *C. difficile* toxin may be a cause of relapse in patients with inflammatory bowel disease. LaMont and Trnka[46] reported 6

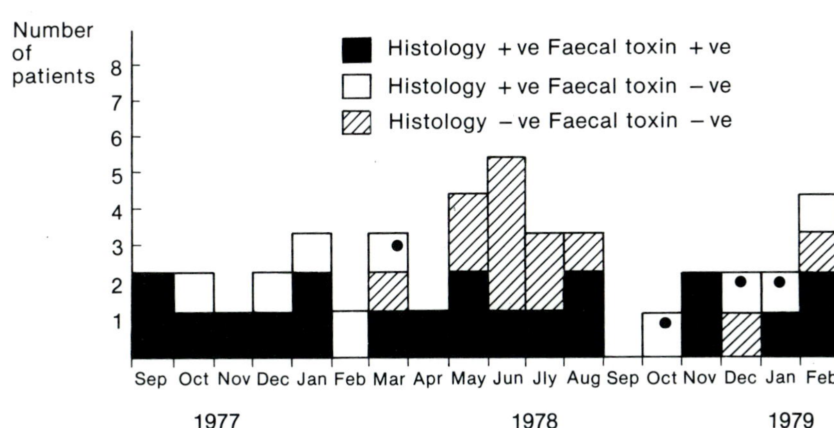

Fig. 6.3 Fluctuation in the appearance of cases in the General Hospital, Birmingham, between September 1977 and February 1979.

patients with symptomatic relapse of inflammatory bowel disease (5 ulcerative colitis and 1 Crohn's disease) associated with *C. difficile* toxin. All of them improved when the toxin disappeared spontaneously (1 case) or following treatment with vancomycin (5 cases). Only 2 of the patients had had an antibiotic recently and none had a pseudomembrane on sigmoidoscopy. It was suggested, therefore, that *C. difficile* toxin might be responsible for relapse of inflammatory bowel disease. Similar findings were observed by Bolton, Sherrif and Read,[47] where clearance of toxin in 5 patients with inflammatory bowel disease in relapse was associated with clinical improvement. Trnka and LaMont[48] subsequently reported that *C. difficile* toxin was present in 9 of 15 patients with severe disease compared with none of the 25 patients with mild disease. Lishmann, Al-Jumaili and Record[49] could not confirm these findings in any of their 28 patients with ulcerative colitis or the 8 with Crohn's disease.

Greenfield and others[50] also found that the incidence of *C. difficile* or its toxin was no higher in patients with ulcerative colitis (13 per cent) or Crohn's disease (14 per cent) than in patients with non-specific diarrhoea (12 per cent). The incidence of *C. difficile* or its toxin was similar in patients in remission (14 per cent) and those in relapse (13 per cent) but it was higher in patients who had recently been exposed to antibiotics. *C. difficile* was not therefore regarded as being responsible for relapse but as a complication of recent exposure to antibiotics.[51] Our own studies support this view:[52] only 4 of 69 patients with inflammatory bowel disease had evidence of *C. difficile* toxin and all had recently received antibiotics. Of the 10 patients with *C. difficile* alone, 2 had recently received antibiotic cover for an operation, 5 were receiving sulphasalazine and 3 had not been recently exposed to antibiotics. Where *C. difficile* was found without toxin, spontaneous disappearance of the organism was observed. In our experience, therefore, *C. difficile* alone is of no pathological significance in inflammatory bowel disease, and its presence is probably merely a reflection of an abnormal intestinal microflora enhancing detection in such subjects. *C. difficile* toxin, on the other hand, does not seem to be related to relapse or disease activity and is usually a complication of antimicrobial therapy. It is unlikely from this evidence that patients with inflammatory bowel disease are more susceptible to PMC than are other individuals.

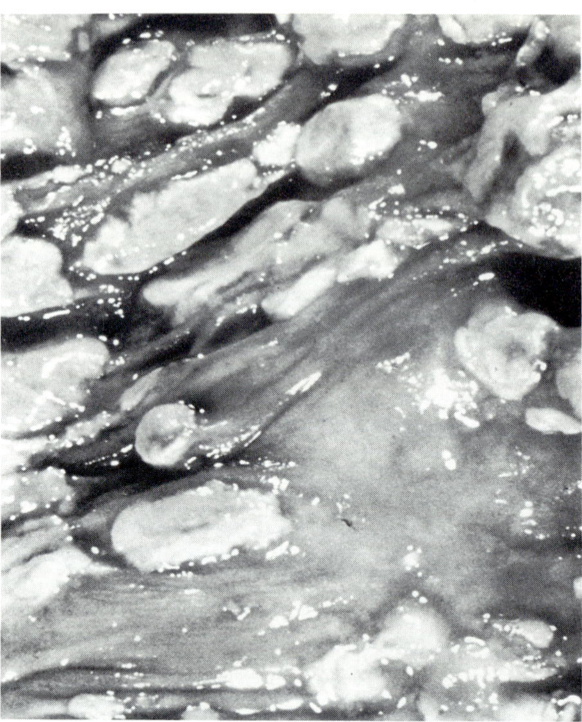

Fig. 6.4 Macroscopic appearances of PMC at post-mortem. Similar lesions can be seen on the rectal mucosa by sigmoidoscopy.

Macroscopic appearances

The typical macroscopic features of the disease are shown in Fig. 6.4. Characteristically there are plaques of white pseudomembrane measuring 2–5 mm in diameter which are multiple, raised and adherent with intervening mucosa which looks relatively normal. The bowel wall is not thickened but occasionally the condition may be associated with toxic dilatation, although free perforation seems to be rare.[53, 54]

There is rarely any evidence of underlying colitis or proctitis. The extent of the disease is variable, with 77 per cent of cases involving the rectal mucosa, and it is unusual for the changes to be present in the right side of the colon alone.[4]

Histology

A biopsy should be taken during sigmoidoscopy or colonoscopy from every patient with suspected

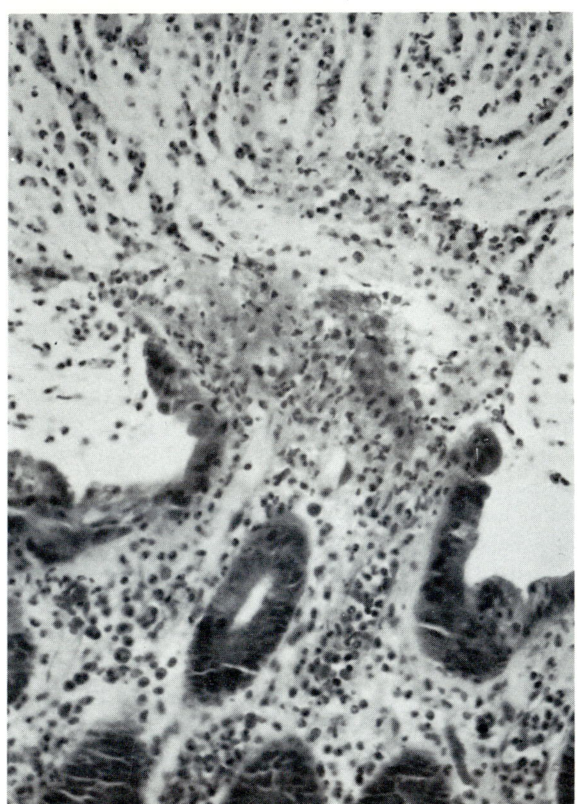

Fig. 6.5 Histological section of an early lesion. The interglandular epithelium and lamina propria are infiltrated by inflammatory cells, and the lesion is capped by a spray of fibrin, polymorphs and epithelial debris.

PMC, preferably from the junction between the normal mucosa and plaque but otherwise from an area of inflammation (Fig. 6.5). Biopsies from patients without macroscopically visible pseudomembrane may reveal characteristic microscopic lesions. The histological criteria of PMC and a scheme for grading the lesions have been described by Price and Davies.[55] It may be difficult, however, to distinguish PMC histologically from ischaemic colitis. The principal diagnostic feature is polymorphs, streaming out from the lamina propria, forming a surface membrane. Other non-specific findings are inflammatory change, disruption of glands distended with mucus and polymorph infiltration of the submucosa. The membrane is formed by fibrin, mucus, polymorphs and epithelial debris. Frozen sections are a reliable alternative to conventional paraffin sections and can provide a rapid diagnosis in patients without visible mucosal plaques.[56]

Clinical features

The clinical features of PMC have been described by Tedesco,[57] Bartlett and Gorbach,[58] Kappas et al.[25] and Mogg et al.[45] The principal symptom is watery diarrhoea which is associated with an intermittent low grade fever in 60 per cent of patients. A few patients have colicky abdominal pain, and in the most severe cases this may simulate an acute abdominal emergency. Toxic megacolon is rare. The stool often contains excess mucus but pus or blood were not found in any of our series of 66 patients. Bloody diarrhoea has been reported, but seems to be uncommon. Nausea and vomiting accompany the diarrhoea in a few cases.

The duration of symptoms in untested patients may be as short as 48 hours or as long as 50 days, but in the majority resolution of symptoms is complete within 10–14 days of stopping antibiotics.[57] Symptoms may begin as early as the second day of antibiotic exposure, but diarrhoea usually starts a few days after completion of the course. The onset is sometimes delayed by as much as 3 weeks. The mortality of PMC was formerly thought to be in the region of 30–40 per cent[25] but this is certainly an exaggeration, partly because the diagnosis was often missed before the faecal cytotoxicity test became available and partly because of a bias introduced by cases which were only recognized at post-mortem. A realistic estimate of mortality before the introduction of specific therapy is 40 per cent in patients over 60 years of age and 10 per cent in those under 60 years of age.[45] Recovery can now be expected in nearly all patients given appropriate therapy.

It is failure to recognize the condition, however, that poses the greatest threat to life. We have recently detected 5 cases from a group of 25 patients where the diagnosis was only made at autopsy. In none of those who died had the diagnosis been considered, despite an episode of diarrhoea. It is also important to recognize that this disorder may occur in the early postoperative period, particularly following an intestinal operation even if only a single dose of antimicrobial has been given. Anyone who develops diarrhoea following intestinal surgery should therefore be investigated by sigmoidoscopy and examination of the stool for *C. difficile* toxin. Many of these patients have fever, suggesting that the diarrhoea is the result of a pelvic abscess. In both conditions the patient is ill and dehydrated and the white cell count is raised. The treatment of an abscess is antibiotics and surgical drainage, whereas if the diarrhoea is due to PMC antibiotics are contraindicated. The problem is compounded if the patient has had a recent colorectal anastomosis. Fever and diarrhoea in these circumstances might suggest an anastomotic leak and under such circumstances sigmoidoscopy might be regarded as invasive and contraindicated. It is absolutely essential, therefore, for stool samples to be examined for cytotoxin in any patient with post-operative diarrhoea, or that antibiotics can be stopped and appropriate therapy started.

Investigations

Laboratory parameters

In our review of 66 patients with PMC 27 (41 per cent) had a leucocytosis greater than 15.0 × 10^6/l. The distribution of white cell counts in these patients is shown in Fig. 6.6. In 15 patients who had counts greater than 20 × 10^6/l, the incidence of anaemia was no greater than one would expect in this surgical population, many of whom had had a recent operation. There were no specific biochemical changes except that the serum albumin was remarkably low, 76 per cent having values less than 30 g/l and 14 per cent with values less than 25 g/l (Fig. 6.7).

Sigmoidoscopy and colonoscopy

Sigmoidoscopic appearances are of small white plaques of membrane adherent to the mucosa, the intervening bowel being relatively normal. When there is profuse diarrhoea or abundant mucus obscuring the rectal mucosa, visualization of the pseudomembrane may be difficult and the findings inconclusive. It is essential, therefore, that suction be available so that the mucosa can be properly examined. If sigmoidoscopy is not diagnostic it should be repeated, at least until the result of the faecal cytotoxin test is available, since the typical morphological appearances of pseudomembrane may not be present at first.[45] The main limitation of sigmoidoscopy is that in some patients with PMC there is sparing of the rectum, with patchy or sometimes extensive involvement of the colon. Such patients can be identified by colonoscopy.[59]

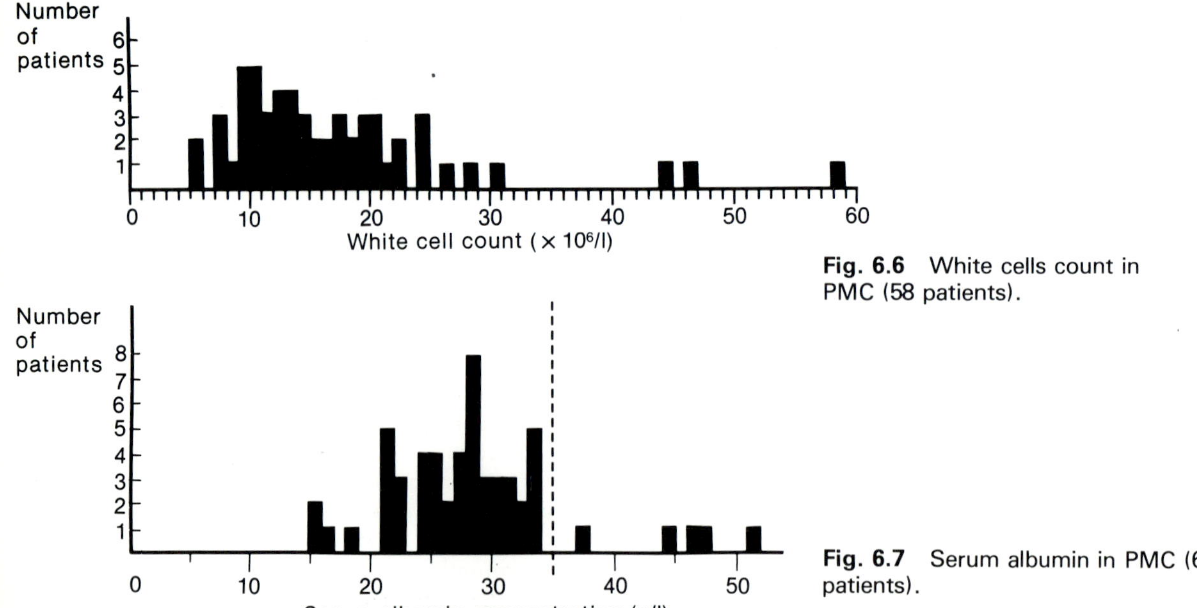

Fig. 6.6 White cells count in PMC (58 patients).

Fig. 6.7 Serum albumin in PMC (60 patients).

Biological investigation

Barium enema has also been recommended as a method for the diagnosis of PMC.[60] The pseudomembrane may be seen on the double contrast examination (Fig. 6.8) but there have been at least 3 patients in our hospital where the barium enema was normal despite good sigmoidoscopic evidence of the disease. Sometimes the radiographic changes are non-specific and merely indicate a diffuse colitis (Fig. 6.9). Of 8 patients who had this investigation in our early review, 2 developed exacerbation of symptoms with severe abdominal pain, surgical emphysema of the abdominal wall, and fever suggestive of perforation.[25] *For all these reasons we do not advise the use of barium enema for diagnosis of PMC.*

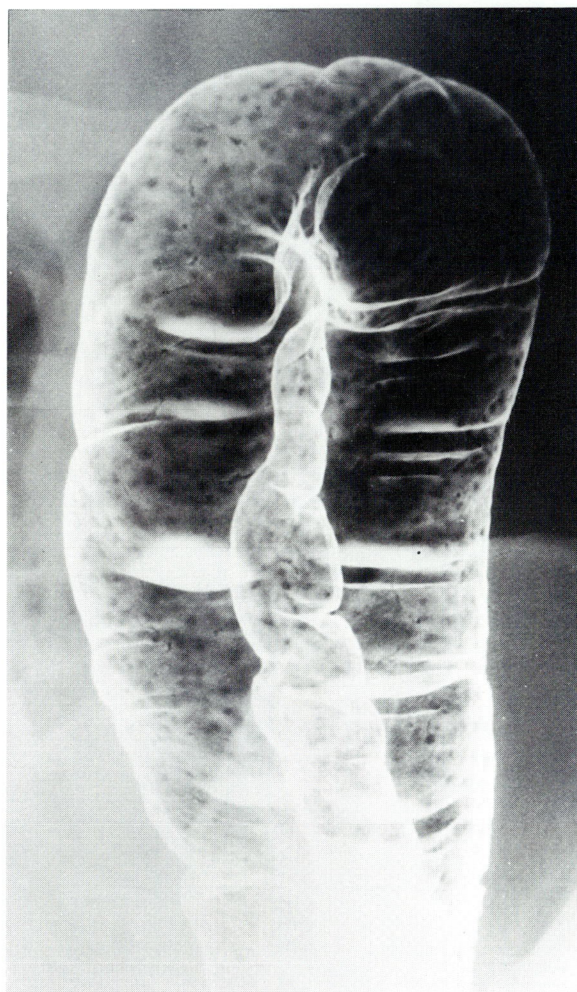

Fig. 6.8 Barium enema showing typical plaques on the colonic mucosa.

Faecal cytotoxin

The discovery of the faecal cytotoxin provided an obvious diagnostic test for PMC. It has the advantage of being simple to perform provided that facilities for tissue culture are available.

Culture of *C. difficile*

The isolation of *C. difficile* from faecal specimens is now relatively easy. Selective media containing the antibiotics cefoxitin and cycloserine are the most suitable for this purpose.[61, 62]

Interpretation of diagnostic findings

The results obtained in 44 of our patients on whom sigmoidoscopy and biopsy were performed and toxin and *C. difficile* were measured are shown in Table 6.4. Rectal pseudomembrane was recorded as present if it was seen at sigmoidoscopy or on histological examination of a biopsy. In most patients with rectal pseudomembrane, both diagnostic criteria were present. Thirty-three had rectal pseudomembrane, and in 25 of these *C. difficile* and cytotoxin were also detected in the faeces. In 7 of them the diagnosis was supported by isolation of *C. difficile*, even though the cytotoxin could not be detected. *In vitro* the *C. difficile* isolated from these patients were all capable of producing cytotoxins. The diagnostic value of the faecal cytotoxin test is limited, therefore, by this failure to detect as many as 20 per cent of patients with PMC. The faeces of 1 patient contained neither *C. difficile* nor cytotoxin, so the aetiology of the intestinal lesion is uncertain in this case.

A further group of patients who present a diagnostic dilemma are those with faecal cytotoxin and *C. difficile* but no rectal pseudomembrane. In this series there were 11 such patients (25 per cent of the whole group). The duration of diarrhoea in patients who have not been given antibiotic therapy for PMC is longer in those with rectal pseudomembrane than in those with rectal sparing.[63] Since the duration of diarrhoea is probably the best clinical indicator of disease severity, sigmoidoscopic or histological evidence of rectal pseudomembrane

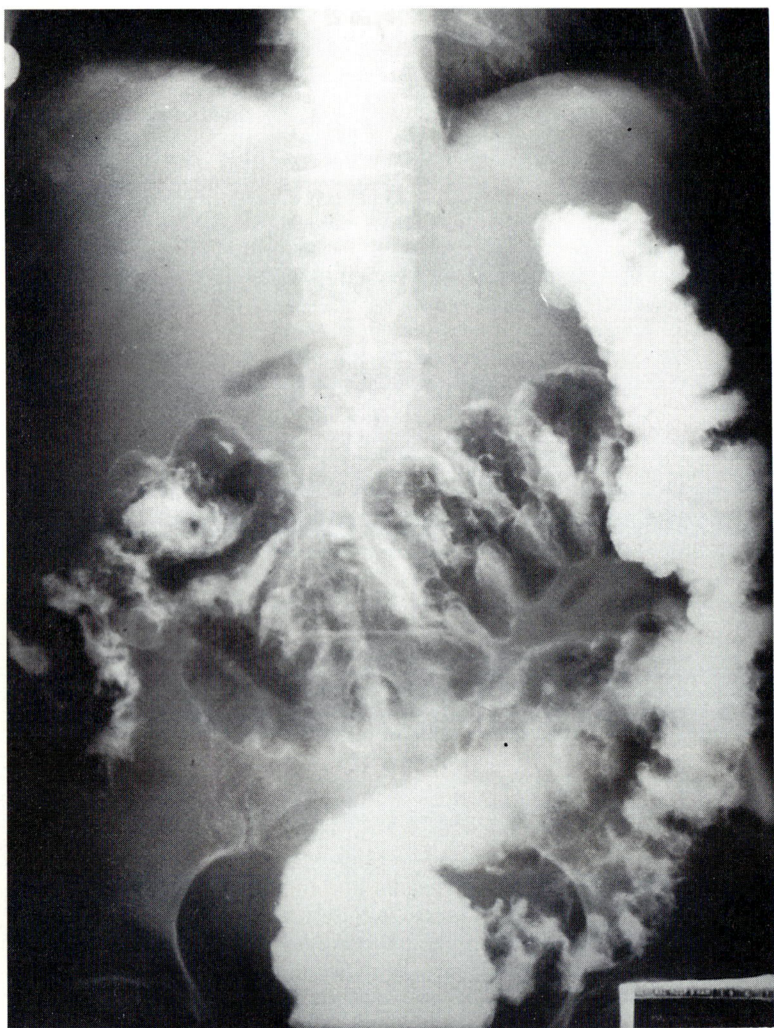

Fig. 6.9 Barium enema in a patient with pseudomembranous colitis but in whom the radiographs have shown a non-specific colitis.

Table 6.4 The relationship between various diagnostic findings in 44 patients (General Hospital, Birmingham)

Number of patients	Rectal pseudomembrane	Faecal cytotoxin	Faecal *C. difficile*
25	Present	Present	Present
7	Present	Absent	Present
1	Present	Absent	Absent
11	Absent	Present	Present

should provide a useful guide to prognosis and to the need for therapy. There was no correlation between faecal toxin titre and the duration of diarrhoea, but the titre was significantly higher in patients with rectal pseudomembrane. Nevertheless, the correlation was imperfect when judged in individual patients and it is impossible to predict the severity of illness by measurement of faecal cytotoxin titre alone. The inadequacy of the cytotoxin test alone is further illustrated by the observation of

Lishman, Al-Jumaili and Record[49] of 4 patients with high faecal cytotoxin titres following antibiotic therapy, none of whom had diarrhoea. In conclusion, there is no single test which is reliable in making a diagnosis of PMC. A satisfactory diagnosis can be reached only by careful consideration of the clinical findings in conjunction with the histological and laboratory data.

Differential diagnosis

With the availability of stool culture, there should be no confusion regarding the diagnosis. However, if this facility is not immediately available, other disorders which might present in the same way must be considered. Amoebic colitis should be distinguished by the presence of bloody diarrhoea together with a history of recent foreign travel and from stool microscopy. Ulcerative colitis causes a diffuse sigmoidoscopic change, there is usually a long-standing history and exacerbations are associated with bloody diarrhoea. Similarly, in Crohn's disease, there is usually a previous history. Other features include perianal disease, linear ulcers and an oedematous rectal mucosa. Ischaemic colitis presents either as gangrene of the colon, which is a much more dramatic and obscure disorder with gross peritonitis, or as a milder form in which bleeding is the dominant symptom. Moreover, the endoscopic appearances are distinctive (Chapter 10). Specific enteropathogens such as Campylobacter, Shigella and Salmonella should be excluded if the history suggests an infective aetiology.

Natural history and relapse

Without treatment, most patients will improve if the antimicrobial therapy responsible for the disorder is discontinued. However, the diarrhoea may continue without specific therapy for up to 5 weeks. Even when symptoms disappear, patients often continue to excrete *C. difficile*, which may pose a threat to the community as a source of further infection.

Relapse is now a well-recognized event, even after apparently successful control of symptoms. Bartlett et al.[64] reported that approximately 14 per cent of all patients treated with vancomycin relapsed. The time interval between resolution of symptoms and relapse ranged from 4 to 21 days after vancomycin therapy had been discontinued. Amongst patients who relapsed, *C. difficile* persisted despite medical therapy significantly more often than in patients who did not relapse. It was concluded that all patients being treated for PMC should be carefully followed up and that failure to eliminate *C. difficile* should alert the clinician to the possibility of this complication.

The mechanism of relapse is not fully understood. It is unlikely that *C. difficile* is resistant to vancomycin since all strains recovered in patients who relapsed were sensitive to the antimicrobial.[65] Spore formation by *C. difficile* is another possibility, and has been observed in animals treated with vancomycin.[66] This mechanism was also suggested as a cause of relapse in 5 of 8 patients reported by Walters et al.[67] Another mechanism is the *in vitro* observation that subinhibitory concentrations of vancomycin increase the toxin production by *C. difficile*.[68] There is now substantial evidence that the normal faecal flora exerts an inhibitory effect on *C. difficile*.[69] Certain strains of Staphylococcus, Pseudomonas, Bacteroides and Lactobacillus inhibit the growth of *C. difficile*. Furthermore, the growth of certain strains of the genera Peptococcus, Peptostreptococcus and Bacteroides were inhibited by *C. difficile*. Hence, if the normal faecal flora is not re-established soon after treatment, the organism may persist and be responsible for relapse. Finally, reinfection from environmental sources is another theoretical possibility. When relapse does occur, it can prove very difficult to completely eradicate the organism. It is of some interest that Walters et al[67] found that a higher dose of vancomycin had been used in patients who relapsed. The treatment of relapse is dealt with later.

Antimicrobial susceptibility of *C. difficile*

The sensitivity of *C. difficile* to antibacterial agents is important in planning treatment. Toxigenic strains of *C. difficile* are invariably resistant to the aminoglycosides and frequently also to penicillin, many of the third generation cephalosporins, clindamycin and tetracycline. All of our strains were sensitive to metronidazole and all were inhibited by 16 mg/l of vancomycin.[70] Vancomcyin given orally is poorly absorbed and provides high faecal levels even using a small dose (i.e. 125 mg q.d.s.), hence this form of treatment has been widely recommended.

Treatment

General measures

The treatment of PMC has been reviewed by George, Rolfe and Finegold.[71] When colitis occurs during antibiotic therapy, the antibiotic should be withdrawn if possible. Tedesco[57] reported that the duration of illness is longer if antibiotic therapy is not stopped and that recovery can be expected in 10–14 days in patients where it is discontinued. If continued antibiotic therapy is essential, there may be an advantage in changing from oral to parenteral administration and in choosing a drug which is poorly excreted in the gut. An alternative strategy is to use a drug different from the one which caused the colitis and to which *C. difficile* is usually sensitive. Possibilities here are penicillin, ampicillin, tetracyline and erythromycin. This might be combined with specific oral vancomycin or metronidazole therapy for *C. difficile* or followed by specific therapy.

The use of constipating drugs such as atropine and diphenoxylate (Lomotil) has been recommended for symptomatic treatment of PMC, but there is the objection that they prolong the retention of clostridial toxins within the gastrointestinal tract. Administration of Lomotil to hamsters with clindamycin-induced caecitis did not influence the outcome.[72]

Steroids also are no longer recommended because of the risk of inducing perforation. Experimental administration of methylprednisolone to hamsters with caecitis conferred no benefit.[72, 73]

Antibiotic therapy

Vancomycin was the first antibiotic to be chosen for treatment of PMC following identification of *C. difficile* as the aetiological agent, partly because of the evidence that it protected hamsters against clindamycin-induced caecitis[7] and also because of the response of patients treated with vancomycin for staphylococcal enterocolitis. *C. difficile* was found to be sensitive to concentrations of vancomycin in the range 0.2–16 mg/l, the majority of strains having minimal inhibitory concentrations (MICs) of 2 mg/l or less.[70, 72] Vancomycin is poorly absorbed from the gut, and so after oral administration high concentrations are achieved in the faeces without risk of toxicity; 125 mg given orally four times daily to patients with diarrhoea resulted in high faecal concentrations.[70] This dosage given for 5 days was evaluated by us[74] in a randomized clinical trial and shown to be effective in patients with PMC (Table 6.5). Other reports, mostly of patients given the higher dosage, have confirmed the efficacy of vancomycin,[75] although some patients have subsequently relapsed.[64, 76, 77] *C. difficile* isolated from the faeces of patients who relapse remain fully sensitive to vancomycin, and a further course is usually followed by remission of symptoms and frequent cure.

Metronidazole has also been successfully used for the treatment of PMC.[17] All strains of *C. difficile* are sensitive, with MICs of 0.4 mg/l or less.[72] Metronidazole is cheap and more acceptable to patients, and has the advantage of being available in intravenous form for those unable to take drugs by mouth. Some patients relapse after metronidazole therapy, and in our experience this happens to the same extent as with vancomycin. This is to be expected since both metronidazole and vancomycin are capable of inducing fatal caecitis in hamsters.[72] A single case of PMC has been reported following metronidazole therapy.[78] Cherry et al.[79] reported relapse in 2 of 13 patients treated with metronidazole but in the remaining patients there was a prompt response to therapy within 1–5 days.

Teasley et al.[80] reported the results of a prospective trial to compare metronidazole with vancomycin for the treatment of *C. difficile* diarrhoea or

Table 6.5 Prospective evaluation of treatment (General Hospital, Birmingham)

C. difficile present	Treatment			
	Placebo	Vancomycin	Colestipol	Metronidazole
Day 1	10	10	10	16
Day 5	10*	1	11*	1
Relapse later	0	0	0	1

* All treated with vancomycin after completion of trial.

colitis; 94 patients entered the trial but only 33 had pseudomembrane and an additional 38 had toxin. There were 2 treatment failures in the 42 who received metronidazole compared with none in the 52 who were given vancomycin. Two relapses occurred with metronidazole compared with 6 following vancomycin. Drug intolerance occurred in 1 patient from each group. The response did not differ in patients with membrane compared with the remaining patients. It was concluded, therefore, that both drugs had equivalent efficacy. However, this conclusion was challenged by Gordon[81] on the grounds that an inadequate number of patients were studied for valid statistical analysis.

Other antibiotics which have been used therapeutically are bacitracin[82] and tetracycline.[83] Bacitracin is of greater interest therapeutically because, like vancomycin, it is not absorbed from the gastrointestinal tract and it is substantially cheaper than vancomycin. *C. difficile* is sensitive to concentrations of 64 units/ml, or less.[65] Of 4 patients treated with bacitracin, 1 relapsed, and it seems unlikely that this problem is avoidable. Relapse might be the result of reinfection but the most likely explanation is the persistence of clostridial spores, against which antibiotics are inactive.

Ion exchange resins

The anion exchange resins cholestyramine and colestipol can bind *C. difficile* toxin *in vitro*,[8, 84] and would appear to have potential as a means of removing clostridial toxins from the gastrointestinal tract. Cholestyramine was reported to be effective therapy for PMC by Kreutzer and Milligan[85] in an uncontrolled study, but this has been disputed. Fekety et al.[72] observed that cholestyramine did not prevent death in hamsters with caecitis although it prolonged the mean survival time. We found no clinical benefit from colestipol as compared with placebo.[86] Moreover, both cholestyramine and colestipol bind vancomycin,[84, 87] so they probably should not be used.

Treatment of relapse

The treatment of relapse is rather empirical and may need to be prolonged. A repeat course of vancomycin was the treatment recommended by Bartlett et al.,[64] and up to three courses of therapy were sometimes needed. The use of vancomycin with cholestyramine was also recommended but this approach seems illogical (see above). Probably the most important aim is to re-establish the normal flora in the colon. In this regard metronidazole is the more rational form of therapy since it has virtually no influence on colonic microflora and can, if necessary, be given intravenously.

Surgery

Although colectomy has been performed for fulminating intractable PMC, this was usually undertaken in the belief that the colitis was a form of inflammatory bowel disease, or in cases where there had been no response to therapy. Now that effective treatment is available, operation need hardly ever be considered. We have never operated for this disorder and none of the fatal cases of PMC seen at post-mortem examination has had evidence of perforation. However, toxic megacolon is a recognized complication, and free perforation has been reported. It is our belief, therefore, that all patients with PMC should be quickly treated and that any failure to respond should be monitored by serial plain x-ray so as to detect megacolon. Operation is indicated only for impending or established perforation.

Prevention

Clindamycin and lincomycin continue to be used in some localities without ill-effect, but should not be given as first choice antibiotics in environments in which PMC is known to occur. Other antibiotics associated with colitis such as the broad spectrum penicillins and particularly the cephalosporins should be prescribed only when there is clear indication for their use. When choosing antibiotics, preference should be given to those which have least effect on the intestinal flora. Oral bowel preparation for gastrointestinal surgery should be abandoned in favour of the equally effective parenteral route, used during operation.

Patients with PMC in hospital should be isolated in single rooms. Contamination of the environment by *C. difficile* can occur but it is not known whether this is a significant source of new infection.[35] Direct transmission from patient to patient is more likely. After infected patients have been discharged, the room in which they were nursed should be thoroughly cleaned, but disinfection is probably unnecessary. Instruments such as sigmoidoscopes and colonoscopes should be carefully disinfected with a sporicidal agent. The recognition of PMC as an infectious disease and the use of preventive measures should reduce its incidence in hospitals.[71]

References

1. Pettet, J.D., Baggenstoss, A.H., Dearing, W.H., Judd, E.S. Post-operative pseudomembranous enterocolitis. *Surg. Gynecol. Obst.* (1954) **98**: 546–52.
2. Goulston, S.M., McGovern, V.J. Pseudomembranous colitis. *Gut* (1965) **6**: 207–11.
3. Ellis, M.E., Watson, B.M., Milewski, P.J., Jones, G. *Clostridium difficile* colitis unassociated with antibiotic therapy. *Br. J. Surg.* (1983) **70**: 242–3.
4. Tedesco, F.J., Corless, J.K., Brownstein, R.E. Rectal sparing in antibiotic-associated pseudomembranous colitis: a prospective study. *Gastroenterology* (1982) **83**: 1259–60.
5. Browne, R.A., Fekety, R., Silva, J., Boyd, D.L., Wax, C.O., Abrams, G.D. The protective effect of vancomycin on clindamycin-induced colitis in hamsters. *John Hopkins Med. J.* (1977) **141**: 183–92.
6. Bartlett, J.G., Onderdonk, A.B., Cisneros, R.L. Clindamycin-associated colitis in hamsters. Protection with vancomycin. *Gastroenterology* (1977) **73**: 772–6.
7. Bartlett, J.G., Onderdonk, A.B., Cisneros, R.L., Kasper, D.L. Clindamycin-associated colitis due to a toxin-producing species of Clostridium in hamsters. *J. Infect. Dis* (1977) **136**: 701–5.
8. Chang, T.W., Bartlett, J.G., Gorbach, S.L., Onderdonk, A.B. Clindamycin-induced enterocolitis in hamsters as a model of pseudomembranous colitis in patients. *Infect. Immun.* (1978) **20**: 526–9.
9. Lusk, R.H., Fekety, R., Silva, J., Browne, R.A., Ringer, D.A., Abrams, G.D. Clindamycin induced enterocolitis in hamsters. *J. Infect. Dis.* (1978) **137**: 464–75.
10. Allo, M. Clostridial toxins in strangulation obstruction and antibiotic related colitis. *J. Surg. Res.* (1980) **28**: 421–5.
11. Larson, H.E., Parry, J.V., Price, A.B., Davies, D.R., Dolby, J., Tyrell, D.A. Undescribed toxin in pseudomembranous colitis. *Br. Med. J.* (1977) **1**: 1246–8.
12. Rifkin, G.D., Fekety, F.R., Silva, J., Sack, R.B. Antibiotic induced colitis. Implication of a toxin neutralized by *Clostridium sordellii* antitoxin. *Lancet* (1977) **2**: 1103–6.
13. Larson, H.E., Price, A.B. Pseudomembranous colitis: presence of clostridial toxin. *Lancet* (1977) **2**: 1312–14.
14. Bartlett, J.G., Chang, T.W., Gurwith, M., Gorbach, S.L., Onderdonk, A.B. Antibiotic-associated pseudomembranous colitis due to toxin-producing clostridia. *N. Engl. J. Med.* (1978) **198**: 531–4.
15. George, R.H., Symonds, J.M., Dimock, E., et al. Identification of *Clostridium difficile* as a cause of pseudomembranous colitis. *Br. Med. J.* (1978) **1**: 695–7.
16. Keighley, M.R.B. Antibiotic associated pseudomembranous colitis: pathogenesis and management. *Drugs* (1980) **20**: 49–56.
17. Pashby, N.L., Bolton, R.P., Sherriff, R.J. Oral metronidazole in *Clostridium difficile* colitis. *Br. Med. J.* (1979) **1**: 1605–6.
18. Keighley, M.R.B., Burdon, D.W., Alexander-Williams, J., et al. Diarrhoea and pseudomembranous colitis after gastrointestinal operations. *Lancet*: (1978) **2**: 1165–7.
19. Peikin, S.R., Galdibini, J., Bartlett, J.G. Role of *Clostridium difficile* in a case of non-antibiotic-associated pseudomembranous colitis. *Gastroenterology* (1980) **79**: 948–51.
20. Wald, A., Mendelow, H., Bartlett, J.G. Non-antibiotic-associated pseudomembranous colitis due to toxin-producing clostridia. *Ann. Intern. Med.* (1980) **92**: 798–9.
21. Cudmore, M., Silva, J., Fekety, R. Clostridial enterocolitis produced by antineoplastic agents in hamsters and humans. In: Nelson, J.D., Grassi, C., eds. *Current Chemotherapy and Infectious Disease.* Washington DC: American Society for Microbiology (1980) 1460–61.
22. Scott, A.J., Nicholson, G.I., Kerr, A.R.R. Lincomycin as a cause of pseudomembranous colitis. *Lancet* (1973) **2**: 1232–4.
23. Tedesco, F.J., Barton, R.W., Alpers, D.H. Clindamycin-associated colitis. *Ann. Intern. Med.* (1974) **81**: 429–33.
24. Keighley, M.R.B., Arabi, Y., Alexander-Williams, J., Youngs, D., Burdon, D.W. Comparison between systemic and oral antimicrobial prophylaxis in colorectal surgery. *Lancet*: (1978) **1**: 894–7.
25. Kappas, A., Shinagawa, N., Arabi, Y., et al. Diagnosis of pseudomembranous colitis. *Br. Med. J.* (1978) **1**: 675–8.
26. Keighley, M.R.B., Crapp, A.R. Short-term prophylaxis with tobramycin and lincomycin in bowel surgery. *Scott. Med. J.* (1976) **21**: 70–72.
27. Hares, M.M., Greca, F., Youngs, D., Bentley, S., Burdon, D.W., Keighley, M.R.B. Failure of anti-

microbial prophylaxis with cefoxitin or metronidazole and gentamicin in colorectal surgery: is mannitol to blame? *J. Hosp. Infect.* (1981) **2**: 127–33.

28. Morris, D.L., Fabricius, P.J., Ambrose, N.S., Scammell, B., Burdon, D.W., Keighley, M.R.B. A high incidence of bleeding is observed in a trial to determine whether addition of metronidazole is needed with latamoxef for prophylaxis in colorectal surgery. *J. Hosp. Infect.* **5**: 398–408.
29. Ambrose, N.S., Johnson, M., Burdon, D.W., Keighley, M.R.B. Influence of single dose intravenous antibiotics in faecal flora and emergence of *Clostridium difficile. J. Antimicrob. Chemother.* (1985) **15**: 319–26.
30. Hill, I.C., O'Toole, E. Intestinal flora in newborn infants. *Am. J. Dis. Child.* (1935) **49**: 390–402.
31. Snyder, M.L. The normal faecal flora of infants between two weeks and one year of age. *J. Infect. Dis.* (1940) **66**: 1–16.
32. Larson, H.E., Honour, P., Price, A.B., Borriello, S.P. *Clostridium difficile* and the aetiology of pseudomembranous colitis. *Lancet* (1978) 1063–6.
33. George, W.L., Sutter, V.L., Finegold, S.M. Toxigenicity and antimicrobial susceptibility of *Clostridium difficile*, a cause of antimicrobial agent-associated colitis. *Curr. Microbiol.* (1978) **1**: 55–8.
34. Larson, H.E., Price, A.B., Boriello, S.P. Epidemiology of experimental enterocaecitis due to *Clostridium difficile. J. Infect. Dis.* (1980) **142**: 408–13.
35. Mulligan, M.E., Rolfe, R.D., Finegold, S.M., George, W.L. Contamination of a hospital environment by *Clostridium difficile. Curr. Microbiol* (1979) **3**: 173–5.
36. Greenfield, C., Burroughs, A., Szawathowski, M., Bass, N., Noone, P., Pounder, R.E. Is pseudomembranous colitis an infectious disease? *Lancet* (1981) **1**: 371–2.
37. Rogers, T.R., Petrou, M., Lucas, C. et al. Spread of *Clostridium difficile* among patients receiving nonabsorbable antibiotics for gut decontamination. *Br. Med. J.* (1981) **283**: 409–10.
38. Mulligan, M.E., George, W.L., Rolfe, R.D., Finegold, S.M. Epidemiological aspects of *Clostridium difficile* induced diarrhoea and colitis. *Am. J. Clin. Nutr.* (1980) **33**: 2533–8.
39. Rolfe, R.D., Finegold, S.M. Purification and characterization of *Clostridium difficile* toxin. *Infect. Immun.* (1979) **25**: 191–201.
40. Aswell, J.E., Ehrich, H., Van Tassell, R.L., Tsai, C.-C., Holdemann, L.V., Wilkins, T.D. Characterization and comparison of *C. difficile* and other clostridial toxins. In: Schlesinger, D., ed. *Microbiology*, Washington DC: American Society for Microbiology (1979) 272–5.
41. Taylor, N.S., Bartlett, J.G. Partial purification and characterization of a cytotoxin from *Clostridium difficile. Rev. Infect. Dis.* (1979) **1**: 379–85.
42. Taylor, N.S., Thorne, G.M., Bartlett, J.G. Separation of an enterotoxin from the cytotoxin of *Clostridium difficile. Clin. Res.* (1980) **28**: 285A.
43. Burdon, D.W., Thompson, H., Candy, D.C.A., Kearns, M., Lees, D., Stephen, J. Enterotoxin(s) of *Clostridum difficile. Lancet* (1981) **2**: 258–9.
44. Libby, J.M., Gartner, B.S., Wilkins, T.D. Effect of the two toxins of *C. difficile* in antibiotic-associated cecitis in hamsters. *Infect. Immun.* (1982) **36**: 822–4.
45. Mogg, G.A.G., Keighley, M.R.B, Burdon, D.W. et al. Antibiotic-associated colitis — a review of 66 cases. *Br. J. Surg.* (1979) **66**: 738–42.
46. LaMont, J.T., Trnka, Y.M. Therapeutic implications of *Clostridium difficile* toxin during relapse of chronic inflammatory bowel disease. *Lancet* (1980) **1**: 381–3.
47. Bolton, R.P., Sherrif, R.J., Read, A.E. *Clostridium difficile* associated diarrhoea: a role of inflammatory bowel disease. *Lancet* (1980) **1**: 383–5.
48. Trnka, Y.M., LaMont, J.T. Association of *Clostridium difficile* toxin with symptomatic relapse of chronic inflammatory bowel disease. *Gasteroenterology* (1981) **80**: 693–6.
49. Lishman, A.H., Al-Jumaili, I.J., Record, C.O. Spectrum of antibiotic associated diarrhoea. *Gut* (1981) **22**: 34–7.
50. Greenfield, C., Aquilar Ramirez, J.R., Pounder, R.E., et al. *Clostridium difficile* and inflammatory bowel disease. *Gut* (1983) **24**: 713–17.
51. Myers, S., Mayor, L., Bottone, E., Desmond, E., Janowitz, H.D. Occurrence of *Clostridium difficile* toxin during the course of inflammatory bowel disease. *Gastroenterology* (1981) **80**: 697–700.
52. Keighley, M.R.B., Youngs, D., Johnson, M., Allan, R.N., Burdon, D.W. *Clostridium difficile* toxin in acute diarrhoea complicating inflammatory bowel disease. *Gut* (1982) **23**: 410–14.
53. Cone, J.B., Wetzel, W. Toxic megacolon secondary to pseudomembranous colitis. *Dis. Colon Rectum* (1982) **25**: 478–82.
54. Templeton, J.L. Toxic megacolon complicating pseudomembranous colitis. *Br. J. Surg.* (1983) **70**: 48.
55. Price, A.B., Davies, D.R. Pseudomembranous colitis. *J. Clin. Pathol.* (1977) **30**: 1–12.
56. Slater, D., Corbett, C., Underwood, J., Richards, D. Rapid frozen section diagnosis of pseudomembranous colitis. *Lancet* (1981) **1**: 1046.
57. Tedesco, F.J. Clindamycin associated colitis: review of the clinical spectrum of 47 cases. *Am. J. Dig. Dis.*

(1976) **21**: 26–32.

58. Bartlett, J.G., Gorbach, S.L. Pseudomembranous enterocolitis (antibiotic related colitis). *Adv. Intern. Med.* (1977) **22**: 455–76.
59. Tedesco, F.J. Antibiotic associated pseudomembranous colitis with negative proctosigmoidoscopy examination. *Gastroenterology* (1979) **77**: 295--7.
60. Shimkin, P.M., Link, P.J. PMC: a consideration in the barium enema differentiated diagnosis of acute generalized ulcerative colitis. *Br. J. Radiol.* (1973) **46**: 437–9.
61. Willey, S.H., Bartlett, J.G. Cultures for *Clostridium difficile* in stools containing a cytotoxin neutralized by *C. sordellii* antitoxin. *J. Clin. Microbiol.* (1979) **10**: 880–84.
62. George, W.L., Sutter, V.L., Citron, D., Finegold, S.M. A differential medium for isolation of *Clostridium difficile. J. Clin. Microbiol.* (1979) **9**: 214–19. 214–19.
63. Burdon, D.W., George, R.H., Mogg, G.A.G., et al. Fecal toxin and severity of antibiotic associated pseudomembranous colitis. *J. Clin. Pathol.* (1981) **34**: 548–51.
64. Bartlett, J.G., Tedesco, F.J., Shull, S., Lowe, B., Chang, T. Symptomatic relapse after oral vancomycin therapy of antibiotic associated pseudomembranous colitis. *Gastroenterology* (1980) **78**: 431--4.
65. George, W.L., Kirby, B.D., Sutter, V.L., Finegold, S.M. Antimicrobial susceptibility of *Clostridium difficile*. In: Schlesinger, D., ed. *Microbiology*, Washington DC: American Society for Microbiology (1979) 267–71.
66. Onderdonk, A.B., Cisneros, R., Bartlett, J.G. Study of *Clostridium difficile* antibiotic mice. *Infect. Immun.* (1980) **28**: 277–82.
67. Walters, B.A.J., Roberts, R., Stafford, R., Seneviratne, E., Relapse of antibiotic associated colitis: endogenous persistence of *Clostridium difficile* during vancomycin therapy. *Gut* (1983) **24**: 206–12.
68. Onderdonk, A.B., Lowe, B.R., Bartlett, J.G. Effect of environmental stress on *Clostridium difficile* toxin levels during continuous cultivation. *Appl. Environ. Microbiol.* (1979) **38**: 637–41.
69. Rolfe, R.D., Finegold, S.M. Inhibitory interactions between normal fecal flora and *Clostridium difficile. Am. J. Clin. Nutr.* (1980) **33**: 2539.
70. Burdon, D.W., Brown, J.D., Youngs, D.J., et al. Antibiotic susceptibility of *Clostridium difficile. J. Antimicrob. Chemother.* (1979) **5**: 307–10.
71. George, W.L., Rolfe, R.D., Finegold, S.M. Treatment and prevention of antimicrobial agent-induced colitis and diarrhea. *Gastroenterology* (1980) **79**: 366–72.
72. Fekety, R., Silva, J., Browne, R.A., Rifkin, G.D., Enright, J.R. Clindamycin induced colitis. *Am. J. Clin. Nutr.* (1979) **32**: 244–50.
73. Bartlett, J.G., Chang, T.W., Onderdonk, A.B. Comparison of five regimens for treatment of experimental clindamycin-associated colitis. *J. Infect. Dis.* (1978) **138**: 81–6.
74. Keighley, M.R.B., Burdon, D.W., Arabi, Y., et al. Randomised controlled trial of vancomycin for pseudomembranous colitis and post-operative diarrhoea. *Br. Med. J.* (1978) **2**: 1667--9.
75. Tedesco, F.J., Markham, R., Gurwith, M., Christie, D., Bartlett, J.G. Oral vancomycin for antibiotic-associated pseudomembranous colitis. *Lancet* (1978) **2**: 226--8.
76. George, W.L., Volpicelli, N.A., Stiner, D.B. et al. Relapse of pseudomembranous colitis after vancomycin therapy. *N. Engl. J. Med.* (1979) **301**: 414–15.
77. Ritchie, P.H., Pennington, C.R. Pseudomembranous colitis. *Scott. Med. J.* (1980) **25**: 278–80.
78. Saginur, R., Hawley, C.R., Bartlett, J.G. Colitis associated with metronidazole therapy. *J. Infect. Dis.* (1980) **141**: 772–4.
79. Cherry, R.D., Portnoy, D., Jabari, M., Daly, D.S., Kinnear, D.G., Goresky, C.C.A. Metronidazole, an alternative therapy for antibiotic associated colitis. *Gastroenterology* (1982) **82**: 849--51.
80. Teasley, D.G., Gerding, D.N., Olson, M.M., Prospective randomised trial of metronidazole versus vancomycin for *Clostridium difficile* associated diarrhoea and colitis. *Lancet* (1983) **2**: 1043–6.
81. Gordon, L.S., Metronidazole or vancomycin for *Clostridium difficile* associated diarrhoea. *Lancet*: (1983) **2**: 1617.
82. Chang, T.W., Gorbach, S.L., Bartlett, J.G., Saginur, R. Bacitracin treatment of antibiotic associated colitis and diarrhea caused by *Clostridium difficile. Gastroenterology* (1980) **78**: 1584–6.
83. DeJesus, R., Peternel, W.W. Antibiotic-associated diarrhea treated with oral tetracycline. *Gastroenterology* (1978) **74**: 818–20.
84. George, R.H., Youngs, D.J., Johnson, E.M., Burdon, D.W. Anion-exchange resins in pseudomembranous colitis. *Lancet* (1978) **2**: 624.
85. Kreutzer, E.W., Milligan, F.D. Treatment of antibiotic-associated pseudomembranous colitis with cholestyramine resin. *Johns Hopkins Med. J.* (1978) **143**: 67–72.
86. Mogg, G.A.G., George, R.H., Youngs, D., et al. Randomised controlled trial of colestipol in antibiotic associated colitis. *Br. J. Surg.* (1982) **69**: 137–9.
87. Taylor, N., Bartlett, J.G. Binding of *Clostridium difficile* cytotoxin and vancomycin by anion-exchange resins. *J. Infect. Dis.* (1980) **141**: 92.

7

Neonatal necrotizing enterocolitis

D.F.M. Thomas

Introduction

Intestinal ischaemia in infancy occurs either because of extrinsic vascular compression (strangulation) or as part of a low flow state which progresses to necrotizing enterocolitis (NEC). Intrinsic vascular disease is virtually unknown in this age group. Strangulation such as occurs in midgut volvulus and external herniae is not considered here, but necrotizing enterocolitis, which is now a major cause of death and morbidity in newborn infants, will be discussed in detail. Some 5 per cent of babies undergoing treatment in neonatal intensive care units develop NEC and, despite advances in therapy, one-third of them die. The radiology (pneumatosis intestinalis) and the pathology (patchy intestinal necrosis) are absolutely characteristic of this infantile disorder.

Although prospects for survival of low birth weight infants have improved dramatically over the last two decades because of more informed neonatal care, the incidence of necrotizing enterocolitis has increased. It is difficult to assess the incidence of NEC before the 1960s. Some reported cases of perforation of the gut probably resulted from underlying NEC, but, although the condition was certainly underdiagnosed at that time, there can be no doubt that it has become much more frequent since.

Case reports of intestinal perforation in the newborn appear sporadically in the literature from the nineteenth and early twentieth centuries. In 1939, Thelander[1] reviewed the world literature and analysed the details of 85 cases: 46 of these involved perforation of the stomach or duodenum and are unlikely to have been due to NEC, but the other 39 cases of ileal and colonic perforation may have been so related. The first surgical success with a neonatal perforation of the ileum must be credited to Agerty, Ziserman and Hollenberger[2] in 1943. Further accounts of enteritis and intestinal perforation appeared in the European literature in the 1940s and 1950s,[3] but it is probable that many of the cases reported in the early literature were complications of conditions other than NEC, such as meconium ileus or unrecognized Hirschsprung's disease. Rickham, [4] reviewing the Liverpool experience of neonatal peritonitis and perforation wrote in 1955, 'we have not encountered a neonate suffering from peritonitis who passed blood per rectum'. Rectal bleeding is such a prominent symptom of NEC (occurring in up to 80 per cent of affected infants) that it seems very unlikely that he was seeing this condition.

In 1961 Singleton, Rosenberg and Samper[5] described the radiological appearances of 'perinatal distress syndrome' and reported 12 cases of non-infectious enterocolitis which were attributed to anoxia of the alimentary tract. Five years later, Mizrahi et al.[6] in New York, published their classic paper defining the clinical and radiological features of NEC in 18 low birth weight infants. The mortality rate quoted at this time was high, and it was not improved by the adoption of surgical treatment. Thus, Touloukian et al.[7] in 1967 reviewed the initial surgical experience with this condition and reported a mortality rate of over 80 per cent. This has now been reduced to around 30 per cent because of the introduction of potent antibiotics and parenteral nutrition, a clearer definition of the indications for operation and, perhaps most importantly, improved understanding of the needs of sick neonates, with corresponding developments in technology.

Aetiology

Clinical and experimental studies suggest that NEC is the result of ischaemia of the bowel wall which in turn permits bacterial invasion and proliferation (see 'Introduction'). Although this concept of NEC as an ischaemic phenomenon is generally accepted, some authors have placed more emphasis upon infection as the central cause.

Intestinal ischaemia

Babies affected by NEC have a high incidence of prematurity, birth asphyxia, respiratory distress and hypoxia. All these factors would be expected to reduce intestinal perfusion.

However, there may be a different mechanism operating here. It has been postulated that intestinal ischaemia occurs as the result of a reflex which redistributes blood away from the gut, related to the 'diving reflex' of certain mammals.[8] In the seal, for example, blood is shunted from the mesenteric and musculoskeletal vascular beds in order to maintan perfusion of more vital structures such as the brain and heart. Scholander,[9] who investigated diving reflexes in detail, described this form of circulatory redistribution as 'a generalized response of vertebrate animals to the threat of asphyxia from any one of a number of quite different circumstances'. He confirmed the existence of such a reflex in human adults. Healthy volunteers, when their faces are immersed in water, develop reflex bradycardia and reduced blood flow through the calf muscles. Lloyd[8] and others have suggested that 'a diving reflex' occurs in newborn human infants in response to hypoxia, and that an exaggerated reaction by the labile mesenteric vasculature could result in ischaemic necrosis as the first step in necrotizing enterocolitis.

Experimental studies

The effects of asphyxia on neonatal gut have been studied by Touloukian, Posch and Spencer.[10] Piglets ranging from 7 to 20 days age were taken and intestinal perfusion measured in different circumstances. The blood flow to various gut segments was determined by the intracardiac injection of indium-111 and perfusion within the bowel wall as studied by fractionation techniques using rubidium. Piglets subjected to asphyxia reacted by a marked reduction in perfusion of the entire alimentary tract, with the exception of the oesophagus. The most pronounced changes occurred in the intestinal mucosa: mucosal perfusion fell to 13 per cent of its normal value in the stomach and 17 per cent of the normal value in the distal colon. Histological examination of the intestine of animals sacrificed during an asphyxial episode showed that the capillary network in the mucosal and submucosal plexuses was collapsed and empty. Animals which were first resuscitated and then sacrificed were found to have mucosal and submucosal lesions consisting of vascular congestion and focal haemorrhage. Touloukian suggested that the human neonate reacts to asphyxia in a similar fashion and that focal mucosal lesions induced by ischaemia progress to necrosis and necrotizing enterocolitis.

The weaknesses of this study (the piglets were not truly neonatal and asphyxia was more extreme than that encountered by human neonates) were largely overcome when Alward et al.[11] repeated the work with piglets 6–96 hours of age and subjected them to less profound asphyxia. In these experiments cardiac output was measured by dye dilution techniques and organ blood flow quantified by the use of labelled microspheres. Mild asphyxia of 30 minutes' duration was found not to influence mesenteric blood flow, but when this degree of asphyxia was maintained for 90 minutes, decreased perfusion was observed in the stomach and upper and lower intestinal tract. Focal vascular lesions resembling those found by Touloukian and his colleagues were also identified following sacrifice of the animals in this study.

In 1974, Barlow et al.[12] described an interesting set of experiments in which two groups of neonatal rats were subjected to repeated near-lethal asphyxia. One group, fed on an artificial formula milk, all succumbed to diarrhoea and intestinal necrosis. The second group were fed on rat breast milk and these animals survived the asphyxial insult. Although some animals in both groups were given an oral inoculum of Klebsiella prior to their exposure to asphyxia, this did not appear to influence suspectibility to enterocolitis. The protective effect of breast milk was later shown to be associated with breast milk leucocytes rather than immunoglobulins. Since the bacterial flora of the

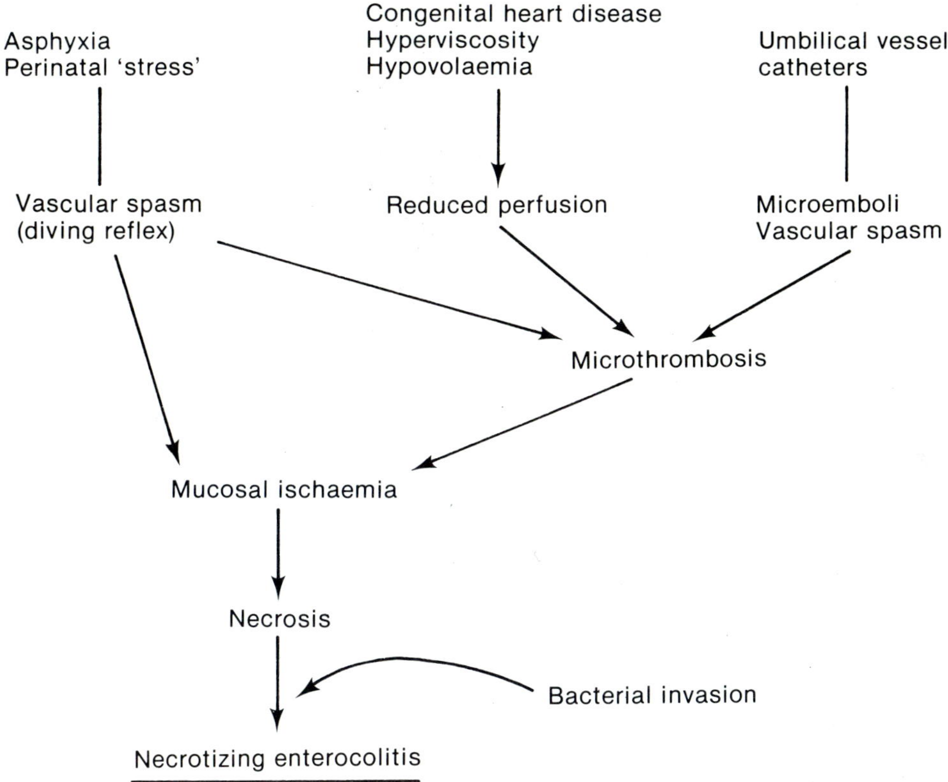

Fig. 7.1 The 'vascular cascade' of factors thought to promote NEC.

neonatal rat gut were not studied in these experiments, it is unclear which organisms were responsible for the enterocolitis. Unfortunately, the relevance of these findings to human NEC is limited. Human breast milk confers little if any protection in clinical practice.[13]

The evolving concept of necrotizing enterocolitis as an ischaemic disease of the bowel was further supported by clinical reports linking the onset of enterocolitis to such factors as the use of umbilical arterial and venous catheters,[14] cyanotic congenital heart disease[15] and hyperviscosity low flow states.[16] A unifying scheme derived from experimental and clinical observations is illustrated in Fig. 7.1.

Critics of the accepted aetiological view have pointed to the fact that birth asphyxia, respiratory distress and other purported risk factors are common events in the perinatal histories of many sick premature neonates, the majority of whom do not develop NEC. The results of controlled studies are conflicting. Some authors[17] have found significant differences in the incidence of risk factors. Wilson et al.[18] have recently suggested that there is a strong association between respiratory distress, polycythaemia and hypocalcaemia and NEC when the disease occurs in full-term babies. Other studies,[19, 20, 21] have failed to identify any differences in the frequency of exposure to 'risk factors' between groups of babies with NEC and unaffected low birth weight controls. If anything, the larger and more carefully controlled prospective studies do not confirm an important role for the majority of the accepted risk factors.

It has been noted that neither Touloukian nor Alward reproduced symptomatic enterocolitis in their animal models. The revelance of their experiments to human NEC remains conjectural. Furthermore, the degree of asphyxia entailed in these studies is rarely encountered in clinical practice.

Despite these and other criticisms, it is nevertheless widely accepted that NEC begins as an ischaemic insult.

Microbiological aspects of NEC
There is broad agreement that the gut microflora play some role in the pathogenesis of NEC, though their importance is still unclear. Specific pathogens such as Salmonella have been incrimated in some outbreaks; faecal and blood cultures in most cases grow commensals such as *Escherichia coli*, Klebsiella and Clostridia. A particular role for Klebsiella was favoured by some American authors in the 1970s, but with the discovery of *Clostridium difficile* as an important cause of pseudomembranous colitis, attention has since shifted to clostridia (Chapter 6).

Clostridium difficile. The presence of this organism in the gut of an adult is usually associated with diarrhoea. Healthy children, however, may tolerate both the organism[22] and low concentrations of its exotoxins[23] in their stools without ill effect. Wide differences have been reported in the isolation rate of *C. difficile* from children's stools, which probably reflect varying degrees of environmental colonization. Several authors have studied the possible involvement of *C. difficile* in the pathogenesis of NEC. Chang and Areson[24] and Stoll et al.[25] failed to identify *C. difficile* toxin in the stools either of affected babies or of healthy control neonates. Cashore et al.,[26] however, have reported finding cytopathic toxin in the stools of babies with NEC significantly more often than in the stools of healthy neonates. Conversely, Sherertz and Sarubbi[27] and Donta and Myers[28] have identified *C. difficile* toxin with equal frequency in the stools of babies with NEC and of controls. We[29] have measured the concentration of *C. difficile* cytopathic toxin in the stools of babies with severe NEC, with mild NEC and in unaffected control neonates. The levels of toxin were found to be equal and uniformly low in all three groups. Thus the bulk of the published evidence does not support a significant aetiological role for *C. difficile*.

In a recent publication, Han and his colleagues from Ontario[30] have described an outbreak of NEC which they attributed to *C. difficile*. The introduction of prophylactic oral vancomycin was associated with a reduction in the incidence of NEC from 25 cases per 1000 live births to around 5 cases per 1000 live births — effectively bringing the outbreak to a halt. Whether this effect was genuinely the result of vancomycin's action on *C. difficile* is unproven. This antibiotic agent has a high degree of activity against other Gram-positive organisms — many of which are less easy to detect than *C. difficile*.

Clostridium perfringens (welchii). This commensal colonizes the normal gut within the first week of life.[31, 32] In 1976, Pederson et al.[33] posed the question 'Is NEC gas gangrene of the bowel?' Some comparative evidence supports this view. *C. perfringens* type C is a cause of necrotizing enteritis and pneumatosis intestinalis in newborn piglets,[34] calves and lambs. Immunization with a toxoid vaccine during pregnancy protects the offspring against these forms of necrotizing enteritis. In addition to the veterinary diseases, there are similarities between neonatal necrotizing enterocolitis and a form of human necrotizing enteritis found in children and adults in the highlands of New Guinea. This disease, known as pig-bel[35] results from overgrowth of toxin-producing strains of *C. perfringens* type C within the intestine following the ingestion of a high protein load. An effective immunization programme against pig-bel has recently been introduced.[36]

In clinical practice *C. perfringens* can be isolated from only a proportion of cases of neonatal NEC. As with *C. difficile*, isolation from the gut cannot be taken as firm evidence of a causative role, since the organisms can also be found in healthy infants. A positive blood culture is evidence of pathological involvement, but may represent secondary invasion from the gut rather than any primary role. Examination of stools from babies with NEC for the α-toxin of *C. perfringens* has yielded negative results.[29]

The T antigen. Certain anaerobes (including *C. perfringens* and *Bacteroides fragilis*) produce a neuraminidase within the host which is capable of digesting *N*-acetylneuraminic acid from red cell membranes to expose an underlying antigen — the T antigen. The exposure of this antigen on red cells can be detected by serological techniques and, when present, is suggestive of anaerobic infection. Seges, Kenny and Bird[36] have reported finding a positive T antigen status in 8 neonates with NEC. Whilst this is further evidence of the involvement of anaerobes, it does not distinguish between primary or secondary infection.

Germ-free animal experiments. In 1982, Lawrence, Bates and Gaul[37] described an animal model of NEC and a series of experiments in support of a new hypothesis. A form of enterocolitis was induced in germ-free neonatal rats by giving them by mouth a strain of commensal bacteria in pure culture. Neither asphyxia nor stress was involved in this model. Colonization with single strains of exotoxin-producing organisms (such as staphylococci or clostridia) resulted in enterocolitis, whereas mono-contamination with *E. Coli* or Klebsiella produced no ill effect. Interestingly, adult germ-free rats were not susceptible to this form of experimental enterocolitis. This difference in susceptibility between newborn and adult animals was attributed by Lawrence, Bates and Gaul to the enchanced permeability of neonatal gut mucosa to intact macromolecules. This property, which allows neonatal rats to acquire maternal immunoglobulins from colostrum, may also permit the absorption of bacterial exotoxins. Lawrence, Bates and Gaul argue that neonatal intensive care units represent a grossly abnormal microbiological environment, and that infants in these units become colonized by a limited number of bacterial strains, which may proliferate unopposed in a fashion resembling the germ-free model. Under normal circumstances, bacterial colonization involves several species and occurs as a balanced process. The human infant acquires immunoglobulins by transplacental transfer during pregnancy rather than by intestinal uptake in the newborn period. There is evidence[38] that the process known as 'gut closure' in humans occurs during the last trimester of pregnancy and that at term the gut mucosa is relatively imperm-eable. The enhanced mucosal permeability of the preterm infant may contribute to the greatly increased susceptibility to NEC in this group.

The origin of intramural gas

Engel et al.[39] sampled blebs of gas from the intestinal wall during operations for NEC. Hydrogen was found in high concentration and the authors concluded that the pneumatosis was of bacterial origin. A number of commensals are capable of producing gas, but the experiments of Yale, Balish and Wu[40] suggest that this may not be true *in vivo*. In the studies by Yale and colleagues, adult germ-free rats were maintained within a sterile environment. The animals were subjected to laparotomy and pure cultures of various bacterial strains were injected into sites in the intestinal wall and the peritoneum. When the animals were subsequently sacrificed, gas-filled cysts were found in the bowel wall and mesentery of the rats given *C. perfringens*, but in none of the animals injected with other species, which included bacteria known to be capable of gas production *in vitro* such as *E. coli, K. pneumoniae, S. aureus, C. sporogenes* and *C. novyi*.

Other causative factors

Feeding In the Engel et al.[39] series of 55 neonates, all had received enteral feeding before the onset of NEC. Krouskop[41] has analysed the feeding histories of 298 infants with NEC — of whom only 3 per cent developed symptoms before their first feed. Pneumatosis was generally absent in these cases. Furthermore, Krouskop identified a significant association between timing of the first feed and the onset of symptoms. It appears, therefore, that whilst mucosal ischaemia may be an essential pre-requisite, a combination of bacteria and a suitable substrate for bacterial growth is required to set the chain of events in motion.

Host immunity In the neonatal period, circulating immunoglobulins consist largely of those acquired from the mother by transplacental transfer during the last trimester. Thus, premature babies are relatively deprived of maternal immunoglobulins and are notoriously prone to infection. Plasma levels of IgA and secretory IgA are frequently low or absent. Lack of this immunoglobulin may be an important factor in lowering host immunity at the mucosal level.

Conclusion

Neither ischaemia nor infection has been identified with certainty as the single cause of necrotizing enterocolitis. The two aetiological views of NEC are not mutually exclusive. A number of factors influence the balance between mucosal resistance and invasion by gut bacteria, and it is not difficult to envisage that ischaemic bowel would create an environment favourable to rapid bacterial overgrowth and invasion. Until the discovery of a single causative mechanism or infective agent (if one exists) the best working hypothesis is that NEC is a disease of multifactorial origin — mucosal ischaemia paving the way for bacterial invasion in the presence of suitable substrate. Whether NEC is the end-result of invasion by a number of different bacterial species or whether clostridia play a central role has yet to be determined.

Table 7.1 Necrotizing Enterocolitis in babies born in Grady Memorial Hospital, Atlanta, in a 20-month period[21]

Weight (g)	Live births	NEC		Ratio/1000 live births	
		Cases	Deaths	Cases	Deaths
< 1000	109	7	4	64.2	36.7
1001–1500	194	13	4	67.0	20.6
1501–2000	314	3	1	9.5	3.2
2001–2500	748	2	0	2.7	0.0
2501 +	7476	3	0	0.4	0.0
TOTAL	8841	28	9	3.2	1.0

Clinical aspects of NEC

Incidence

An accurate figure is difficult to establish since the criteria for the diagnosis of mild cases are poorly defined. In addition, it is now clear that the incidence varies from centre to centre and from time to time within one centre.[42] The most important data came from the USA. Stoll et al.[21] analysed 8841 deliveries and arrived at an incidence of 3.2 cases per 1000 live births (Table 7.1). From a survey of 31 hospitals, Sweet[43] derived an incidence of 1.2 cases per 1000 live births. In the UK, Bunton et al.[17] at University College Hospital, London, reported an incidence of 2 cases per 1000 live births.

Within neonatal intensive care units, the incidence is considerably higher than amongst newborn infants at large. Stoll's figures typify the particular susceptibility of low birth weight infants. A limited survey of the literature[17, 18, 19, 20, 21] suggests that between 2 and 5 per cent of babies in intensive care units develop NEC.

Clinical presentation

Vomiting or gastric stasis (poor absorption of nasogastric tube feeds), abdominal distension and rectal bleeding are the clinical hallmarks of NEC. Up to 80 per cent of cases present in this fashion. In addition to these more obvious features, the majority of affected neonates are also lethargic, hypotonic and prone to episodes of apnoea. As the disease progresses, the abdominal wall becomes shiny and erythematous in reaction to the underlying bacterial peritonitis. Thrombocytopenia supervenes, resulting in spontaneous bleeding or oozing from venepuncture sites. At this stage the outlook is grave and only extensive resection of necrotic bowel is likely to redeem the situation. At the opposite end of the spectrum there are mild, radiologically unconfirmed cases, exhibiting only gastric stasis and a minor degree of abdominal distension, without rectal bleeding. Most paediatricians will now treat such episodes as potential NEC by withholding feeds and administering antibiotics. Once treatment has been started, it becomes impossible to distinguish those infants who would have progressed to develop frank NEC from those with a low-grade self-limiting functional obstruction which would have resolved spontaneously. Functional intestinal obstruction undoubtedly exists as a separate entity in this age group, and may be clinically identical to the initial stages of NEC. The absence of generally agreed criteria for the diagnosis of mild or early NEC may be an explanation of the variations in clinical presentation and survival figures reported in different clinical studies.

Radiological features (Figs. 7.2–7.4)

Pneumatosis intestinalis is pathognomonic of the condition. In the absence of pneumatosis it may be difficult to distinguish NEC from functional intestinal obstruction. As the disease progresses, the radiological features are:

1. Generalized gaseous distension affecting several loops of intestine.
2. Distension of discrete bowel loops with thickening of the bowel wall.
3. Pneumatosis intestinalis, giving a frothy

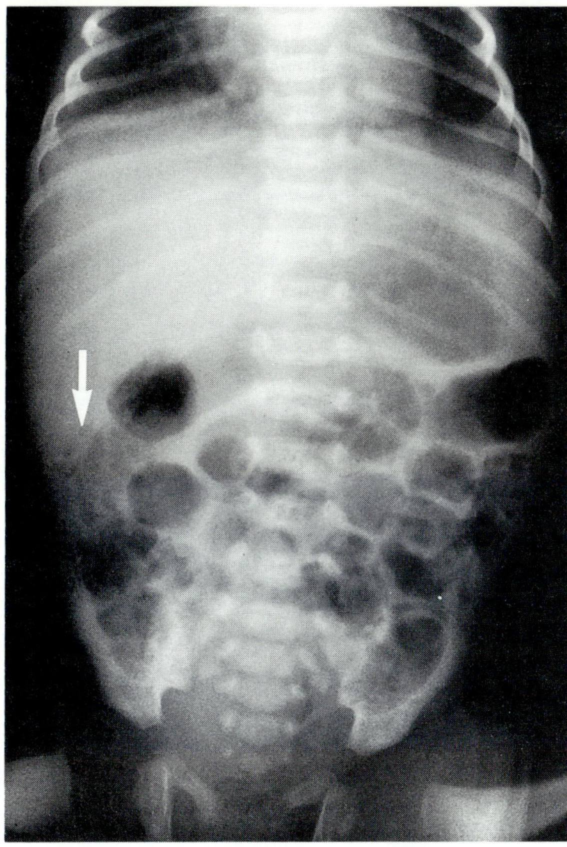

Fig. 7.2 Mild necrotizing enterocolitis. The arrow indicates an area of intestinal pneumatosis in the right iliac fossa. In this case there was a prompt response to medical treatment — with resolution of pneumatosis and symptomatic improvement within 24 hours. (By courtesy of Professor L. Spitz.)

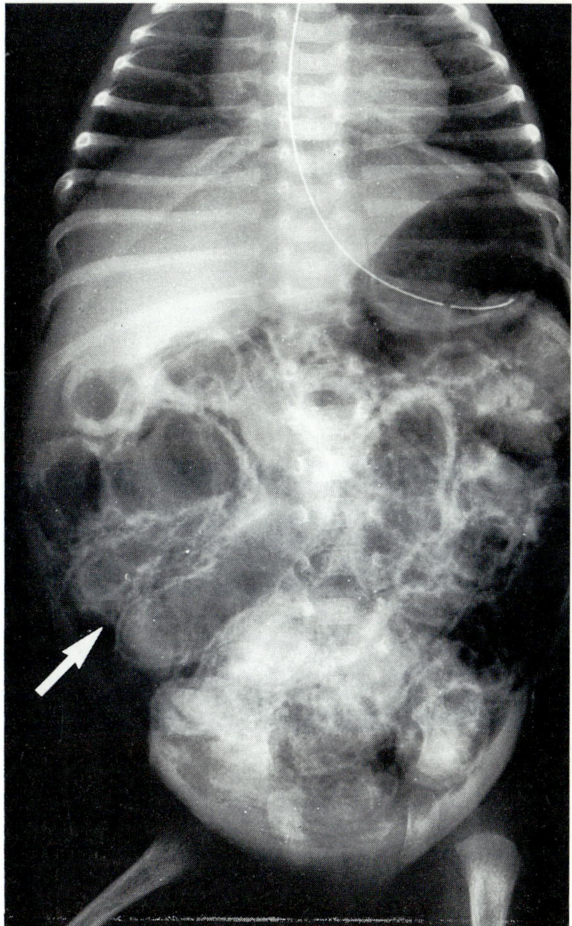

Fig. 7.3 Severe and extensive necrotizing enterocolitis. At operation both small and large intestine were found to be involved. In this radiograph the radiolucent rings of intramural gas are best seen in the region identified with an arrow.

appearance to the bowel, and later radiolucent rings within the bowel wall when viewed 'end on'.

4. Pneumoperitoneum.
5. Gas in the portal veins.

In 5–10 per cent of cases an acute episode of nectrotizing entercolitis leads to the development of a colonic stricture. The radiological features are those of a low intestinal obstruction (usually developing between 2 and 6 weeks after the initial episode) and the diagnosis can be confirmed by contrast enema.

Pathology

The macroscopic appearances at the post-mortem examination (Fig. 7.5) add little to the findings at operation (see later, 'Surgical treatment'). The histological appearances usually consist of areas of necrosis (frequently haemorrhagic), extending in size and severity as the disease progresses. Focal mucosal lesions progress to transmural necrosis with haemorrhage and pneumatosis. Bacteria may be identified within the bowel wall. The distribution of the necrotic lesions around the circumference of the bowel wall does not appear to correspond to any vascular pattern. The typical histological features are illustrated in Fig. 7.6.

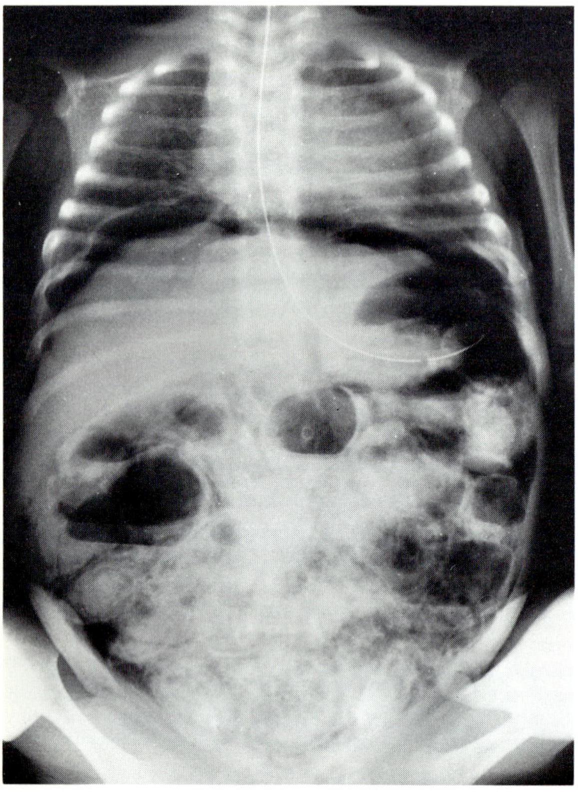

Fig. 7.4 Pneumoperitoneum. Erect radiograph of the same patient as in Fig. 7.3. Free gas below the diaphragm indicates the presence of intestinal perforation resulting from necrosis.

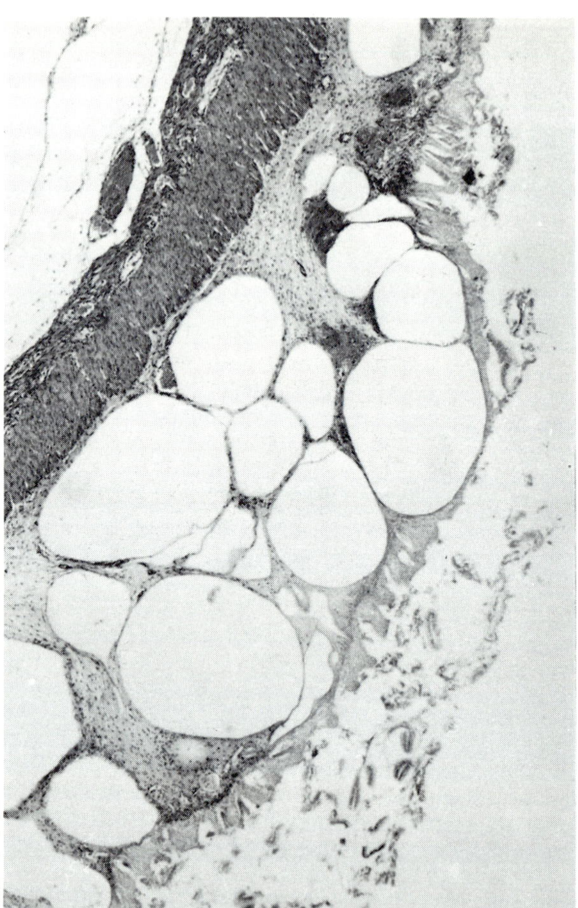

Fig. 7.5 Photomicrograph demonstrating the typical histological features of necrotizing enterocolitis. The intestinal mucosa is disrupted and sloughing. Large gas-filled spaces are clearly evident within the bowel wall and there is extensive necrosis and inflammatory infiltration. (By courtesy of Dr E. Alibone.)

Management

Intensive medical therapy is effective in 60–70 per cent of babies with NEC, but the rest require surgery. There are, however, some very low birth weight infants in whom NEC is merely one of several complications of prematurity, and in such cases surgical intervention may be neither feasible nor desirable. In the early stages of the disease it is important that the child be reviewed frequently (by a paediatric surgeon if possible) to assess the response to treatment and to review the need for operation.

Medical treatment

Cessation of feeds

Total parenteral nutrition is instituted after the acute phase has resolved — usually within 48 hours. Intravenous nutrition is usually maintained for 7–10 days, and after this time enteral feeding can be reintroduced. A reversible lactose intolerance is commonly acquired by these infants, so that many paediatricians now use a lactose-free preparation when feeds are restarted.

Antibiotic therapy

Regardless of any theories regarding a possible causative role for certain bacteria, there is no doubt that a wide range of secondary invaders, both aerobic and anaerobic, may be encountered. Potent broad spectrum cover is required, and in the UK, penicillin, gentamicin and metronidazole have, until recently, been favoured. In some centres the

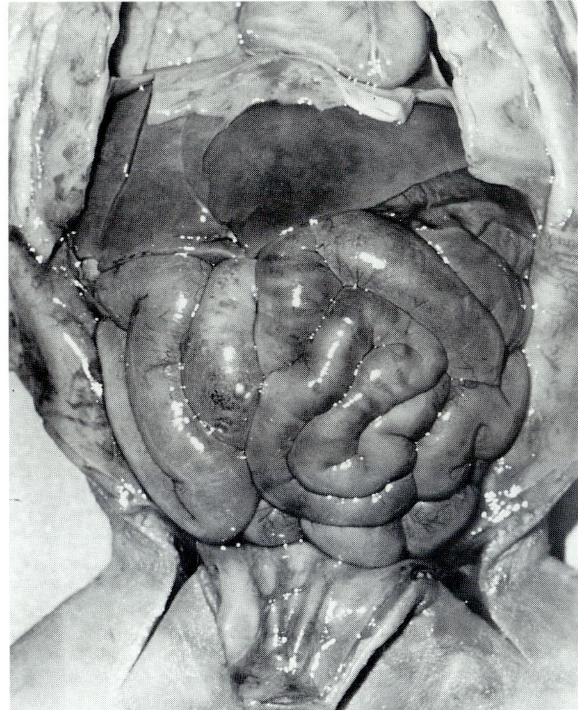

Fig. 7.6 Gross *post mortem* appearances. Necrotizing enterocolitis in this preterm infant was one of several major complications of prematurity. At post-mortem examination the entire small intestine was found to be grey, dilated and friable. Bubbles of subserosal gas can just be seen in one of the central small bowel loops. (By courtesy of Dr E. Alibone.)

aminoglycosides are being replaced by the newer synthetic penicillins and cephalosporins which do not carry the same risk of ototoxicity. Vancomycin has recently been reported to be an effective prophylactic agent,[30] but as yet there are no controlled studies on its use in the established disease.

Supportive therapy

Transfusion of whole blood or of fresh frozen plasma or platelet concentrate may be required to correct hypovolaemia and certain specific coagulation defects. Tissue oxygenation may be improved by ventilatory support (but in any event many of the premature babies are already receiving intermittent positive pressure ventilation). Hydrocortisone, dopamine and naloxone have all been used, but none has been subjected to formal controlled trials.

Indications for surgical intervention

These vary from centre to centre, but there is general agreement that pneumoperitoneum is evidence of perforation and should be treated by laparotomy. The decision that medical treatment is failing is usually made on more subjective criteria such as deterioration in the general condition, increasing erythema and tenderness of the abdominal wall and the development of thrombocytopenia. Many surgeons regard the persistence of discrete dilated loops of intestine on serial plain x-rays as evidence of necrosis and thus an indication for surgery.

Surgical treatment (Figs 7.7 and 7.8)

A transverse supraumbilical incision affords the best access. On opening the peritoneum, free gas may be encountered and there is invariably free fluid, either discoloured by haemolysed blood or frankly purulent. The intestinal lesions vary in appearance, and although usually patchy, they may become confluent at some sites. Some consist simply of areas of oedema with discoloration and intramural haemolysis. There may be white or grey zones of overtly necrotic tissue or the bowel may be so thinned and necrotic that the contents are contained only by a shell of serosa. Bubbles of gas may be seen within the bowel wall, the mesentery and the mesenteric vessels. In a recent review of 33 surgical

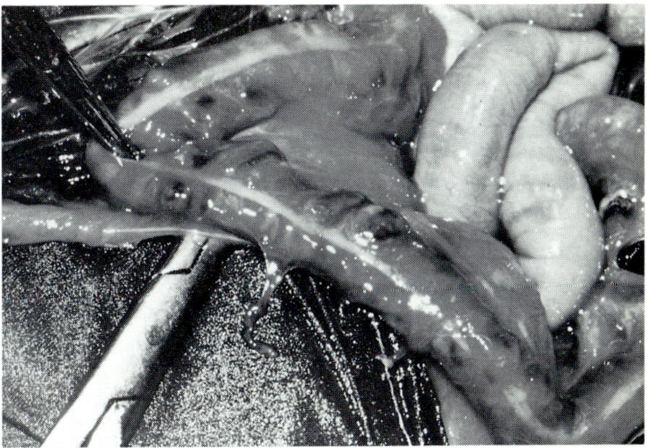

Fig. 7.7 Transverse colon at laparotomy. Laparotomy in this infant revealed extensive oedema and haemorrhage within the wall of the large bowel. In the transverse colon (illustrated) patches of discoloration and necrosis were also present. (By courtesy of Mr H.H. Nixon.)

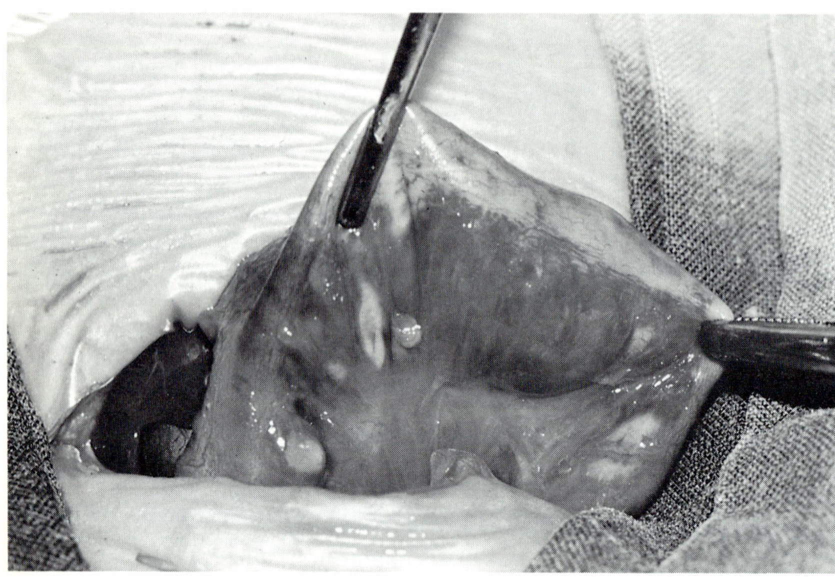

Fig. 7.8 Sigmoid colon. Deteriorating general condition prompted operation in this neonate. Areas of full-thickness necrosis were found in the sigmoid colon. The intestine was otherwise spared.

cases,[44] the lesions were confined to the small bowel in 9 patients, involved both small and large bowel in 12 and colon only in a further 12. The options open to surgeons are as follows.

Resection and temporary cutaneous enterostomy

This is undoubtedly the safest course of action. Affected bowel is resected and a terminal enterostomy and distal mucous fistula created. Problems arise if the lesions are very extensive. At least 50 cm of intact small intestine is required for survival and it may sometimes be better to risk leaving some damaged bowel rather than embark on a massive resection which will subsequently entail many months of intravenous nutrition and an uncertain outcome. Closure of the enterostomy may be undertaken whenever contrast studies of the distal loop have excluded the development of a colonic stricture (usually after 6 weeks). Early closure is particularly helpful if fluid and electrolyte losses from the ileostomy are proving difficult to manage.[45] If total colectomy has been performed at the initial operation, the subsequent ileorectal anastomosis is probably best left for 6–9 months if possible, in view of the technical difficulties of performing this anastomosis in very small children.

Resection and primary anastomosis

Although this may occasionally be safe in selected cases, most paediatric surgeons distrust the viability of bowel in the acute phase and prefer to perform a defunctioning operation until the risk of further necrosis has passed. In contrast, colonic strictures developing after NEC can be safely dealt with by resection and primary anastomosis in one stage.

Defunctioning loop enterostomy

Martin and Neblett[46] have advocated a high defunctioning loop enterostomy for those exceptional cases in which there is extensive pneumatosis without evidence of frank necrosis.

Results of treatment

The comparison of mortality statistics is an unsatisfactory exercise since the criteria for the diagnosis of mild cases are difficult to establish. Furthermore, the majority of deaths occur in babies under 1500 g birth weight and the proportion of such infants in a clinical series will influence the figures. A review of the more recent literature indicates that the overall mortality in necrotizing enterocolitis is around 30 per cent.[19, 21, 44, 47] Approximately one-third of affected babies require surgery and in this group the mortality is between 40 and 50 per cent. Of the two-thirds of neonates with NEC who are managed medically, about 20 per cent die (these are mainly very premature babies with multiple complications of immaturity).

Morbidity

There have been few long-term followed-up studies. Stevenson et al.[47] assessed 40 survivors of NEC at 3 years of age and compared the outcome with a similar group of low birth weight controls. Four children (10 per cent) had alimentary tract sequelae related to NEC: 1 developed a colonic stricture requiring resection, 2 had short gut syndrome and 1 was discovered to have malabsorption of fat. Despite these problems, the growth pattern of all four children was within normal limits. Development delay or mild neurological deficit was a feature of 21 of the 40 children, but the frequency and the degree of this minor handicap did not differ significantly from the finding in the control group. More long-term studies would be helpful, but the limited evidence available so far suggests that intestinal dysfunction will not prove to be a major problem.

Prevention

Since necrotizing enterocolitis is largely a disease of premature infants, the single most effective measure would be to prevent premature labour, which is not at present practicable. Advances in obstetric and neonatal medical practice have undoubtedly reduced the incidence of severe perinatal hypoxia, but this benefit has been offset by the ability of paediatricians to resuscitate and keep alive more low birth weight babies — who run the highest risk of developing NEC. There are good reasons for wishing to limit the use of umbilical vascular catheters, but whilst helpful this would certainly not eradicate the problem.

Modification of feeding practices may offer some scope for prevention. Brown and Sweet[48] have reported a highly significant reduction in the incidence of NEC following the introduction of a feeding regimen for low birth weight neonates. These authors advocate the delayed introduction of enteral feeds and a gradual increase in their volume and concentration. Following the introduction of such a regimen, Brown and Sweet encountered only 2 cases of NEC amongst 5518 admissions to their neonatal nursery in a period of 7½ years. Other authors support this approach. Eyal et al.[49] have recently documented a reduction in the incidence of NEC following a change in feeding policy. 'At risk' neonates appeared to be less prone to NEC if they were fed intravenously for the first 2–3 weeks of life and if enteral feeds were then introduced gradually. Wilson et al.[50] have, however, suggested that intravenous feeding may merely delay the onset of NEC. Events surrounding the introduction of enteral feeds appear to be important.

The value of prophylactic antiobotics is controversial. Systemic antibiotics do not appear to prevent the development of NEC. Trials of oral prophylactic kanamycin[51] and gentamicin[52, 53] have been reported to exert a protective effect, but some studies have failed to confirm any benefit from these agents.[54, 55] The use of oral vancomycin as a prophylactic, as reported by Han et al.[30] is theoretically attractive and merits further investigation.

Conclusion

Necrotizing enterocolitis is now endemic within high technology units caring for sick and premature newborn infants. Despite the distinctive clinical, radiological and pathological features of this disease, no single causative mechanism nor infective agent has yet been identified. It is widely believed that ischaemia plays a crucial role, but that other factors are also implicated. Although there may be some scope for advance in the medical and surgical management of NEC, the disease often presents and progresses so rapidly that the potential for treating the established case is limited. Further research is needed, but the existing evidence suggests that useful preventative measures include skilled neonatal care, modification of feeding practices and the use of oral vancomycin as a prophylatic agent.

References

1 Thelander, H.E. Perforation of the gastrointestinal tract in the newborn infant. *Am. J. Dis. Child.* (1939) **58**: 371–93.

2 Agerty, H.A., Ziserman, A.J., Hollenberger, C.L. A case of perforation of the ileum in a newborn infant with operation and recovery. *J. Pediatr.* (1943) **22**: 233.

3 Schmid, K.O. Uber eine besonder schwer verlaufende form von enteritis beim saugling 'Enterocolitis ulcerosa necroticans' I. Pathologisch-anatomische Studien. *Österr. Z. Kinderheilk.* (1952) **8**: 114–36.

4 Rickham, P.P. Peritonitis in the neonatal period. *Arch. Dis. Child.* (1955) **30**: 23–31.

5 Singleton, E.B., Rosenberg, H.M., Samper, L. Radiologic considerations of the perinatal distress syndrome. *Radiology* (1961) **76**: 200–12.

6 Mizrahi, A., Barlow, O., Berdon, W., et al. Necrotizing enterocolitis in premature infants. *J. Pediatr.* (1965) **66**: 697–706.

7 Touloukian, R.J., Berdon, W.E., Armoury, R.A., Santulli, T.B. Surgical experience with necrotizing enterocolitis in the infant. *J. Pediatr. Surg.* (1967) **2**: 389–401.

8 Lloyd, J.R. The etiology of gastrointestinal perforations in the newborn. *J. Pediatr. Surg.* (1969) **4**: 77–84.

9 Scholander, P.F. The master switch of life. *Sci. Am.* (1963) **109**: 92–106.

10 Touloukian, R.J., Posch, J.N., Spencer, R. The pathogenesis of ischemia in asphyxiated neonatal piglets. *J. Pediatr. Surg.* (1972) **7**: 194–205.

11 Alward, C.T., Hook, J.B., Helmrath, T.A., Mattson, J.C., Bailie, M.D. Effects of asphyxia on cardiac output and organ blood flow in the newborn piglet. *Pediatr. Res.* (1978) **12**: 824–7.

12 Barlow, B., Santulli, T.V., Heird, W.C., Pitt, J., Blanc, W.A., Schullinger, J.N. An experimental study of acute neonatal enterocolitis — the importance of breast milk. *J. Pediatr. Surg.* (1974) **9**: 587–94.

13 Reisner, S.H. Garty, B. Necrotising enterocolitis despite breast feeding. *Lancet* (1977) **2**: 507.

14 Corkery, J.J., Dubowitz, V., Lister, S. Colonic perforation after exchange transfusion. *Br. Med. J.* (1968) **4**: 345–9.

15 Dickinson, D.F., Galloway, R.W., Wilkinson, J.L., Arnold, R. Necrotising enterocolitis after neonatal cardiac catheterisation. *Arch. Dis. Child.* (1982) **6**: 431–3.

16 Hakanson, D.O., Oh, W. Necrotizing enterocolitis and hyperviscosity in the newborn infant. *J. Pediatr.* (1977) **90**: 458–61.

17 Bunton, G.L., Durbin, G.M., McIntosh, N., et al. Necrotising enterocolitis: controlled study of three years' experience in a neonatal intensive care unit. *Arch. Dis. Child.* (1977) **52**: 772–7.

18 Wilson, R., del Portillo, M., Schmidt, E., Feldman, R.A., Kanto, W.P. Risk factors for necrotizing enterocolitis in infants weighing more than 2000 grams at birth: a case control study. *Pediatrics* (1983) **71**: 19–22.

19 Kleigman, R.M., Hack, M., Jones, P., Fanaroff, A.A. Epidemiologic study of necrotizing enterocolitis among low birth weight infants. *J. Pediatr.* (1982) **100**: 440–44.

20 Frantz, I.D., L'Heureux, P., Engel, R.R., Hunt, L.C.E. Necrotizing enterocolitis. *J. Pediatr.* (1975) **86**: 259–63.

21 Stoll, B.J., Kanto, W.P., Glass, R.I., Nahmias, M.D., Brann, A.W. Epidemiology of necrotizing enterocolitis: a case control study. *J. Pediatr.* (1980) **96**: 447–51.

22 Larson, H.E., Barclay, F.E., Honour, P., Hill, I.D. Epidemiology of *Clostridium difficile* in infants. *J. Infect. Dis.* (1982) **146**: 727–33.

23 Rietra, P.J.G.M., Slaterus, K.W., Zanen, H.C., Meuwissen, S.G.M. Clostridial toxin in faeces of healthy infants. *Lancet* (1978) **2**: 319.

24 Chang, T.W., Areson, P. Neonatal necrotizing enterocolitis: absence of enteric bacterial toxins. *N. Engl. J. Med.* (1978) **299**: 424.

25 Stoll, B.J., Nahmias, A.J., Wickliffe, C., Brann, A.W., Dowell, V.R., Whaley, D.N. Bacterial toxin and neonatal necrotizing enterocolitis. *J. Pediatr.* (1980) **96**: 114–15.

26 Cashore, W.J., Peter, G., Lavermann, M., Stonestreet, B.S., Oh, W. Clostridia colonization and clostridial toxin in neonatal necrotizing enterocolitis. *J. Pediatr.* (1981) **98**: 308–11.

27 Sherertz, R.J., Sarubbi, F.A. The prevalence of *Clostridium difficile* and toxin in a nursery population: a comparison between patients with necrotizing enterocolitis and an asymptomatic group. *J. Pediatr.* (1982) **100**: 435–9.

28 Donta, S.T., Myers, M.G. *Clostridium difficile* toxin in asymptomatic neonates. *J. Pediatr.* (1982) **100**: 431–4.

29 Thomas, D.F.M., Fernie, D.S., Bayston, R., Spitz, L. Clostridial toxins in neonatal necrotizing enterocolitis. *Arch. Dis. Child.* (1984) **59**: 270–72.

30 Han, V.K.M., Sayed, H., Chance, G.W., Brabyn, D.G., Shaheed, W.A. An outbreak of *Clostridium difficile* necrotizing enterocolitis: a case for oral vancomycin therapy? *Pediatrics* (1983) **71**: 935–41.

31 Kindley, A.D., Roberts, P.J., Tulloch, W.H. Neonatal necrotising enterocolitis. *Lancet* (1977) **1**:649.

32 Rotimi, V.O., Duerden, B.I. The deveopment of the bacterial flora in normal neonates. *J. Med. Microbiol.* (1981) **14**: 51–62.

33 Pedersen, P.V., Hansen, F.H., Halveg, A.B., Christiansen, E.D., Justensen, T., Høgh, P. Necrotising enterocolitis of the newborn. Is it gas gangrene of the bowel? *Lancet* (1976) **2**: 715–16.

34 Høgh, P. Necrotizing infectious enteritis in piglets caused by *Clostridium perfringens* type C. *Acta Vet. Scand.* (1967) **8**: 301–23.

35 Lawrence, G., Shann, F., Freestone, D.S., Walker, P.D. Prevention of necrotising enteritis in Papua New

Guinea by active immunisation. *Lancet* (1979) **1**: 227–30.

36 Seges, R.A., Kenny, A., Bird, G.W.G. Pediatric surgical patients with severe anerobic infection. Report of 16 T antigen positive cases and possible hazards of blood transfusion. *J. Pediatr. Surg.* (1981) **16**: 905–10.

37 Lawrence, G., Bates, J., Gaul, A. Pathogenesis of neonatal necrotising enterocolitis. *Lancet* (1982) **1**: 137–9.

38 Roberton, D.M., Pagnelli, R., Dinwiddie, R., Levinsky, R.J. Milk antigen absorption in the preterm and term neonate. *Arch. Dis. Child.* (1982) **57**: 369–72.

39 Engel, R.R., Virnig, N.L., Hunt, C.E., Levitt, M.D. Origin of mural gas in necrotizing enterocolitis. *Pediatr. Res.* (1973) **7**: 292.

40 Yale, C.E., Balish, E., Wu, J.P. The bacterial etiology of pneumatosis intestinalis. *Arch. Surg.* (1974) **109**: 89–94.

41 Krouskop, R.W. Influence of feeding practices. *Neonatal Necrotizing Enterocolitis,* In: Brown, E.G., Sweet, A.Y., eds. New York: Grune & Stratton (1980) 57–68.

42 Book, L.S., Overall, J.C., Herbst, J.J., Britt, M.R., Epstein, B., Jung, A.L. Clustering of necrotizing enterocolitis: interruption by infection-control measures. *N. Engl. J. Med.* (1977) **297**: 984–6.

43 Sweet, A.Y. Informal review of mortality of necrotizing enterocolitis. In: Brown, E.G, Sweet, A.Y., eds. *Neonatal Necrotizing Enterocolitis*, New York: Grune & Stratton (1980) 13–15.

44 Anon. *Communicable Disease Report.* Public Health Laboratory Service (1983) June.

45 Rothstein, F.C., Halpin, T.C., Kliegman, R.J., Izant, R.J. Importance of early ileostomy closure to prevent chronic salt and water losses after necrotizing enterocolitis. *Pediatrics* (1982) **70**: 249–53.

46 Martin, L.W., Neblett, W.W. Early operation with intestinal diversion for necrotizing enterocolitis. *J. Pediatr. Surg.* (1981) **16**: 252–5.

47 Stevenson, D.K., Kerner, J., Malachowski, N., Sunshine, P. Late morbidity among survivors of necrotizing enterocolitis. *Pediatrics* (1980) **66**: 925–7.

48 Brown, E.G., Sweet, A.Y. Neonatal necrotizing enterocolitis. *Pediatr. Clin. North. Am.* (1982) **29**: 1164–7.

49 Eyal, F., Sagi, E., Arad, I., Avital, A. Necrotising enterocolitis in the very low birthweight infant: expressed breast milk feeding compared with parenteral feeding. *Arch. Dis. Child.* (1982) *57*: 274–6.

50 Wilson, R., Kanto, W.P., McCarthy, B.J., Feldman, R.A. Age at onset of necrotizing enterocolitis: risk factors in small infants. *Am. J. Dis. Child.* (1982) **136**: 814–16.

51 Egan, E.A., Mantilla, G., Nelson, R.M., Eitzman, D.V. A prospective controlled trial of oral kanamycin in the prevention of neonatal necrotizing enterocolitis. *J. Pediatr.* (1976) **89** 467–70.

52 Rowley, M.P., Dahlenburg, G.W. Gentamicin in prophylaxis of neonatal necrotising enterocolitis. *Lancet* (1978) **2**: 532.

53 Grylack, L.J., Scanlon, J.W. Oral gentamicin therapy in the prevention of neonatal necrotizing enterocolitis. *Am. J. Dis. Child.* (1978) **132**: 1192–4.

54 Nelson, J.D. Commentary. *J. Pediatr.* (1976) **89**: 471.

55 Boyle, R., Nelson, J.S., Stonestreet, B.S., et al. Alterations in stool flora resulting from oral kanamycin prophylaxis of necrotizing enterocolitis. *J. Pediatr.* (1978) **93**: 857–61.

8

Chronic intestinal ischaemia

Introduction

The concept of abdominal pain originating from chronic obstruction of the intestinal arteries, analogous to angina pectoris or calf claudication, is appealingly simple and has been mentioned in medical writing since the beginning of this century.[1, 2, 3] The pattern of symptoms has been given various names, such as 'abdominal claudication' and 'mesenteric angina', but the term 'intestinal angina' (IA) originally developed by Mikkelsen[4] has been most generally accepted. Although such a phrase still begs the question by assuming the reality of a syndrome which needs to be evaluated, it is a useful shorthand and will be used here, recognizing its limitations. Intestinal arterial occlusion (IAO), however, refers to lesions *seen on an angiogram*, with no assumption as to their significance, and this concept is much more firm.

Although IA has been discussed for some time in the European literature, a firm clinical basis was not available until Dunphy's[5] classic paper published in 1936. Dunphy showed that, of 12 patients dying from intestinal infarction, 7 gave a prodromal history of a characteristic abdominal pain, occurring in close relation to meals. He showed that this prodrome was usually less than 2 years, and went on to suggest that if such patients could be identified early in the course of their disease, then not only might their pain be relieved but perhaps also a lethal infarction could be prevented by timely reconstruction of the arteries involved.

It has been known for over a hundred years that a blockage of the visceral artieries which builds up slowly enough to permit a collateral circulation to develop, may be well tolerated, and indeed be asymptomatic. Chiene[6] reported the body of a 65-year-old woman received in 1868 for dissection at Edinburgh University Medical School which contained an aortic aneurysm, involving complete occlusion of the CA and SMA, the bowel being supplied by extracoelomic vessels and by a superior haemorrhoidal artery which was enlarged to the size of the femoral. The incidence and distribution of blockages in the visceral arteries have been established by many autopsy studies such as those of Maljatzkaja,[7] Johnson and Bagenstoss,[8] Carucci,[9] Derrick, Pollard and Moore[10] and Reiner.[11] Our group have reviewed this problem[12] and have corrected the earlier data on the basis of 203 unselected autopsies, the largest series hitherto reported (Fig. 8.1). The present state of knowledge can be summarized as follows:

1. Atherosclerosis of the visceral arteries is common, and is usually confined to the first 4 cm of the vessel. The frequency increases with age. However, most of these lesions are of minor degree, and 'critical stenosis' as defined by careful analysis of external and internal diameters, in relation to accepted estimates of flow, is unusual, amounting to some 6 per cent of the subjects studied.
2. The coeliac axis and the SMA are affected in roughly equal proportions, the IMA rather less so.
3. The gross appearance of the bowel is the same, whether or not such arterial lesions are present.
4. No relation can be found between the degree of arterial occlusion as seen post mortem and alimentary symptoms experienced during life.

Thus, stenoses and occlusions of the visceral arteries are easily demonstrated on an angiogram or at post-mortem, but intestinal angina is a rare symptom. It

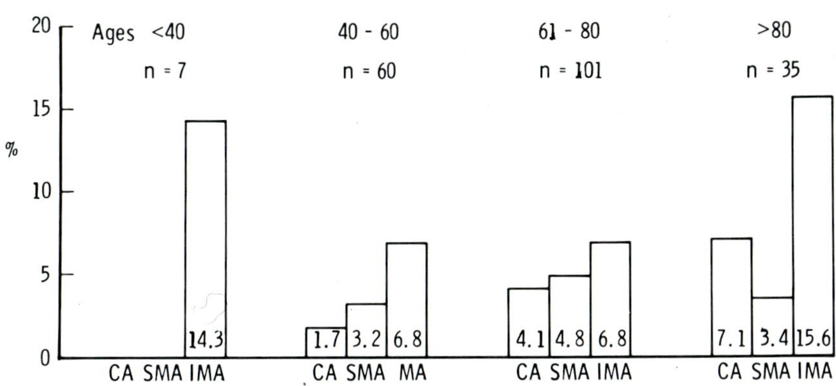

Fig. 8.1 The incidence of critical stenosis (> 50 per cent) of the visceral arteries as demonstrated at 203 unselected autopsies. (From Croft, Menon and Marston[12] by kind permission of the Editor, *British Journal of Surgery*.)

is, nevertheless, one which it is important to identify, not only because of the severe distress it causes but also because it implies a direct threat to life. A test designed to pick out the type of arterial occlusion which poses such a threat is badly needed but is not at present available.

The diagnosis of obscure abdominal pain forms a major part of every clinician's daily work. The patient presents with chronic distressing symptoms but without corroborative physical signs, and conventional diagnostic methods fail to reveal an anatomical fault. This situation is particularly common in the middle aged and the elderly, who are at the same time prone to various types of cardiovascular illness. To assign their symptoms to vascular disease of the alimentary tract is a convenient short-cut to accurate diagnostic thinking, but may at the same time carry considerable danger to the patient, who may be subjected to intensive investigation and even perhaps to an ambitious but inappropriate surgical operation. It is the purpose of this chapter to examine critically the concept of chronic intestinal ischaemia, and to consider what it has to offer in practical terms.

Clinical picture of intestinal angina

Symptoms

As conventionally described, the patient with one or more occluded visceral arteries complains of cramping abdominal pain occurring in very strict relationship to meals, and usually between 20 and 50 minutes after ingestion of food. The pain is centred on the epigastrium but radiates all over the abdomen, and is described as cramping or colicky in nature. It is sometimes relieved by standard analgesic agents and by 'vasodilator' drugs. As the disease progresses, the pain intensifies so that the patient becomes terrified of eating (the classic symptom of 'food fear') and loss of weight inevitably follows. This weight loss is almost certainly due to diminished intake rather than to interference with absorption.[13]

Together with the pain and the weight loss, there is a disturbance in bowel habit. Most authors report initial constipation, due to diminished bulk intake, which is later followed by diarrhoea secondary to malabsorption of fat. However, study of the literature[14, 15, 16, 7] discloses no consistent pattern of bowel symptomatology.

Many patients (indeed, perhaps the majority) present as an emergency, when an incidental crisis precipitates their chronic intestinal ischaemia into necrosis.[18] In these cases the prodromal syndrome of pain, loss of weight and disturbance of bowel habit will often have been dismissed as a neurotic complaint, or misinterpreted as malignant disease. Associated cardiovascular problems, such as a past history of myocardial infarction, episodes of left ventricular failure, arterial hypertension and chronic renal failure, or occlusive disease of the aortofemoral segment leading to symptoms in the legs, are commonly found.

Physical signs

The patient is described as presenting a picture of emaciated misery, with the scars of several previous

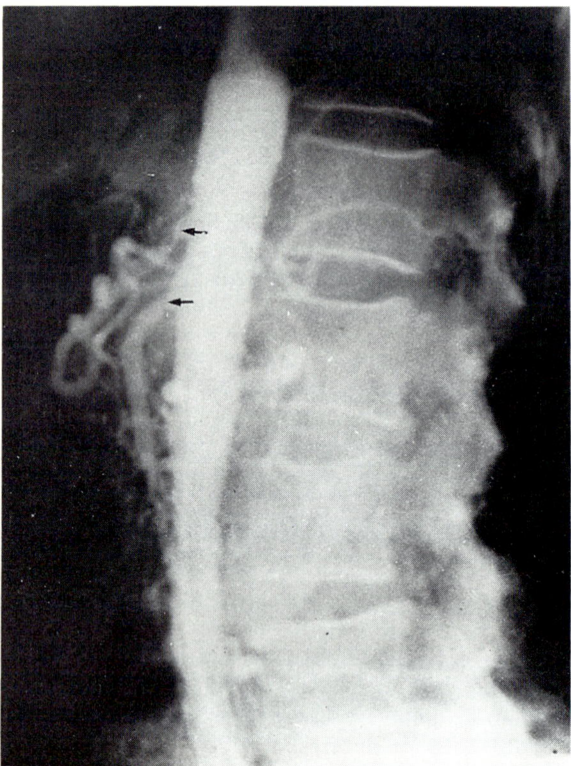

Fig. 8.2 Stenosis of the CA and the SMA (lateral view).

ineffective abdominal operations.

The physical sign which is most constantly referred to in the medical literature is the finding of a loud systolic bruit in the upper abdomen, midway between the umbilicus and the xiphisternum, and corresponding to the position of the SMA. This was found, for instance, in 21 out of the 24 patients reported by Reul et al.[19] However, this physical sign is of (to say the least) doubtful validity. Not only is such a bruit a frequent accompaniment of atheromatous roughening of the aorta (which is very common in this age group), but it can also in fact be heard in a large proportion of young men and women.[20] The other physical sign which has been mentioned is the finding of exaggerated bowel sounds following meals. Once again, however, this is clearly a highly subjective finding which is difficult to confirm or to reproduce.

Radiological appearances

In practice, the diagnosis is made by exclusion. This is to say, the patient presents with a non-specific picture of obscure abdominal pain and weight loss, and is then subjected to the normal gamut of examinations designed to exclude organic disease of the upper gastrointestinal tract. These will include ultrasonography, fibrendoscopy of the stomach, duodenum and colon, with screening of the oesophagus and gravitational search for reflux, and perhaps conventional contrast studies of the stomach and bowel. Additionally, an oral chole-

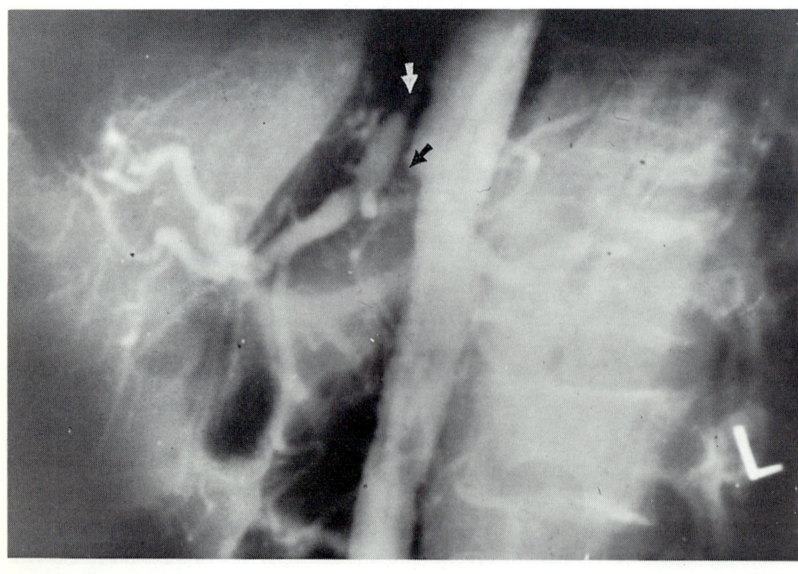

Fig. 8.3 Stenosis of the CA with complete occlusion of the SMA (lateral view).

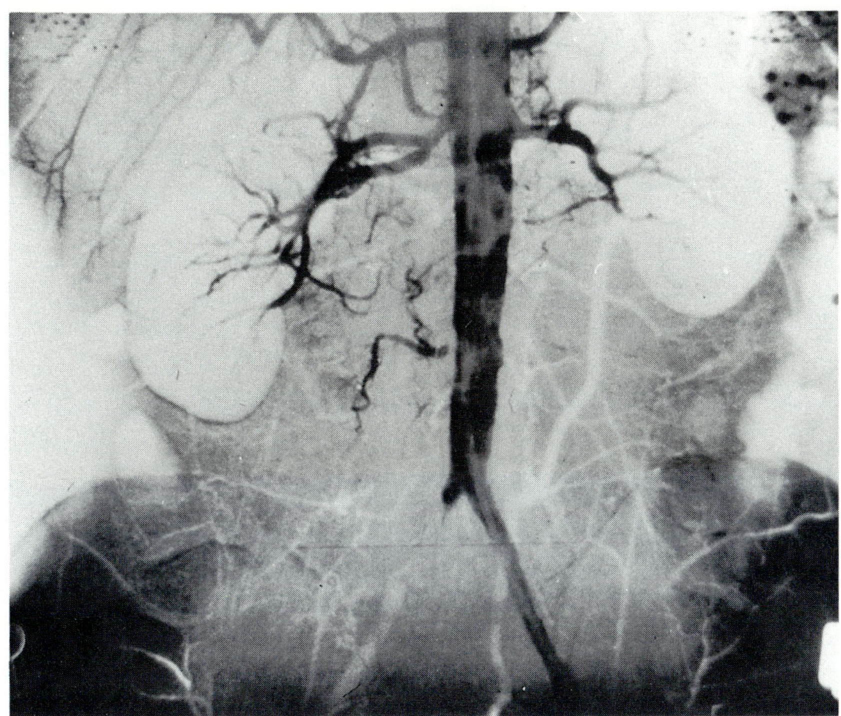

Fig. 8.4 Occlusion of the SMA (end face view). Subtracted angiogram to show dilated marginal artery to the colon in the late phase. (Note also the occlusion of the right common iliac artery.)

cystogram will have been carried out with negative results, and many patients will have had a intravenous urogram. These negative examinations will have prompted the need for aortography.

The diagnosis of IA depends on the correlation of clinical symptoms with aortographic findings. It is essential to examine the contrast-filled aorta in both anteroposterior and lateral projections, and also to carry out selective examination of the three main visceral trunks. A varying pattern of occlusion, roughly corresponding to the post-mortem findings outlined above, will be demonstrated. These appearances are illustrated in Figs. 8.2–8.6. However the demonstration of a stenosis on an x-ray film is in fact of little help in explaining a patient's symptoms, and still less in recommending a line of treatment.

As already pointed out, the human body has great capacity for building collateral flow around a blocked visceral artery, and the incidence of asymptomatic stenosis is high. Dick et al.[21] studied 1000 aortograms obtained from patients with and without abdominal symptoms, in order to provide some idea of the relationship between blood flow (as estimated by the summed cross-sectional areas of the arteries) and symptomatology. Eleven of their patients had undergone aortography because of suspected intestinal angina and, of these, 6 were found to have other diseases common to this age group. The remaining 5 had variable symptoms which suggested mesenteric vascular disease. Of these 5 patients the fact of chronic intesinal ischaemia was proven in 2, of whom 1 had complete relief of symptoms following arterial reconstruction. (See also Fig. 8.1).

Intestinal function

It seems logical to suppose that reduction in blood supply to the alimentary tract would produce absorptive or exsorptive abnormalities which could be measured in the clinical laboratory. In fact, studies of this nature are not easy to come by, and tend to disagree. Thus while some workers[22, 23, 24] were unable to demonstrate any functional abnormality in intestinal ischaemia, others[25, 26] found steatorrhoea which disappeared following arterial reconstruction. A study by Webb and Hardy[27] demonstrated abnormal absorption of carbohydrate and fat, measured respectively by the

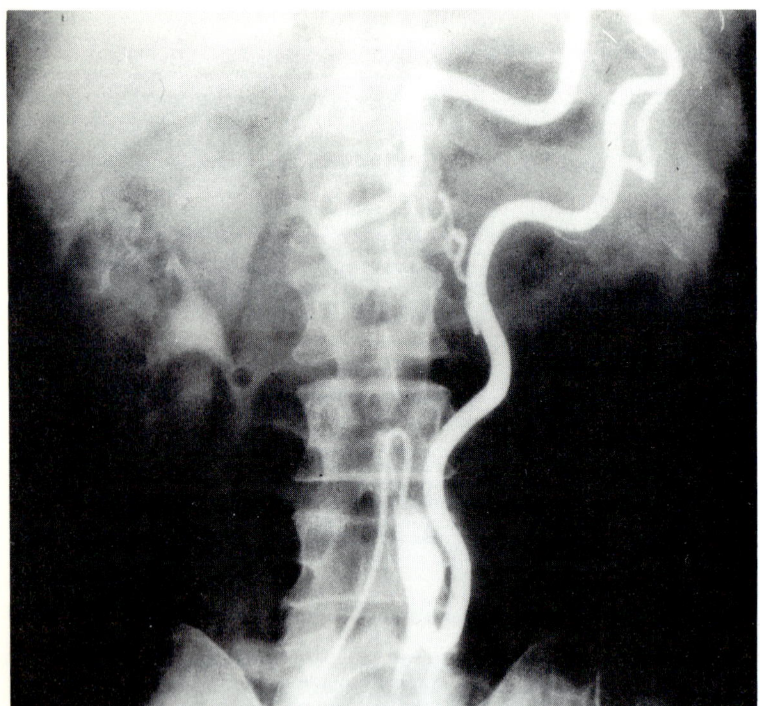

Fig. 8.5 Occlusion of the CA and the SMA, with stricture and poststenotic dilatation of the IMA, and retrograde flow in the marginal artery. (By courtesy of Dr R. Dick, Royal Free Hospital.)

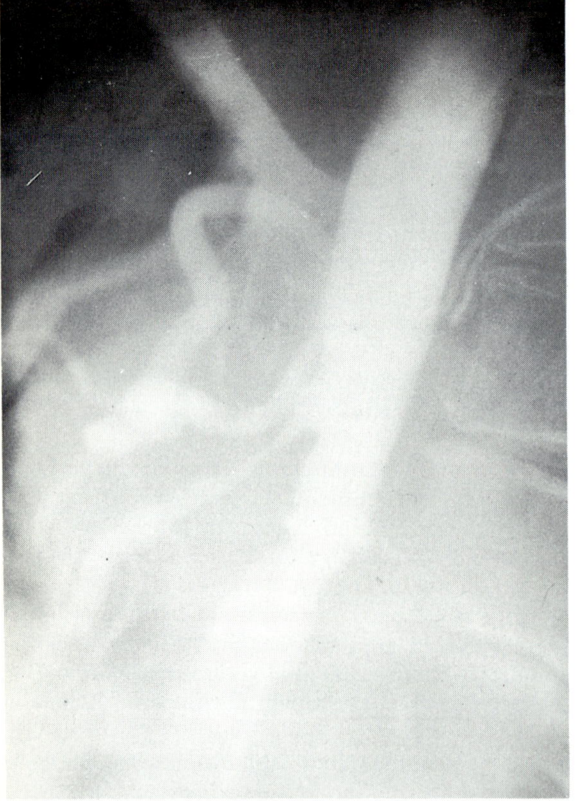

Fig. 8.6 Occlusion of the CA and long stenosis of the SMA. (This patient had a carcinoma of the pancreas proven by needle biopsy.)

d-xylose and ^{131}I-triolein techniques, which was corrected by aorto-SMA bypass. Larson, Spittel and Kirklin[28] reported abnormal serum carotene levels and increase in faecal fat, and Dardik et al.[29] confirmed abnormal preoperative serum carotene values, delayed absorption of radioiodinated triolein and impaired *d*-xylose absorption in their patient with SMA stenosis, which reverted to normal following operation.

Because of the lack of knowledge of the relationship between radiologically demonstrated lesions of the visceral arteries (IAO) and the symptoms and physiological variables in the individual patient, a prospective study of the problem was started in 1965 in the Department of Surgical Studies of The Middlesex Hospital,[13] and the data reported here extend to January 1984.

From 1962 to 1984 approximately 100 patients with abdominal pain were referred to our group as possible cases of treatable IAO. This total is necessarily inexact because, as already reported,[30] a number of these patients were not investigated further and are now untraceable, either because

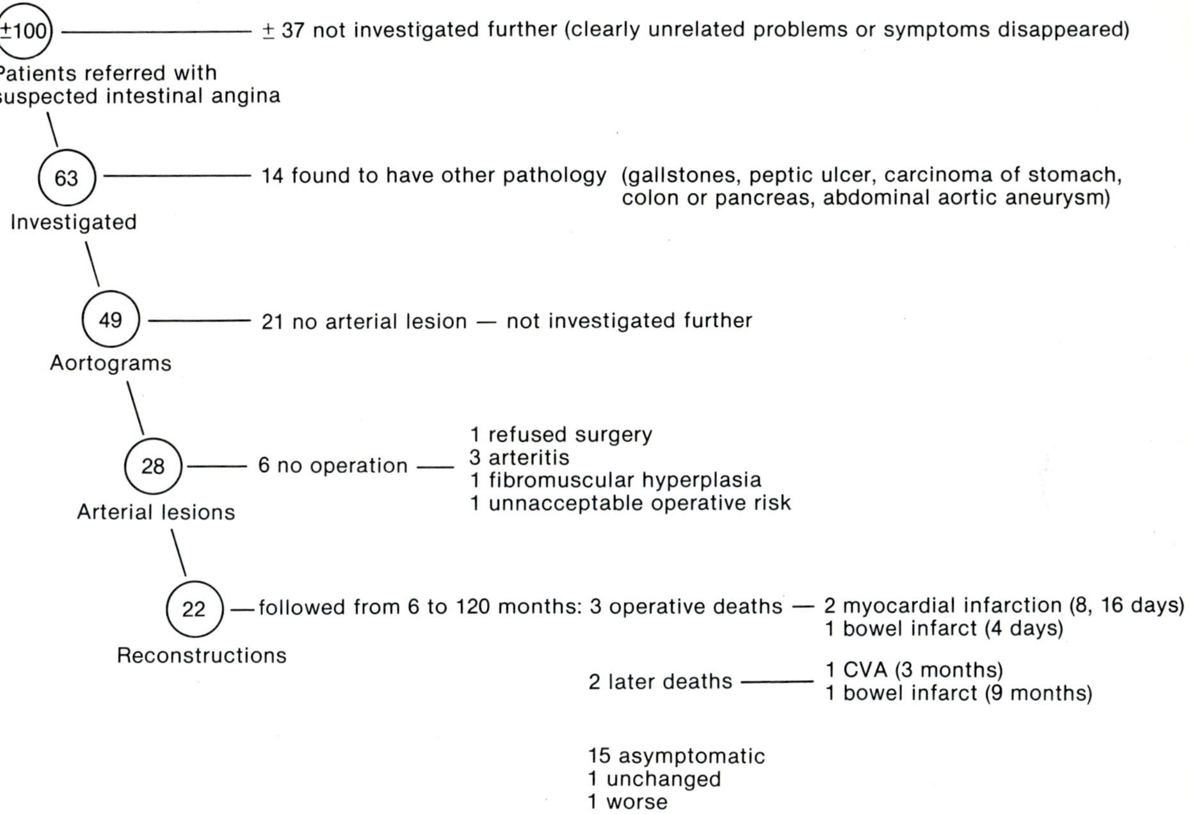

Fig. 8.7 Analysis of clinical experience of intestinal arterial occlusion (IAO) at The Middlesex Hospital, 1962–1984. (From Marston et al.[13] by kind permission of the Editor, *Gut*.)

their symptoms had disappeared when they arrived at the clinic or because their problems did not seem in any way to resemble those related to IAO and hence were not followed up. A further group were found on investigation to have other causes of abdominal pain, as is shown in Fig. 8.7; these patients were not submitted to angiography. Once these conditions had been excluded, angiography was carried out. In 21 the findings were normal. If the angiogram showed stenosis or occlusion of the main visceral arteries, it seemed ethical to submit the patient to a more exacting diagnostic procedure, in order to justify major surgery. Because all patients in this series presented with abdominal pain, this study does not relate to other reports in which IAO was found incidentally on angiograms carried out for different reasons, nor to arterial operations performed on patients without alimentary symptoms.

Table 8.1 shows the total group of patients studied. They were evaluated as follows.

Clinical appraisal

Symptoms All the patients, by definition, complained of adbominal pain related to meals and reported loss of weight and an alteration in bowel habit (either constipation or diarrhoea). Nausea and vomiting was noted in 9 and 20 gave a history relating to vascular occlusion elsewhere in the body.

Physical signs The 20 patients with arterial symptoms had objective evidence of arterial disease, as evidenced by absent lower limb pulses or by asymptomatic arterial bruits. An abdominal systolic bruit, although not always specifically sought, was found in 14. The significance of this sign is in any case doubtful.[27] Apart from weight loss, there were no other relevant abnormalities on examination.

Baseline investigation Physical evaluation was followed by baseline tests comprising chest x-ray,

Table 8.1 Intestinal function studies in chronic arterial disease

Case no.	Sex and age	Date of presentation	Duration of symptoms (months)	Arterial lesion			Associated vascular disease	Abnormalities detected	Operation	Course
				CA	SM	IM				
1	M54	1962	24	O	○	•	Bilateral claudication angina	Diabetic GTT	Ileocaecal-aortic Anastomosis	Symptom-free for 4 years. Death from myocardial infarction. anastomosis patent at autopsy
2	M60	1967	9	○	O	O	Nil	Nil	Patch CA	Pain persisted following surgery. Lost to follow-up after 1 year
3	F61	1969	6	○	•	O	Myocardial infarction	Protein loss (2.3%)	Aorto-SMA anastomosis	Alive and well 8 years after operation. Faecal protein loss reverted to normal post operation
4	M48	1970	24	•	○	O	Nil	Nil	Patch CA	Symptoms persist at 9 years
5	F65	1971	18	O	•	O	Mitral stenosis	Glucose (8 mmol/l) GTT (diabetic) Protein loss (2.19%)	None	Refused operation. Alive with same symptoms at 10 years
6	M27	1971	12	○	○	O	Nil	Ischaemic stricture seen on barium study	Patch CA	Symptom free 10 years after operation
7	M61	1972	12	•	•	•	Angina	Nil	Aorto-SMA anastomosis	Symptom free for 6 months, then death from cerebrovascular accident
8	F38	1974	6	•	•	•	Hypertension Carotid & vertebral stenosis	Nil	Aorto-SMA anastomosis	Death from bowel infarct 1 week after operation
9	M64	1974	9	○	•	O	Hypertension Claudication	Nil	Aorto-SMA anastomosis	Symptom free at 6 years
10	M51	1976	24	○	○	O	Nil	Nil	None	Alive and well at 3 years, some persistent symptoms
11	M40	1977	36	○	•	○	Ileal infarct resected previously	Faecal fat (8 g per day) Carotene (0.69 μmol/l) *d*-Xylose (25%) Previous resection on barium study	Aorto-SMA anastomosis	Further laparotomy 1979— blind loop resected. Symptom free 6 years post reconstruction
12	F44	1977	24	○	O	O	Nil	Nil	None	Subsequent psychiatric referral following suicide attempt
13	F46	1977	42	○	○	O	Nil	Nil	Freeing CA	Symptom free at 6 months — subsequently lost to follow-up
14	M44	1977	12	O	○	O	Myocardial infarction	Nil	Aorto-SMA anastomosis	Death 3 days post operation from myocardial infarct

15	F23	1980	24	Small vessel disease	Polyarteritis nodosa	Nil	None	Symptoms controlled on steroids at 2 years. Renal function deteriorating
16	F35	1981	30	○ O O	Nil	Nil	Patch angioplasty CA	Symptom free 1 year post operation
17	F45	1981	18	○ • •	Angina Claudication Below-knee amputation	Fe (12 μmol/l) TIBC (103 μmol/l)	Patch angioplasty SMA	Symptom free for 6 months, then reocclusion, infarction, resection, fistula, death 9 months post operation
18	M47	1981	30	○ ○ •	Splenic flexure resected for ischaemia	Nil	Laparotomy only	Symptom free for 6 months, then recurrence of mild discomfort
19	F56	1981	24	• ○ O	Hypertension	Nil	Patch angioplasty CA	Symptom free 2 years post operation
20	F61	1981	18	• • O	Claudication Below-knee amputation	Nil	Patch angioplasty CA & SMA	Symptom free 2 years post operation
21	F38	1981	48	○ • O	Aortitis Previous SMA surgery	Nil	None	Severe distal arteritis. Symptoms persist on steroids
22	F65	1981	12	• • O	Type II aortic dissection	*d*-Xylose (16%) gallstones on ultrasound	Reimplantation of SMA	Symptoms relieved. Lost to follow-up a few weeks post operation
23	M54	1981	6	• • ○	Hypertension	Duodenal ulcer on endoscopy, gallstones on ultrasound	Patch angioplasty CA & IMA	Reoperation for small bowel volvulus at 1 week. Cholecystectomy at 6 months. Symptom free at 1 year
24	M73	1982	12	○ O ○	Hypertension Angina Myocardial infarction	Nil	None	Symptoms continue at 1 year. Considered unacceptable operative risk
25	F77	1983	6	○ ○ •	Angina	Nil	None	Symptoms continue at 6 months
26	M61	1983	18	• • ○	Previous aortic surgery, angina	Fe (6 μmol/l) TIBC (105 υmol/l)	Patch angioplasty SMA	Symptom free at 6 months
27	F66	1983	12	○ • ○	Hypertension	Pyloric ulcer on endoscopy	Aorto-SMA bypass	Symptom free for 9 months. Graft then occluded and pain recurred. Patency restored and confirmed angiographically. Well to date
28	M55	1984	36	○ • ○	Previous aortic surgery	Faecal fat (13 g per day) *d*-Xylose (10%)	Patch SMA	Died at 10 days — myocardial infarction

O = normal vessel; ○ = stenosis; • = occlusion.
GTT, glucose-tolerance test; TIBC, total iron-binding capacity.
Reproduced from *Gut* (1985) by kind permission of the Editor.

Table 8.2 Reported cases of coeliac axis compression

Reference	No. of patients		Operations		Follow-up period (months)	Results
	Male	Female	Decompression	Reconstruction		
35	(2)		2		Unstated	2 symptomless
36	1	1			"	
37	2		2		"	2 symptomless
38	(27)		13 (+2)			Unstated
44	(17)		1	1	Unstated	2 unchanged
57		2	2		"	2 symptomless
58	1	3				
59	3	13	11		6–50	9 symptomless 3 improved 1 unchanged
60	3	27	25		12–48	18 symptomless 4 improved 3 unchanged
61	3	9	4	8	"	11 symptomless 1 unchanged
62	1		1		8	1 symptomless
63	1	2	1		Unstated	1 symptomless
64	1	1	2		"	2 symptomless
65	5	1	6	2	"	6 symptomless
66	(37)		Unstated		"	(good)
67		1	1		"	1 symptomless
68	2	4	3		"	3 symptomless
20	2	5	Unstated		"	2 symptomless
69		1		1	15	1 symptomless
70	3	2	5		Unstated	5 improved
71	5	10	12	1	"	7 symptomless 2 unchanged 2 worse
72						
50	10	40	47		6	39 symptomless 8 unchanged
39	4	4	6	1	6–50	4 symptomless
73	(30)		Unstated		12–48	20 symptomless 6 improved 4 unchanged
Totals	47 (113) =286	126	144 (+2)	14		131 symptomless 18 improved 26 unchanged or worse

ECG, blood film with indices and routine serum biochemistry in order to eliminate concomittant disease and to determine fitness for possible surgery.

Arteriography
In the first years of the study this was by the translumbar route. Subsequently the preferred technique was retrograde cathereterization via the femoral artery, with free injection into the aorta and selective opacification of the visceral turnks (see Figs. 8.2–8.5).

Tests of intestinal function
Once an arterial obstruction had been identified, the patient was further studied with regard to intestinal function. The tests applied necessarily reflect a series which has extended over 20 years (see Fig. 8.7), and nowadays would be modified in the light of recent experience. The following functions were investigated:

1. *Iron metabolism and vitamin B_{12} absorption* comprising serum iron concentration (Fe), total iron-binding capacity (TIBC), B_{12} and folate levels and the Schilling test for B_{12} absorption.

2. *Fat metabolism* comprising serum β-lipoprotein and fasting triglyceride levels, mean daily faecal fat excretion over 5 days, and also serum carotene concentrations, which, as mentioned above, have been reported[28, 29] as reflecting malabsorption of vitamin A in chronic intestinal ischaemia.

3. *Liver function*, by means of serum albumin and globulin levels, bilirubin, alkaline phosphatase and aspartate transaminase (AST).

4. *Carbohydrate absorption and metabolism*, comprising random blood glucose concentration, glucose tolerance test (GTT) following a 50 g dose and *d*-xylose excretion following a 25 g dose.

5. *Intestinal protein loss*, by measurement of faecal activity, following an intravenous dose of ^{51}Cr-labelled albumin.

6. *Barium studies.* These were initially by conventional upper gastrointestinal series, later by the intubated duodenal technique.

7. *Imaging.* The series was begun before fibrendoscopy of the alimentary tract or ultrasound examination were easily available, but later patients were studied with these techniques.

The results are set out in Table 8.1. It will be seen that the great majority of our patients had normal absorptive and exsorptive function as measured by the tests employed. Abnormalities did occur (deficient fat absorption in 2, carbohydrate absorption in 4 and an exudative protein-losing enteropathy in 2), but these were sporadic and bore no consistent relation to symptoms or to the arterial lesion. Because of this, it seemed pointless to repeat the tests following operation.

As in all previous case series, management was decided on clinical criteria, as no laboratory test gave sufficient discrimination. In practice this meant that significant IAO (i.e. that requiring operation) was identified by exclusion, so that only those patients who continued to complain of pain in the presence of a known arterial block, when a full clinical assessment had not produced any other explanation, were submitted to surgery.

This full evaluation of every case not only helps the individual patient but may perhaps in the future also provide us with a working profile of the disease which will enable us to identify others at risk. A corollary of this is that such information should be pooled so that the contribution of each individual clinician can be added to a common data bank.

It must be admitted that surgical enthusiasm has, to an extent, outrun science in the management of this condition. There have been many series of operations reported in the literature, designed rather to correct an aortographic appearance than to improve physiological disturbance. Nevertheless, following this pathway of evaluation, a core of patients will be identified who might benefit from surgery, and the techniques chosen need to be discussed.

Operative techniques

These may be direct or indirect.

1. *Direct attack* on the ostial lesion is the only possible method in the case of the CA, because of the situation of the artery. It is also used for the SMA (although there are alternatives). The reconstruction may take the form of patch,[31] reimplantation[31, 32, 33] or endarterectomy[33, 34] (see Fig. 8.8).

2. The other method comprises an *indirect attack* on the mesenteric system, avoiding the difficult territory of the origin of the SMA and having the advantage that it can be accomplished through a purely abdominal operation.

These will be discussed separately.

Direct exposure of the visceral trunks

This is best and most safely accomplished via a thoracoabdominal incision[30] (Fig. 8.9) which allows a complete and safe exposure of the supra-and infradiaphragmatic aorta, the median arcuate ligament, the origin of the coeliac axis, the mouth of the SMA, the neck of the pancreas and both renal arteries.

With the patient in an appropriate half-lateral position, the incision is developed along the line of the eighth rib, crosses the costal margin and is prolonged downwards into the left rectus sheath. The muscle layers are divided with diathermy, and the ribs spread apart with a Finochietto-type rib spreader. The abdominal contents are then carefully checked over in order to exclude non-vascular pathology. The diaphragm is incised circumferentially, to avoid dividing terminal branches of the phrenic nerve, to an extent which allows complete exposure of the thoracoabdominal

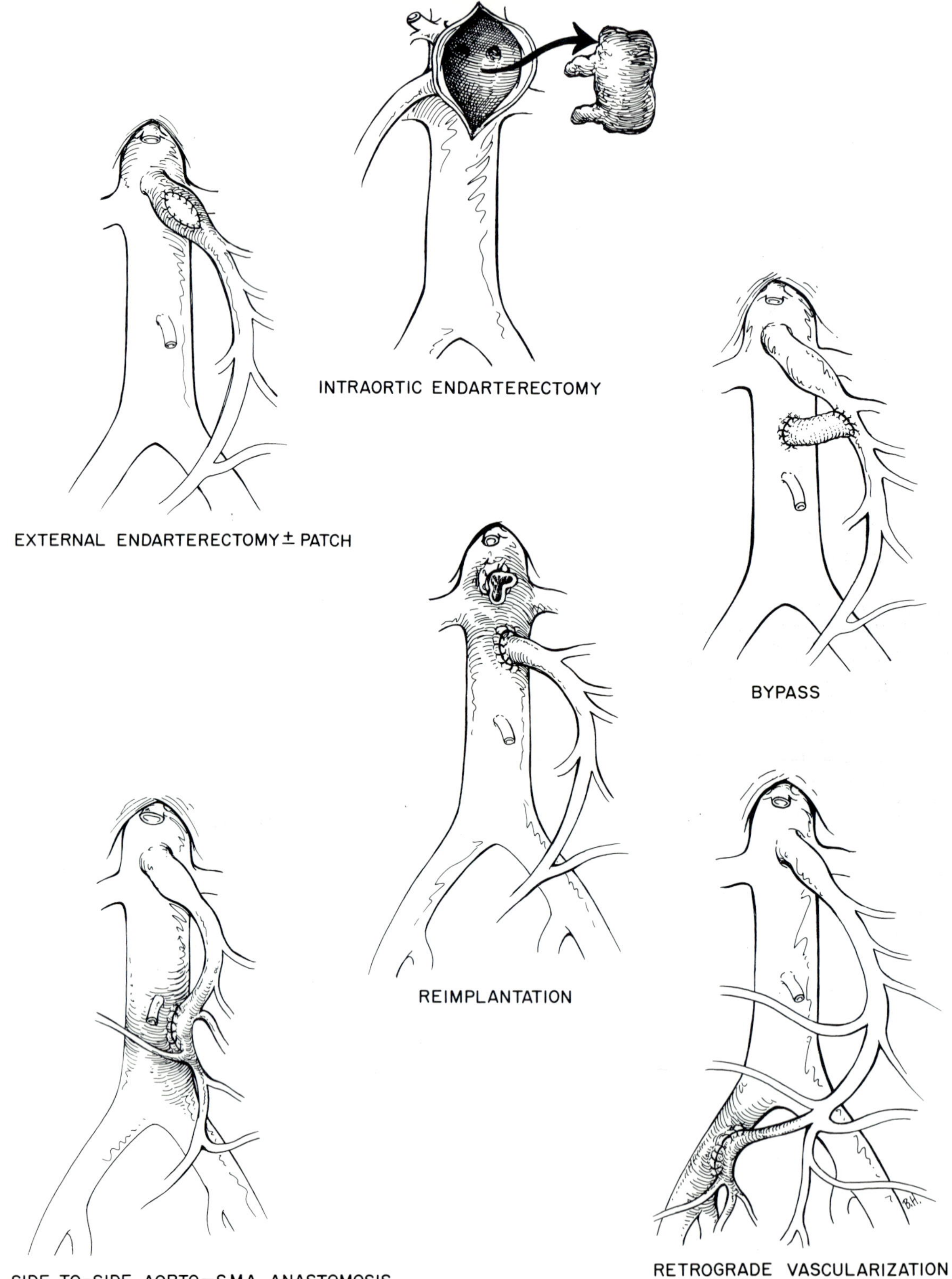

Fig. 8.8 Techniques for reconstruction of the intestinal circulation.

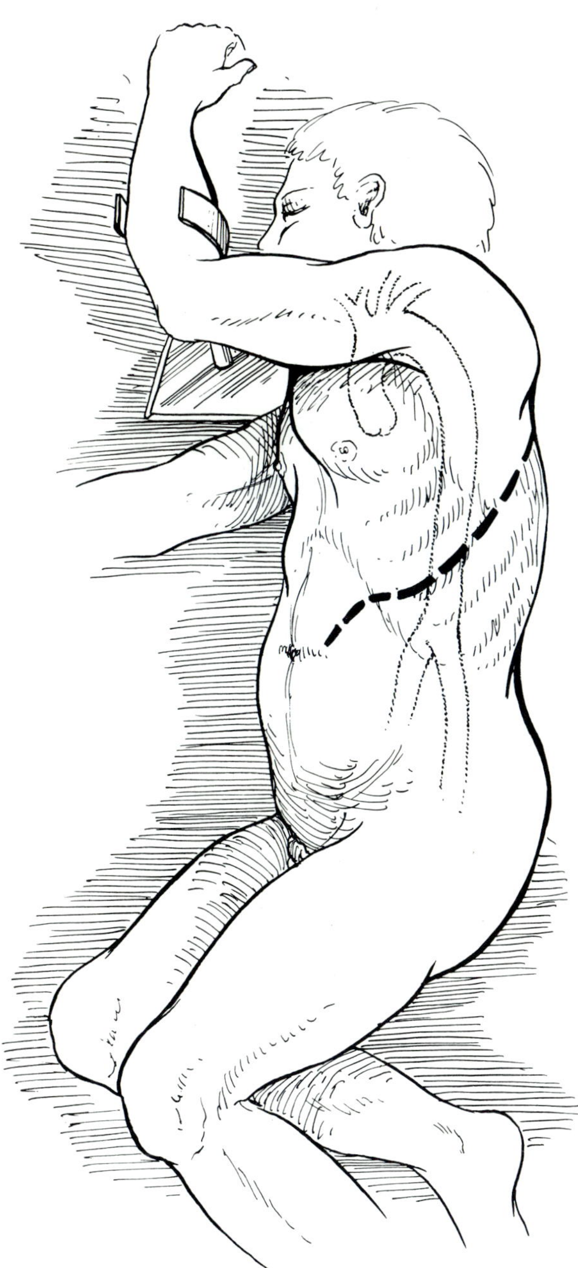

Fig. 8.9 The thoracoabdominal approach to the great vessels.

cavities. The peritoneum behind the spleen is incised and the spleen, the splenic vessels and the tail of the pancreas are mobilized over to the right, carrying with them the fundus of the stomach, until the aorta is clearly seen. Careful dissection with forward mobilization of the lymph nodes and vessels will expose the origin of the coeliac axis as it emerges from beneath the median arcuate ligament. Keeping close to the wall of the aorta, a plane of dissection can be developed which leads directly downards to the origin of the SMA (Fig. 8.10) which usually lies between 1 and 2 cm below that of the coeliac axis. Lateral clearance of the aorta brings into view the origins of the renal arteries, which are identified for their later preservation.

Having inspected and palpated the obstructing lesions, pressure measurements are taken in order to determine whether a significant gradient exists. A needle connected to a standard transducer and display device is inserted into the aorta, the coeliac axis and the SMA, and pressures are recorded at a stable state (Fig. 8.11). If an electromagnetic or Doppler flowmeter is available, it is conveniently applied at this stage.

The exact form of reconstruction will clearly depend on the symptomatology, the aortographic appearances and the recorded pressure and flow profile. Available techniques are as follows:

1. Division of the median arcuate ligament of the diaphragm, freeing the origin of the coeliac axis. This is discussed in detail below.
2. Patch angioplasty. This requires application of a side-clamp to the aorta (Fig. 8.12) and coeliac axis, followed by a longitudinal incision across the origin of the vessels, and insertion of a patch of Teflon, Dacron or previously removed distal saphenous vein to broaden the origin.
3. Transaortic endarterectomy, by which the origins of the CA, SMA and, if necessary, both renal arteries can be opened. This is the technique developed in San Francisco by Dr R.J. Stoney and his colleagues[33] (see Fig. 8.8).
4. Alternatively, the vessels can be detached and reimplanted, following similar application of a side-clamp to the aorta (see Fig. 8.8).

The same techniques are applicable to both the CA and the SMA, with the proviso that great care must be taken not to occlude the origins of the renal arteries when the clamp is applied low down. Following reconstruction, the pressure gradient is again measured or the flow probe reapplied, in order to verify or check the improvement.

Indirect approach

By this is meant procedures designed to revascularize the intestine which do not encroach on the origin

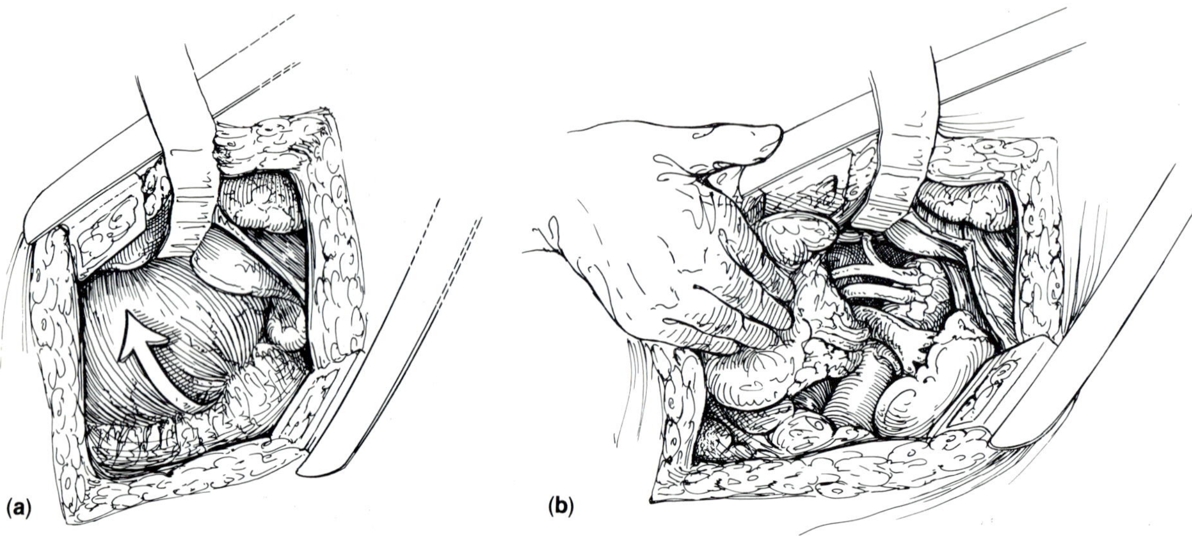

Fig. 8.10 The stomach, spleen and pancreas are mobilized to the right.

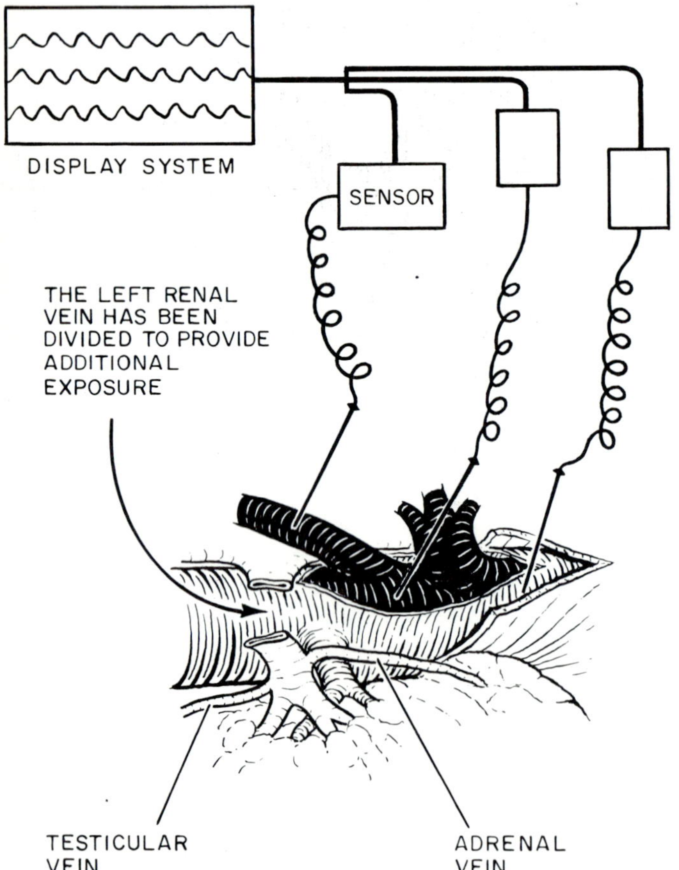

Fig. 8.11 Measurement of pressure gradients in the great vessels.

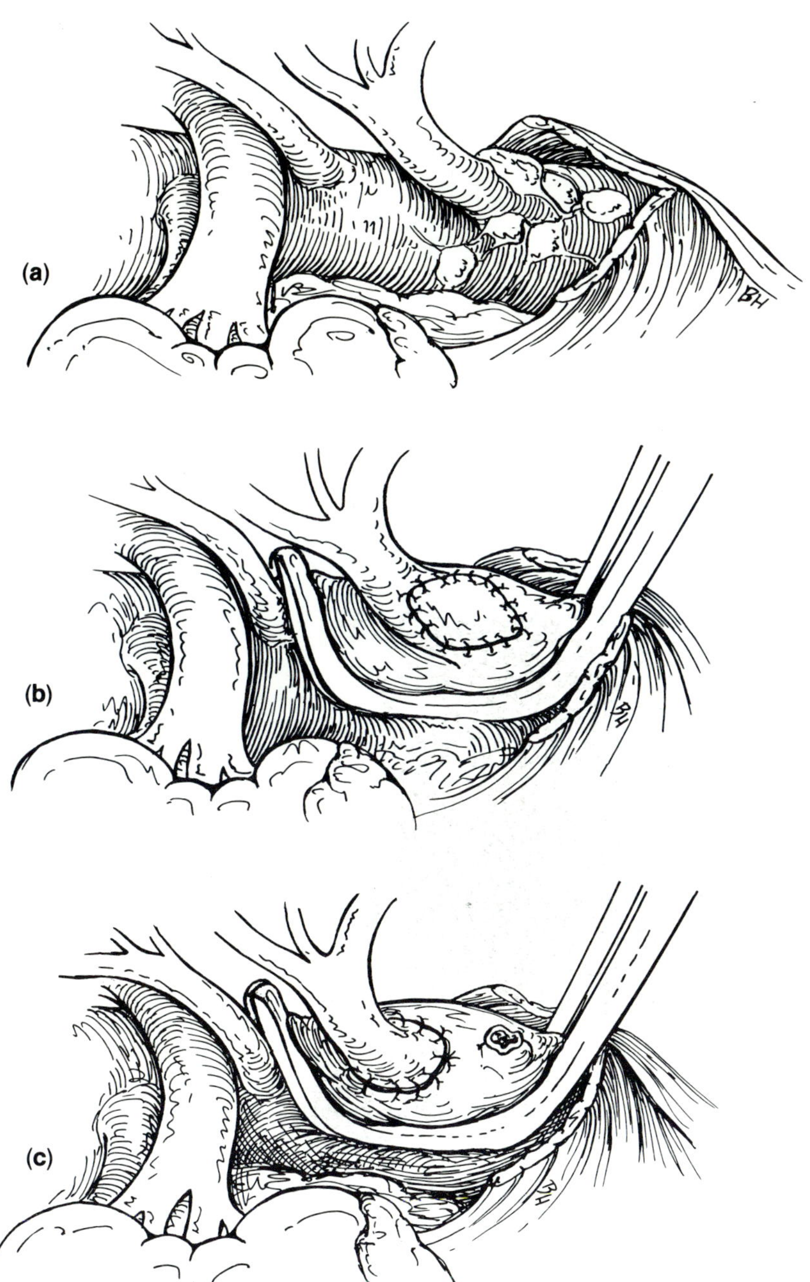

Fig. 8.12 (**a** and **b**) Applying a patch to the CA. (An identical technique can be used for the SMA.) (**c**) Reimplantation of the CA.

of the coeliac axis or the SMA. These have the great advantages of avoiding the need to open the chest, and at the same time steering clear of the difficult anatomical territory around the origin of the great vessels.

The standard incision is a long left paramedian, extending from just to the left of the xiphistenum to a point halfway between the umbilicus and the symphysis pubis. The peritoneum is opened and the abdominal contents are carefully explored in the standard order.

Assuming that no other lesion has been found and that all is well within the peritoneal cavity, the revascularization proceeds according to the site of the main lesion.

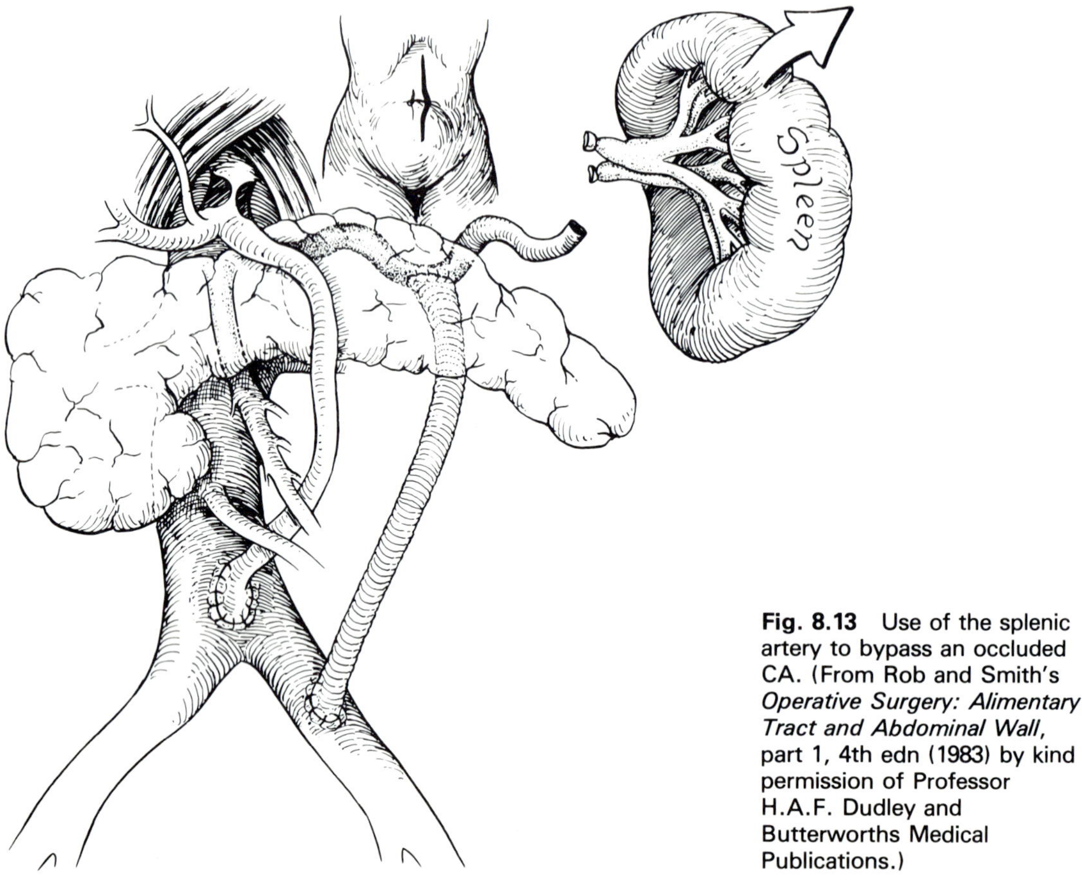

Fig. 8.13 Use of the splenic artery to bypass an occluded CA. (From Rob and Smith's *Operative Surgery: Alimentary Tract and Abdominal Wall,* part 1, 4th edn (1983) by kind permission of Professor H.A.F. Dudley and Butterworths Medical Publications.)

Occlusion of the coeliac axis

This is dealt with by utilizing the splenic artery which, following removal of the spleen, is a convenient channel for retrograde irrigation of the coeliac territory. The artery may be implanted into the aorta, or a bypass may be inserted between it and the aorta or common iliac artery. In either case, the object is achieved of perfusing the coeliac axis distal to the occlusion or stenosis from an area of higher pressure (Fig. 8.13).

A more usual situation is stenosis or occlusion of the SMA. In fact, if normal arterial pressure is restored to the SMA territory, a coexistent lesion of the coeliac axis can often be ignored, as the collaterals will have been developed to such an extent that adequate perfusion of the upper zone is assured. However, some reports[34] deny this and insist on the need to restore patency to all occluded vessels.

There are various methods of revascularization of the SMA, all of which require the same exposure (see Fig. 8.14). To achieve this, the transverse colon is lifted upwards out of the wound and its mesentery incised over the origin of the middle colic artery. This vessel is then followed upwards to the main trunk of the SMA, which is then carefully freed from its companion vein. The SMA is mobilized up and down over some 3–4 cm, carefully preserving each intestinal artery as it is encountered, until a sufficient length has been mobilized for it to lie comfortably against the aorta.

The peritoneum overlying the abdominal aorta is then incised and reflected medially and laterally so as to expose the whole circumference of the vessel for 5 cm. If the aorta is of large calibre (4 cm or more in diameter) then it will usually be possible to effect the side-to-side anastomosis by application of a side-clamp to the aorta, without interrupting flow (see Fig. 8.12). Usually, however, the diameter of the aorta is not big enough to allow the anastomosis to be performed comfortably in this way, and it is necessary to occlude it completely. This involves

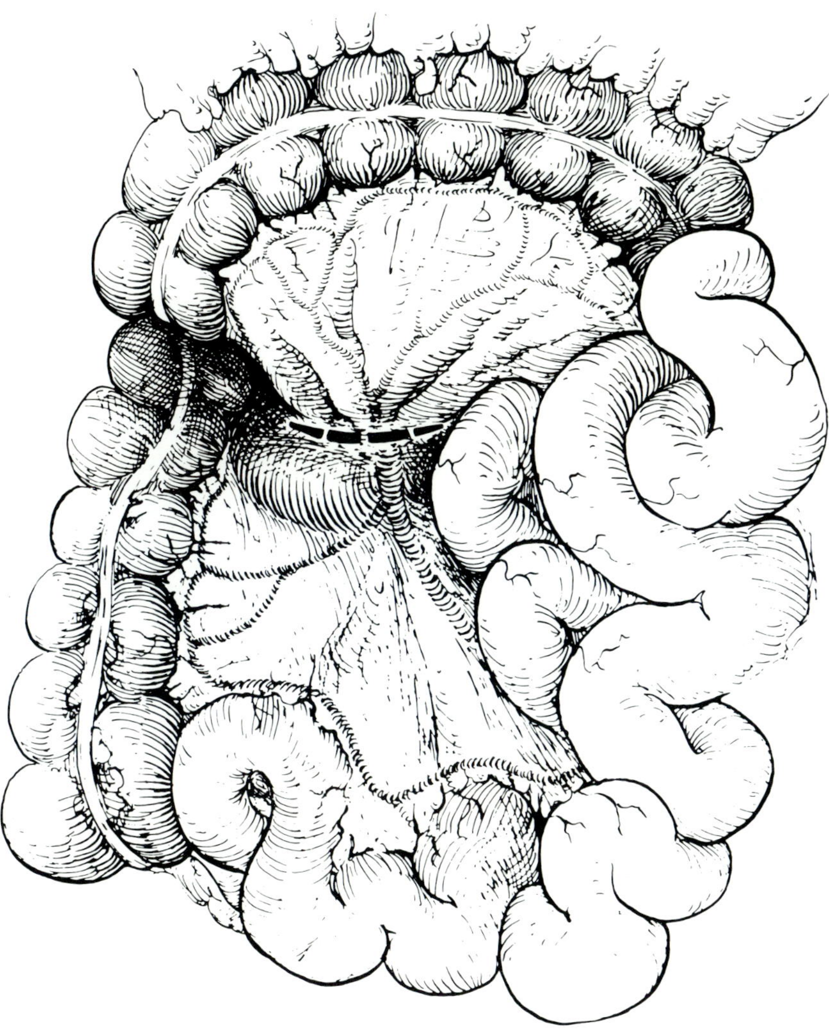

Fig. 8.14 Approach to the origin of the SMA from below. (From Rob and Smith's *Operative Surgery: Alimentary Tract and Abdominal Wall*, part 1, 4th edn (1983), by kind permission of Professor H.A.F. Dudley and Butterworths Medical Publications.)

circumferential dissection of a 5 cm length, the lumbar branches being controlled with thread snares or bulldog clips (Fig. 8.15).

Whenever the aorta is completely occluded, the renal circulation is protected by transfusing 20 g of mannitol intravenously.

Having controlled the aorta and the SMA, the two vessels are approximated without tension by manipulating the controlling clamps, and a 2 cm longitudinal arteriotomy is made in each of them (Fig. 8.16a). A stay-suture of 4/0 synthetic material connects the arteriotomies at each end, and a continous running suture completes the posterior layer (Fig. 8.16b). As the end of this layer is reached, the suture is tied and the anterior layer then completed (Fig. 8.16c). Before final closure, clamps are briefly released from the aorta and the SMA in order to flush out any accumulated clot or debris. The anastomosis is then rapidly closed and the clamps removed, following which pressure measurements are again recorded.

An interesting finding during the performance of this type of anastomosis is that whereas the aorta is usually thickened and atheromatous, the part of the SMA used for the anastomosis, which lies distal to the block, is thin, supple and healthy. This illustrates the protective effect of a proximal arterial stenosis on the distal arterial tree, and helps to explain the relative rarity of atheromatous stenoses in the intestinal vessels themselves. There is some

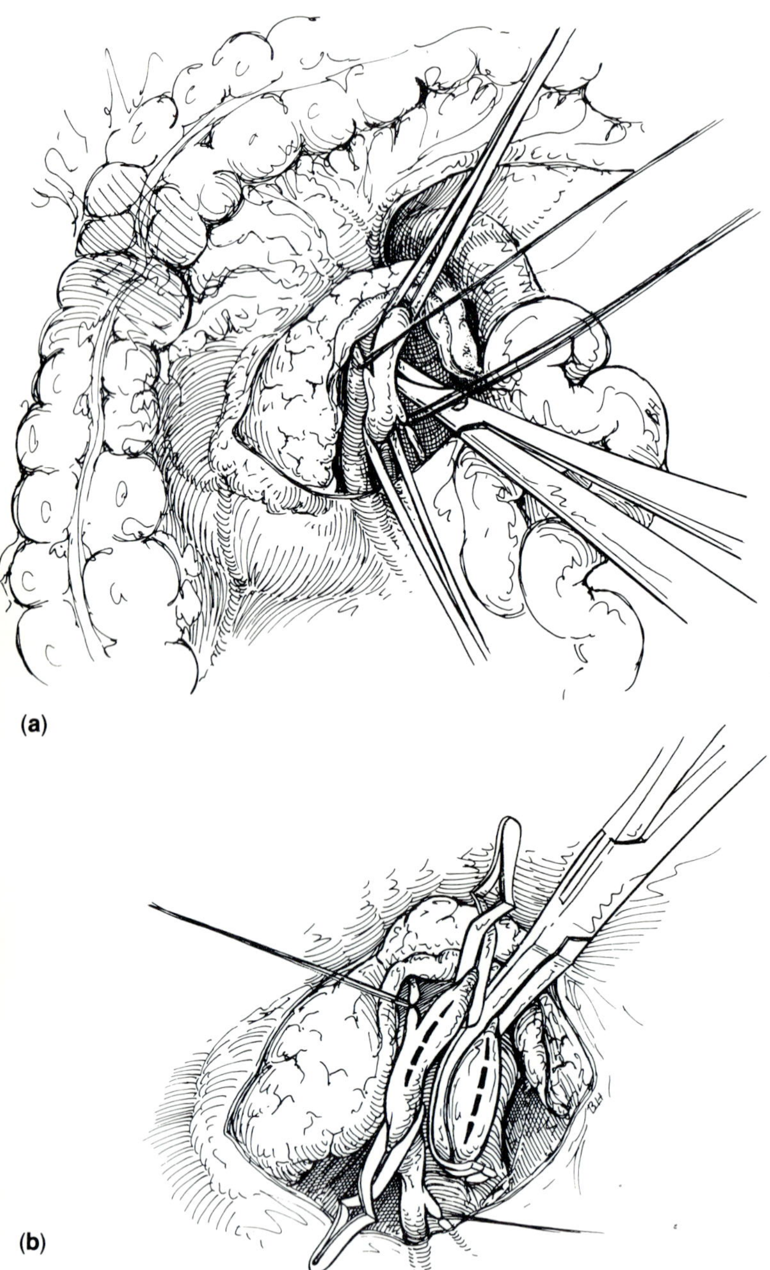

Fig. 8.15 Exploring and mobilizing the SMA. (From Rob and Smith's *Operative Surgery: Alimentary Tract and Abdominal Wall*, part 1, 4th edn (1983), by kind permission of Professor H.A.F. Dudley and Butterworths Medical Publications.)

evidence to suggest that, in the lower limb, restoration of a normal distal pressure by means of an arterial reconstruction deprives the smaller vessels of this type of protection, so they begin to develop plaques of atheroma. There is as yet no information forthcoming as to whether this process operates in the mesenteric circulation.

This operation (side-to-side aorto-SMA anastomosis) is safe and simple to carry out, and is of wide general applicability. The size of the stoma which can be obtained is illustrated in Fig. 8.17, and is comparable with that following patch grafts (Fig. 8.18).

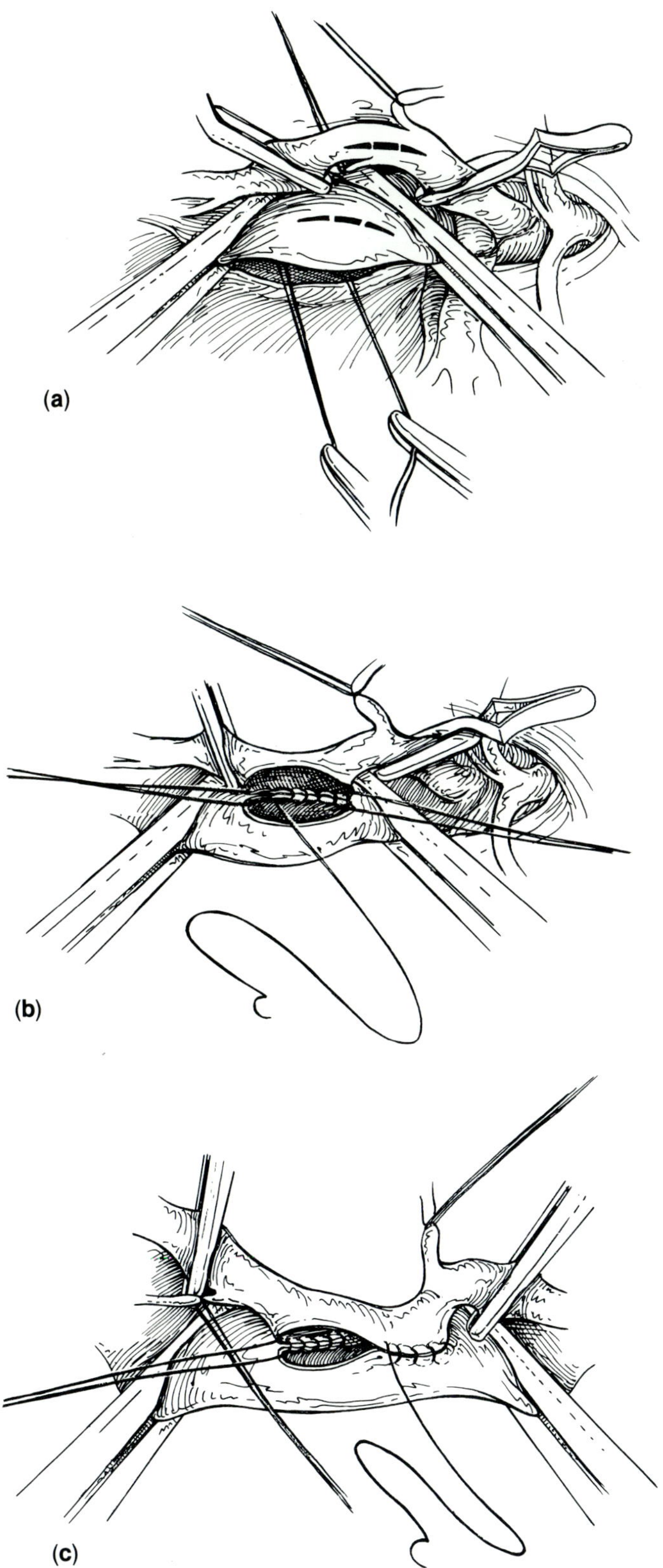

Fig. 8.16 The side-to-side aorta-SMA anastomosis. (From Rob and Smith's *Operative Surgery: Alimentary Tract and Abdominal Wall*, part 1, 4th edn (1983), by kind permission of Professor H.A.F. Dudley and Butterworths Medical Publications.)

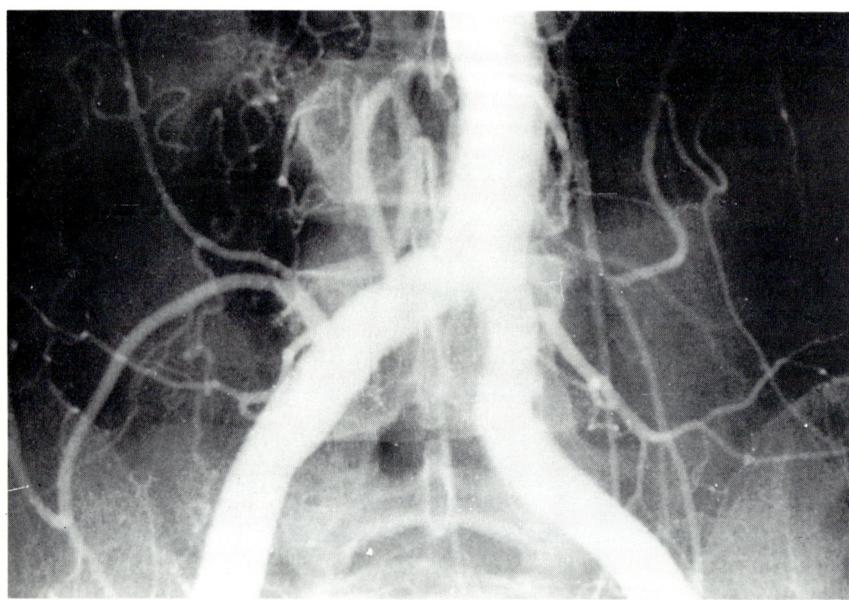

Fig. 8.17 Postoperative angiogram showing the result of side-to-side aorto-SMA anastomosis. (By courtesy of Mr R.W. Marcuson.)

The coeliac axis compression syndrome (Fig. 8.19)

In 1963 Harjola[35] reported from Finland the case of a 57-year-old man who had complained for 10 years of colicky epigastric pains following meals and who was found on clinical examination to have an arterial bruit in the upper abdomen. A lateral aortogram demonstrated stenosis of the origin of the coeliac axis. At operation it was found that the artery itself was normal but that it was compressed by the fibres of the median arcuate ligament of the diaphragm. Division of these fibres abolished the palpable thrill and audible bruit, and was followed by complete relief of the patient's pain when he was seen 2 months later.

Harjola was impressed by the similarity of this pain to 'classic' intestinal angina as described above, but was careful not to impute the symptoms to a reduction of blood supply, postulating rather a neural origin, due to fibrosis of the coeliac ganglion.

The concept of coeliac axis compression causing ischaemia of the upper abdominal viscera quickly caught on, however, and further cases were brought to light and operated upon. Thus Vollmar et al.[36] and Gautier, Barrie and Sarrazin[37] each treated 2 patients by division of fibrous tissue, muscular bands and sympathetic nerves, with complete relief of symptoms. Dunbar et al.[38] then described a series of 21 patients, all of whom had epigastric pain after meals, associated with a systolic bruit. In 15 of these a lateral aortogram disclosed compression of the coeliac axis and this was confirmed in 13 at laparotomy. Although no very high pressure gradients were recorded across the stenoses, it was felt that there was impairment of flow, and indeed all these patients were relieved of their symptoms after division of the median arcuate ligament.

Following this work, there have been a large number of cases reported in the literature, in which the coeliac axis (and, more rarely, the SMA) has been 'freed up', with relief of pain. Some authors have gone further than this and have actually carried out a reconstruction of the origin of the coeliac axis[39] (Fig. 8.20) if simple division of the ligament did not appear to bring about adequate improvement in pressure and flow. This case material is summarized in Table 8.2.

In an attempt to validate the concept of coeliac axis compression leading to ischaemia, there have been a number of laboratory studies. Thus Anderson et al.[40] studied the effect of graded occlusion of the coeliac axis with a Goldblatt clamp in a number of dogs, and demonstrated that, as the lumen was progressively reduced, ulceration of the stomach and duodenum, and later actual infarction of the small bowel, occurred with increasing frequency. The number of survivors corresponding-

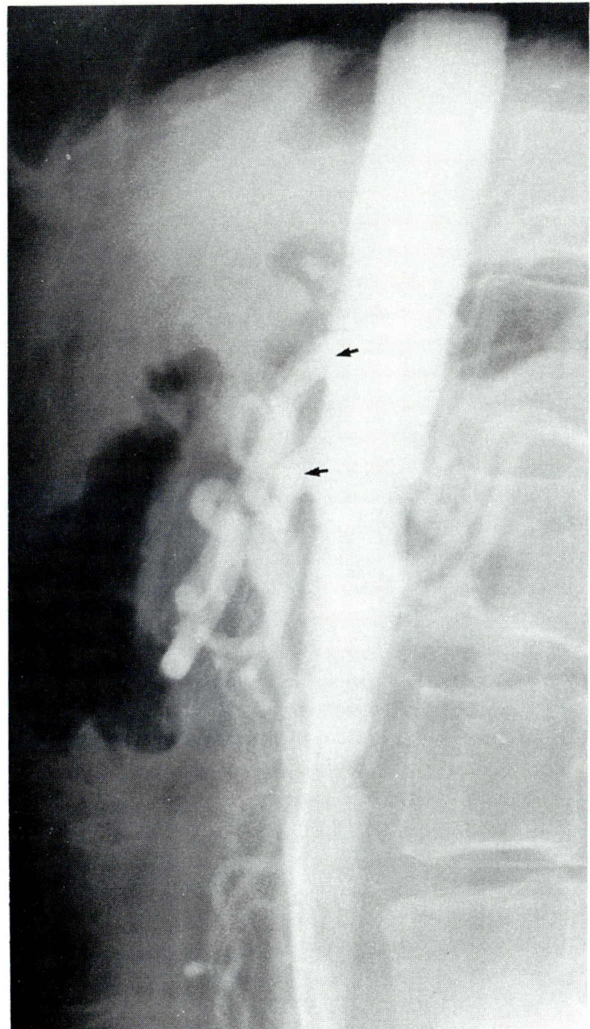

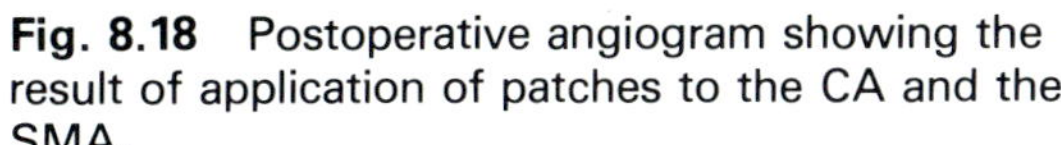

Fig. 8.18 Postoperative angiogram showing the result of application of patches to the CA and the SMA.

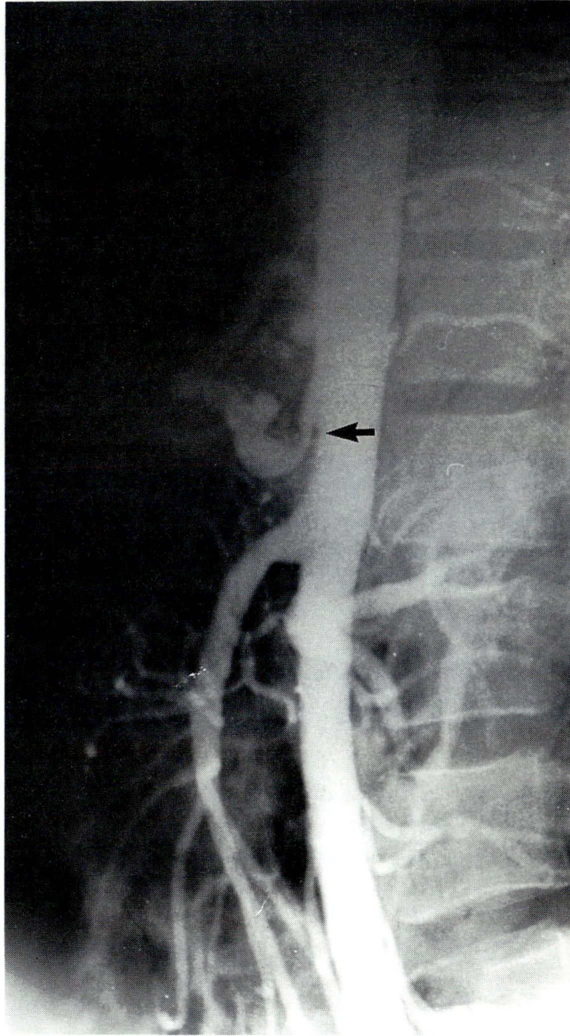

Fig. 8.19 Coeliac axis compression.

ly declined, so that with a 75 per cent occlusion one-third of the animals had died at 2 days, and of 5 dogs undergoing a total occlusion, none survived. Stanley and Fry[41] studied the effect of chronic coeliac axis occlusion on *d*-xylose absorption following the challenge of a meat meal. It is already known that no change in xylose absorption occurs under standard conditions following complete chronic occlusion of the SMA[42] but the authors felt that in the postabsorptive state the situation might be different, and indeed were able to demonstrate some impaired absorption in the 7 dogs they studied.

The challenge

Whilst there remains a substantial body of surgical opinion which is convinced that the coeliac axis compression syndrome is a genuine entity, which can be completely relieved by division of the median arcuate ligament, others do not share this view. The

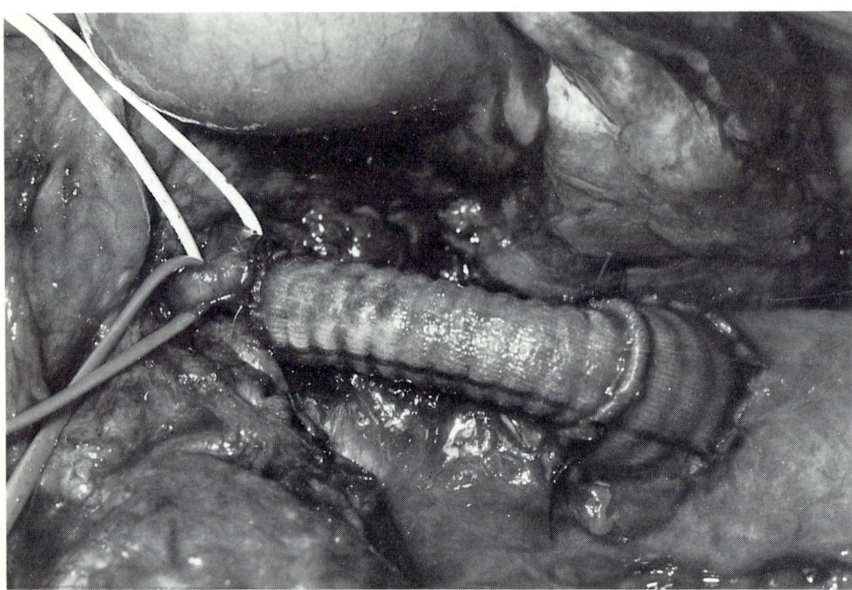

Fig. 8.20 Aortocoeliac bypass. (By courtesy of Mr R.W. Marcuson.)

earliest note of caution was struck by Reuter,[43] reporting from Lund, who examined 720 aortograms carried out between 1959 and 1965 in their department: 17 cases of coeliac axis stenosis or occlusion were picked out, of whom 5 had no abdominal symptoms and 7 had other types of pathology to account for their abdominal pain. Of the remaining 5 patients, 2 had cirrhosis and 1 was thought to have a peptic ulcer; the other 2 demonstrated stenosis of the inferior mesenteric artery as well as of the coeliac axis, and, largely by exclusion, are presumed to be genuine cases of visceral ischaemia.

The following year, Drapanas and Bron[44] reported their 17 patients with coeliac axis stenosis or occlusion, of whom 6 were asymptomatic and 6 were suffering from gross intra-abdominal surgical pathology. Of the remaining 5, 1 patient underwent splenoaortic anastomosis, with no effect on the symptoms; in another, the coeliac axis was freed up by division of adhesions, but again the symptoms continued unabated. The other 3 patients all had extensive psychiatric problems. Bron and Redman, in a later paper,[45] reported a 17 per cent incidence of CA and SMA stenosis in 713 aortograms, all of which were asymptomatic. Edwards et al.[20] found that, of 200 healthy medical students, 13 had epigastric bruits of whom 1 complained of dyspepsia, whereas of 25 dyspeptics 1 had a bruit; 7 patients who had pain, bruit and a positive angiogram were offered operation, of whom 2 refused. Of the 5 patients operated upon, 2 lost their symptoms but the remainder were unchanged or worse. The authors were the first to measure pressure and flow during the operation, and were unable to correlate these with either preoperative symptoms or postoperative result. The frequency of asymptomatic stenosis of the coeliac axis has been further confirmed by Cornell[46] and Colapinto, McLoughlin and Weisbrod.[47]

A powerful onslaught on the whole idea of coeliac axis compression was mounted by Szilagy et al.[48] who, following an extensive review of the literature, pointed out the variable nature of the symptoms described, the uncertainty of its relationship to 'true' intestinal angina resulting from SMA occlusion, and the lack of objective measurements recorded in the literature. These authors emphasized the fact that the postulated fault in coeliac compression was ischaemia, and consequent dysfunction, of the small bowel. No one had seriously suggested that there was any disturbance in function of the stomach, as this organ has an abundantly rich collateral blood supply, and it is within the experience of every general surgeon that it can be extensively devascularized without any impairment of function.[49] The theory is that the collateral vessels which develop as a result of coeliac artery stenosis 'steal' blood from the midgut loop, thus causing intestinal angina. However, the symptoms reported in the literature are of extreme variability, even if they are adequately described, which is by no means always the case. The only constant symptom is abdominal pain, but this is of quite unpredictable character, duration and relationship to meals. The so-called 'typical' pain is in fact reported in only 40 per cent of the total number of patients. Similarly, weight loss and diarrhoea are rare, and malabsorption, when sought, is almost never present. The results of pressure and flow studies are equally equivocal. It is noteworthy that among the patients described there is a high incidence of psychological problems and of multiple previous abdominal explorations. Furthermore, a number of patients had additional, more mundane, abdominal problems such as peptic ulcer and gall-bladder disease, which might well have contributed to or even been entirely responsible for the symptoms, and certainly treatment of these conditions is as plausible a reason for the disappearance of pain as is the (possibly irrelevant) division of the median arcuate ligament.

Szilagy and his associates went on to analyse their own clinical material. Examination of 200 000 new hospital admissions from 1965 to 1971 failed to reveal any case of supposed coeliac artery compression syndrome which satisfied them as showing a combination of angina, radiologically demonstrated coeliac artery stenosis and weight loss, and which was reversed by division of the median arcuate ligament. They did, however, find 24 cases in which coeliac axis compression had been considered as causing pain, other abdominal pathology having been ruled out. Additionally, on reviewing 157 unselected abdominal angiograms, they found a 49 per cent incidence of coeliac axis stenosis. Interestingly, the incidence of stenosis was more or less evenly distributed between patients with and without abdominal pain and with and without gastrointestinal disease.

Evans[50] carried out a long-term evaluation of the 'coeliac band syndrome', studying 71 patients aged from 13 to 68 treated between the years 1963 and 1971. All of these patients had had a long history of abdominal pain, and 70 per cent of them had undergone previous abdominal surgery. Of the 59 patients traced from the original 71, 47 had undergone division of the median arcuate ligament (in 3 a cholecystectomy had been performed in addition) and 12 had been treated conservatively. At the initial follow-up examination which was carried out less than 6 months after the operation, 39 patients were free of symptoms and in 8 the situation was unchanged. However at the later follow-up of 40 of these patients carried out at 3–11 years after the surgical procedure, the picture was very different. Of 18 patients who were asymptomatic, 13 had been reoperated upon for other abdominal conditions such as gall-bladder disease, peptic ulcer or subacute obstruction, leaving only 5 who ascribed their maintained improvement to the operation on the arcuate ligament. There were 4 patients who still had some symptoms although were somewhat improved, and 22 in fact reverted to this original preoperative condition; 2 of these were subsequently rid of their pain by cholecystectomy.

Of the 12 patients not subjected to surgery, 9 were asymptomatic, 1 was improved and 2 had retained their symptoms. It was interesting that there was no correlation between the condition of the patient at the original presentation and the achieved result at late follow-up.

The mesenteric steal syndrome

The question arises as to whether, in patients with severe occlusive disease of the lower aorta where the legs are supplied by the mesenteric system (usually via the marginal artery of the colon), intestinal angina can arise on exercise (Chapter 5). This had been called the aortoiliac steal syndrome[51] but perhaps the mesenteric steal syndrome would be a better term, blood being 'stolen' from the gut due to decreased peripheral resistance in the legs. Although Strandness and Sumner[52] on closely argued haemodynamic grounds, have postulated that this does not occur, other authors[53, 54] have reported convincing examples. Harris and Charlesworth[53] describe a 51-year-old patient who complained of severe abdominal pain on eating or exercise, which was corrected by the insertion of an aortobifemoral bypass. This patient had a dilated marginal artery through which the SMA supplied both legs. (Fig. 8.21).

Discussion

The diagnosis of chronic intestinal ischaemia remains a challenge. Dunphy in 1936[5] demonstrated that 7 out of 12 patients dying from acute occlusion of the SMA gave a prodromal history of abdominal pain. Others[18] have reported that

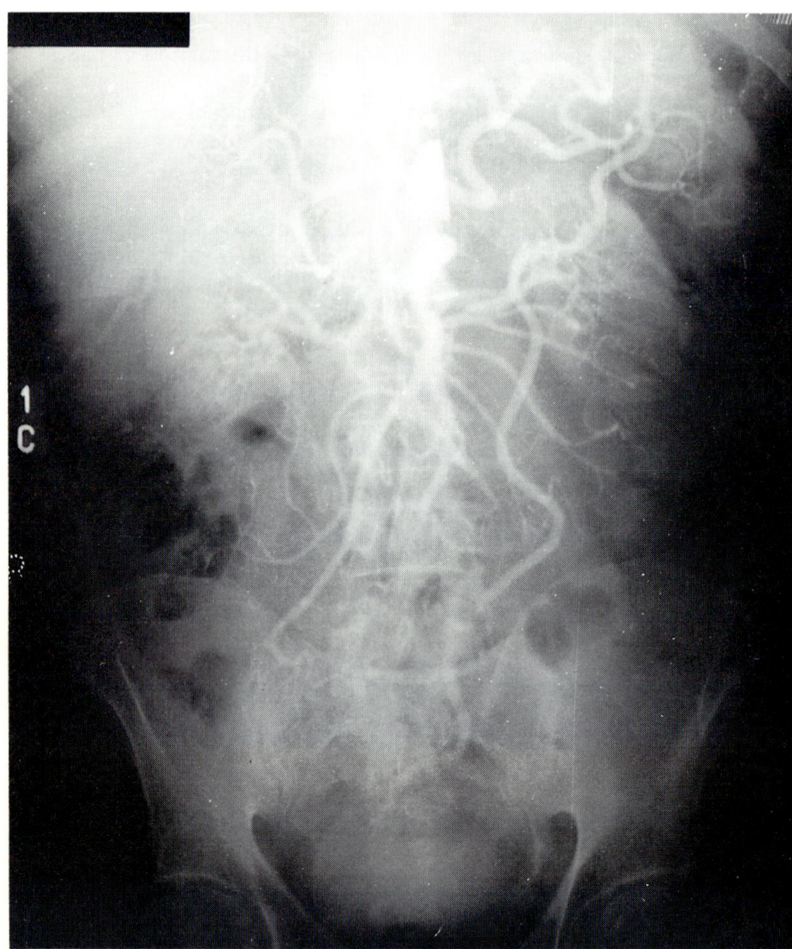

Fig. 8.21 The mesenteric steal syndrome. Note the enlarged marginal artery to the colon, supplying the lower limbs. (From the *Journal of Cardiovascular Surgery* (1974) **15**: 122, by kind permission of Mr David Charlesworth.)

asymptomatic patients with occluded main visceral arteries may be precipitated into acute intestinal infarction by a fall in central arterial pressure, however caused. Some surgeons therefore favour prophylactic correction of any such occlusion seen on an angiogram, whilst others would operate only on those who are symptomatic.

Clearly, diagnostic tests which could accurately identify the patient who is at risk of infarction would be valuable. Arteriography reveals the vascular lesion, but the clinical relevance of such appearances are not certain enough to allow a surgical decision to be made. This is because asymptomatic lesions are common[11, 12] and how much they constitute a threat to life has yet to be decided. Almost certainly, resting blood flow in such patients is within normal range, and the pain which some of them experience after eating represents failure of the gut to produce the hyperaemia which the processes of propulsion and digestion require. This would equate with what is being observed as happening in other vascular territories such as the heart and the legs. There is ample evidence that resting blood flow in the claudicating limb is normal, and the deficiencies appear only when the circulation is challenged by exercise. If this obtains in the alimentary tract, it is not at all surprising that tests of intestinal function carried out in hospital are found to be quite normal, even with gross mesenteric arterial occlusion.

By means of various compensatory mechanisms to redistribute blood flow in the wall, the absorptive area appears capable of working satisfactorily virtually to the point of irreversible damage. Because of available collateral circulation (particularly in the coeliac and inferior mesenteric territories), major occlusion in the visceral arteries can be compensated for, to the extent that the gut is not ischaemic and no symptoms occur. This compensation may additionally be effected by internal switching mechanisms at submucosal level[55] and by the operation of the countercurrent exchange mechanism within the villus. In any event, the tips of the villi, which are the main absorptive area, receive only some 8 per cent of total flow. As arterial input is reduced still further, then pain arises from the ischaemic muscle which does not receive the increased flow required by the peristalsis initiated by food, but still the mucosal flow remains normal and insorptive/exsorptive capacity is unimpaired. Hansen et al.[56] showed that total splanchnic flow rises in (arteriographically) normal subjects following a meal, and that this rise fails to occur in patients with IAO but can be restored by suitable surgery.

As vascular disease progresses, resting flow eventually falls below the level required to maintain the mucosal defences against osmolar and bacterial challenge, and infarction (focal or massive) results. One might postulate four stages:

0 Normal.
1 An arterial lesion is present but compensated so that both resting and postcibal flow are unimpaired and there are no symptoms.
2 The arterial disease has progressed to the point where resting flow is normal but reactive hyperaemia cannot occur. This is signalled by the occurrence of postcibal pain.
3 The blood supply is so deficient that resting flow is reduced and perhaps minor impairments of cellular function and small focal infarcts are occurring. This is analogous to 'rest pain' in the ischaemic limb.
4 The bowel is infarcted.

It is the identification of stage 3 which has been the subject of so much clinical and laboratory endeavour over the last eighty years, since Schnitzler[1] first postulated the concept of 'abdominal claudication', and it must be admitted that little progress has been made. Many authors have commented that tests of intestinal function have little predictive value, although no formal prospective study had up till now been carried out. Nevertheless, it has often been stated that chronic IAO is associated with malabsorption. Our data suggest that this is not the case, and that the weight loss which occurs is due to diminished intake. Quite different, of course, is the patient who sustains an acute ischaemic episode and is rescued by emergency surgery from a threatened infarction.

Conclusions

It is clear from the statistics in Fig. 8.7 and Table 8.2, as well as from a considerable amount of unpublished anecdotal material, that a number of patients with a combination of upper abdominal pain, epigastric bruit and narrowed origin of their visceral arteries do express gratitude following arterial reconstriction or division of the median arcuate ligament of the diaphragm. However, it is difficult to go beyond this point and to prove that the pain is caused by diminished blood flow, that this interferes with function and that the symptoms and the dysfunction are cured by surgery.

The placebo effect of a major operation, particularly when carried out by an attentive, enthusiastic and positive-minded surgeon, is enormous. It is fallacious to suppose that an operation is curative simply because the patient feels better after it, and the history of surgery is littered with inappropriate procedures which have been evaluated in this way. Surgical success can be evaluated only on strict criteria.

1. There must be a constant and definite syndrome, so that all can agree that they are treating the same problem. The 'atypical' case, therefore cannot, by definition, exist. This certainly does not apply to chronic intestinal ischaemia, in which the published series have included patients with widely differing modes of presentation and complaint.

2. There must be a constant and definite structural or functional abnormality which it is intended to correct. Extensive anatomical and radiological studies have shown that narrowing of the visceral arteries is a common finding in all manner of people with and without symptoms, and must therefore be considered as much an anatomical variant as a pathological abnormality. Also, no consistent pattern of dysfunction has ever been demonstrated in the alimentary tract, resulting from such lesions. This applies both to haemodynamic studies and to measurements of absorption and excretion.[13]

3. The abnormality must be eliminated following the operation. It is not enough to cure the symptoms. What is necessary is to show a measurable disturbance of function which has been

corrected. Such has yet to be found in chronic SMA occlusion, and this applies with even more force with regard to the coeliac artery compression syndrome.

Because of these fundamental objections, the tide of surgical opinion has now swung strongly against the concept that isolated narrowing of the origin of the coeliac axis is responsible for symptoms, or that operations designed to relieve it retain validity. To prove a negative is impossible, and indeed it cannot be said that division of the median arcuate ligament is in every case an irrelevant operation. However, the burden of proof that this major surgical intervention is beneficial rests with its proponents.

Atheromatous occlusion of the SMA, particularly in combination with other arterial stenoses, is in a different category because there is much circumstantial evidence that such lesions can be dangerous. However, they are not always so, and it remains difficult to distinguish the life-threatening from the clinically irrelevant mesenteric arterial block.

References

1 Schnitzler, J. Zur Symptomatologie des Darmartevienverschlüsses. *Münch. Med. Wochenschr.* (1901) **98**: 5.

2 Meyer, J. Intermittent claudication involving the intestinal tract. *J.A.M.A.* (1924) **83**: 1414–5.

3 Sedlacek, R.A., Bean, W.B. Abdominal angina. The syndrome of intermittent ischemia of the mesenteric arteries. *Ann. Intern. Med.* (1957) **46**: 148–52.

4 Mikkelsen, W.P. Intestinal angina — its surgical significance. *Am. J. Surg.* (1957) **94**: 262–7.

5 Dunphy, J.E. Abdominal pain of vascular origin. *Am. J. Med. Sci.* (1936) **192**: 109–12.

6 Chiene, J. Complete obliteration of the coeliac and mesenteric arteries. *J. Anat. Physiol.* (1869) **3**: 65–72.

7 Maljatzkaja, M.I. Über die Atherosklerose der Baucharterien. *Beitr. Path. Anat.* (1934) **98**: 81–90.

8 Johnson, C.C., Baggenstoss, A.H. Mesenteric vascular occlusion. *Proc. Mayo Clin.* (1949) **24**: 649–56.

9 Carucci, J.J. Mesenteric vascular occlusion. *Am. J. Surg.* (1953) **85**: 47–51.

10 Derrick, J.R., Pollard, H.S., Moor, R.M. The pattern of arteriosclerotic narrowing of the celiac and superior mesenteric arteries. *Ann. Surg.* (1959) **149**: 684–90.

11 Reiner, L. Mesenteric arterial insufficiency and abdominal angina. *Arch. Intern. Med.* (1964) **114**: 765–72.

12 Croft, R.J., Menon, G.P., Marston, A. Does intestinal angina exist? A critical study of obstructed visceral arteries. *Br. J. Surg.* (1981) **68**: 316–18.

13 Marston, A., Clarke, J.M.F., Garcia Garcia, J., Miller, A.L. Intestinal function and intestinal blood supply. *Gut* (1985) **26**: 656–66.

14 Ranninger, K., Scheiner, D.L. Experimental bowel ischemia. *Arch. Surg.* (1967) **95**: 768–70.

15 Delmont, J.P. L'Insuffisance artérielle dans les territoires du tronc céliaque et des mésenteriques supérieure et inférieure. *J. Chir.* (1965) **101**: 213–36.

16 Bergan, J.J., Dry, L., Conn, J. Trippel, O.H. Intestinal ischemic syndromes. *Ann. Surg.* (1969) **169**: 120–26.

17 Marston, A., Kieny, R., Szilagyi, D.E., Taylor, G.W. Intestinal ischemia: a panel by correspondence. *Arch. Surg.* (1976) **111**: 107–12.

18 Marston, A. The bowel in shock. *Lancet* (1962) **2**: 365–70.

19 Reul, G.J., Wukasch, C., Sandiford, F.M., Chiarillo, L., Hallman, G.L., Cooley, D.A. Surgical treatment of abdominal angina. Review of 25 patients. *Surgery* (1974) **75**: 682–9.

20 Edwards, A.J., Hamilton, J.D., Nichol, W.D., Taylor, G.W., Dawson, A.M. Experience with coeliac axis compression syndrome. *Br. Med. J.* (1970) **1**: 342–5.

21 Dick, A.P., Graff, R., Gregg, McC., Peter, N., Sarner, M. Arteriography study of mesenteric arterial disease. *Gut* (1967) **8**: 206–20.

22 Rampal, P., Delmont, J.-P. La malabsorption d'origine ischémique existe-t-elle? *Chirurgie des Artères Digestives.* Paris: Expansion Scientifique (1975) 11–23.

23 Zelenock, G.B., Graham, L.M., Whitehouse, W.M., et al. Splanchnic arterial disease and intestinal angina. *Arch. Surg.* (1980) **115**: 479–501.

24 Hollier, L.H., Bernatz, P.E., Pairolero, P.C., Payne, W.S., Osmundson, P.J. Surgical management of chronic intestinal ischemia. *Surgery* (1981) **90**: 940–6.

25 Brandt, L.J., Boley, S.J. Ischemic intestinal syndromes. *Adv. Surg.* (1981) **15**: 1–45.

26 Morgan, R.J., Russell, R.I., Imrie, C.W., Pollock, J.G. Chronic small bowel ischaemia presenting as chronic pancreatitis. *Postgrad. Med. J.* (1982) **58**: 121–2.

27 Webb, W.R., Hardy, J.D. Relief of abdominal angina by vascular graft. *Ann. Intern. Med.* (1962) **57**: 289–94.

28 Larson, R.E., Spittel, J.A., Kirklin, J.W. Insuffi-

ciency of superior mesenteric artery. *Proc. Mayo. Clin.* (1963) **38**: 436–40.

29 Dardik, H., Scheidenberg, B., Parker, J.G., Hurwitt, E.S. Intestinal angina with malabsorption treated by elective revascularization. *J.A.M.A.* (1965) **194**: 1206–10.

30 Marston, A. *Intestinal Ischaemia.* London: Edward Arnold (1977) 111–12.

31 Crawford, E.S., Morris, G.C., Myhre, H.O., Roehm, J.F. Celiac axis, superior mesenteric and inferior mesenteric artery occlusion: surgical considerations. *Surgery* (1977) **82**: 856–66.

32 Marston, A. Stenosis of the coeliac axis and superior mesenteric artery. *Ann. R. Coll. Surg. Engl.* (1972) **50**: 327–8.

33 Stoney, R.J., Ehrenfeld, W.K., Wylie, E.J. Revascularization methods in chronic visceral ischemia, caused by atherosclerosis. *Ann. Surg.* (1977) **186**: 486–70.

34 Hollier, L.H. Revascularization of the visceral artery using the pantaloon vein graft. *Surg. Gynecol. Obst.* (1982) **155**: 415–6.

35 Harjola, P.R. A rare obstruction of the celiac artery — report of a case. *Ann. Chir. Gyneac. Fenn.* (1963) **52**: 547–50.

36 Vollmar, J., Hartnet, H., Hasse, M., Schröder, E., Coerper, H.G. Das Chronische Verschluss-syndrom der Eingweide — Schlagadern. *Langenbecks Arch. Klin. Chir.* (1964) **305**: 473–90.

37 Gautier, R. Barrie, J., Sarrazin, R. Les angors abdominaux non-athéromateux. *Lyon Chir.* (1965) **61**: 893–4.

38 Dunbar, J.D., Molnar, W., Berman, F.F., Marable, S.A. Compression of the celiac trunk and abdominal angina. *Am. J. Roentgenol.* (1965) **95**: 731–6.

39 Beger, H.G., Mevers, M., Apitzch, D., Kraas, E., Bittner, R. Diagnose und operative Behandlung bei Arteria Coeliaca Kompression. *Dtsch. Med. Wochenschr.* (1975) **100**: 464–71.

40 Anderson, M.C., Schiller, W.R., Suwa, M., Geurking, R.E. Morphologic effects of graded celiac artery ischemia. *Bull. Soc. Int. Chir.* (1968) **27**: 468–77.

41 Stanley, J.C., Fry, W.J. Median arcuate ligament syndrome. *Arch. Surg.* (1971) **103**: 252–8.

42 Marston, A. *Intestinal Ischaemia.* London: Edward Arnold (1977) Table 6.2.

43 Reuter, S.R. Accentuation of celiac compression by the median arcuate ligament of the diaphragm during deep expiration. *Radiology* (1971) **98**: 561–4.

44 Drapanas, J., Bron, K.M., Stenosis of the celiac artery. *Ann. Surg.* (1966) **164**: 1084–91.

45 Bron, K.M., Redman, H.C. Splanchnic artery stenosis and occlusion. *Radiology* (1969) **92**: 323–8.

46 Cornell, S.H. Severe stenosis of the celiac axis. *Radiology* (1971) **99**: 311–19.

47 Colapinto, R.F., McLoughlin, M.J., Weisbrod, G.L. The routine lateral aortogram and the celiac compression syndrome. *Radiology* (1972) **103**: 557–61.

48 Szilagyi, D.E., Rian, R.L., Elliott, J.P., Smith, R.F. The celiac artery compression syndrome: does it exist? *Surgery* (1972) **72**: 849–63.

49 Lord, R.S.A., Stoney, R.J., Wylie, E.J. Celiac axis compression. *Lancet* (1968) **2**: 795–8.

50 Evans, W.E. Long term evaluation of the celiac band syndrome. *Surgery* (1974) **76**: 867–71.

51 Trippel, O.H., Jurayi, M.N., Midell, A.L. The aorto-iliac steal. *Arch. Surg.* (1971) **175**: 454–6.

52 Strandness, D.E., Sumner, D.E. (editors) *Hemodynamics for Surgeons.* New York: Grune & Stratton (1975) 376–8.

53 Harris, P.L., Charlesworth, D. Chronic intestinal ischaemia due to aorto-iliac steal. *J. Cardiovasc. Surg.* (1974) **15**: 122–4.

54 Granger, D.N., Richardson, P.D.I., Kvietys, P.R., Mortillaro, N.A. Intestinal blood flow. *Gastroenterology* (1980) **78**: 837–63.

55 Jodal, M., Haglund, V., Lundgren, O. Countercurrent exchange mechanisms in the small intestine. In: Shepherd, A.P., Granger, D.N., eds. *Physiology of the Intestinal Circulation.* New York: Raven Press (1984) 83–96.

56 Hansen, H.J.B., Engell, H.C., Ring-Larsen, H., Ranek, L. Splanchnic blood-flow in patients with abdominal angina before and after arterial reconstruction. *Ann. Surg.* (1977) **186**: 216–20.

57 Snyder, M.A., Mahoney, E.B., Rob, C.G. Symptomatic celiac artery stenosis due to constriction by the neurofibrous tissue of the celiac ganglion. *Surgery* (1967) **61**: 372–6.

58 Schmidt, H., Schimanski, K. Die Stenose der Arteria Coeliaca — ihre Diagnose und Klinische Bedeutung. *Fortschr. Röntgenstr.* (1967) **106**: 1–12.

59 Harjola, P.T., Lahtihaju, A. Celiac axis syndrome. *Am. J. Surg.* (1968) **115**: 864–9.

60 Marable, S.A., Kaplan, M.F., Berman, F.M., Molnar, W. Celiac axis compression syndrome. *Am. J. Surg.* (1968) **115**: 97–100.

61 Lord, R.S.A., Stoney, R.J., Wylie, E.J. Coeliac axis compression. *Lancet* (1968) **2**: 795–8.

62 Fadhli, H.A. Congenital diaphragmatic obstruction of the aorta and celiac artery. *J. Thorac. Cardiovasc. Surg.* (1968) **55**: 431–3.

63 Deutsch, V. Compression of the celiac trunk and the angiographic evaluation of its hemodynamic significance. *Clin. Radiol.* (1968) **19**: 309–14.

64 Carey, J.P., Stemmer, E.A., Connolly, J.E. Median arcuate ligament syndrome. *Arch. Surg.* (1969) **99**: 441–6.

65 Olivier, C., Rettori, R., Dimaria, G. Sténoses non-atheromateuses et compressions du tronc céliaque. *Chirurgie* (1970) **96**: 471–81.

66 Hivet, M., Legadec, B., Poilleux, J. Les sténoses chroniques du tronc coéliaque. *Chirurgie* (1970) **96**: 483–6.

67 Jamieson, A., Greig, J.H. Isolated celiac axis compression as a cause of visceral angina. *Can. Med. Ass. J.* (1970) **103**: 374–5.

68 Cormier, J.M., Fontaine, P. Sténose extrinsèque du tronc celiaque. *Chirurgie* (1970) **96**: 453–6.

69 Curl, J.H., Thompson, W.N., Stanley, J.L. Median arcuate ligament compression of the celiac and superior mesenteric arteries. *Ann. Surg.* (1971) **173**: 320.

70 Mulder, D.S., Rubush, J., Lawrence, M.S., Ehrenheft, J.L. Celiac axis compression syndrome. *Can. J. Surg.* (1971) **14**: 123–6.

71 Stanley, J.C., Fry, W.J. Median arcuate ligament syndrome. *Arch. Surg.* (1971) **103**: 252–8.

72 Heberer, G., Dostal, G., Hoffman, K. Zur Erkennung und operativen Behandlung der Chronischen Mesenterialarterieninsuffizienz. *Dtsch. Med. Wochenschr.* (1972) **97**: 750–54.

73 Kieny, R., Cinqualbre, J., Eisenmann, B., Tongio, J. Ischémie mésentérique chronique. *Ann. Radiol.* (1976) **19**: 371–5.

9

Focal ischaemia of the small intestine

Introduction

The fact that insufficiency of arterial supply can produce, first, inflammation and, later, ulceration and stenosis of a loop of small intestine has been known since the eighteenth century.[1,2] It was confirmed in the laboratory in 1909 by Bolognesi,[3] who demonstrated that interference with small vessels led to oedema of the intestinal wall and infiltration of small round cells into the submocusa, later followed by the formation of a fibrous stricture. During this century there has been a great increase in the incidence both of inflammatory bowel disease and of degenerative conditions of the vascular system, and interest has begun to focus on ischaemia as a pathological process which can evoke a spectrum of responses in the small bowel, which may mimic Crohn's disease and other similar conditions.

The whole subject was carefully reviewed by Raf,[4] who examined the records of 12 surgical services in the Stockholm area over the period 1954–1965. He was able to trace 9536 patients with non-malignant small bowel disease, of whom 95 (1 per cent) had presented with a non-inflammatory stricture. Of these patients, 59 had cardiovascular problems and had been under treatment for arterial hypertension and 14 had received radiotherapy to the pelvis, while the remainder had histories of strangulated hernia, abdominal trauma, internal haemorrhage or mesenteric vascular occlusion. In 1 case no cause could be found, and it is worthwhile noting that Thaker, Weingarten and Friedman[5] have drawn attention to the fact that non-occlusive ischaemia can give rise to intestinal stricture formation.

Causation

The following have been described in the literature as important causes of focal ischaemia of the small intestine:

1. Strangulation by external hernia or bands.[6,7,8,9]
2. Trauma to the abdominal wall.[10,11]
3. Acute ischaemia due to occlusion of the SMA, embolization to the small vessels or 'non-occlusive' mechanisms[5,12,13] (see Chapter 5).
4. Inflammatory disease of the vessels of the gut wall.[14,15,16,17]
5. Carcinoid tumours.[15,16]
6. Radiation injury.[18,19]
7. Action of enteric-coated potassium or other drugs acting directly on the mucosal circulation.[20]
8. Oral contraceptive agents.[21]

Strangulation (Fig. 9.1)

The first description is probably that of Garengoet,[1] who described some narrowing of the bowel associated with hernia, which he attributed to pressure from an ill-fitting truss. The condition was successfully operated upon by Vincent.[2] However, credit for the first definitive description of ischaemic damage following a strangulated hernia undoubtedly belongs to Guignard,[22] who described thickenings, constricting rings and loss of mucosa encountered at the time of operation for strangulated hernia. In 1892 Garré[23] produced his classic paper which contains the first description of delayed intestinal obstruction. The patient was a 27-year-old man who, 6 weeks after an operation for strang-

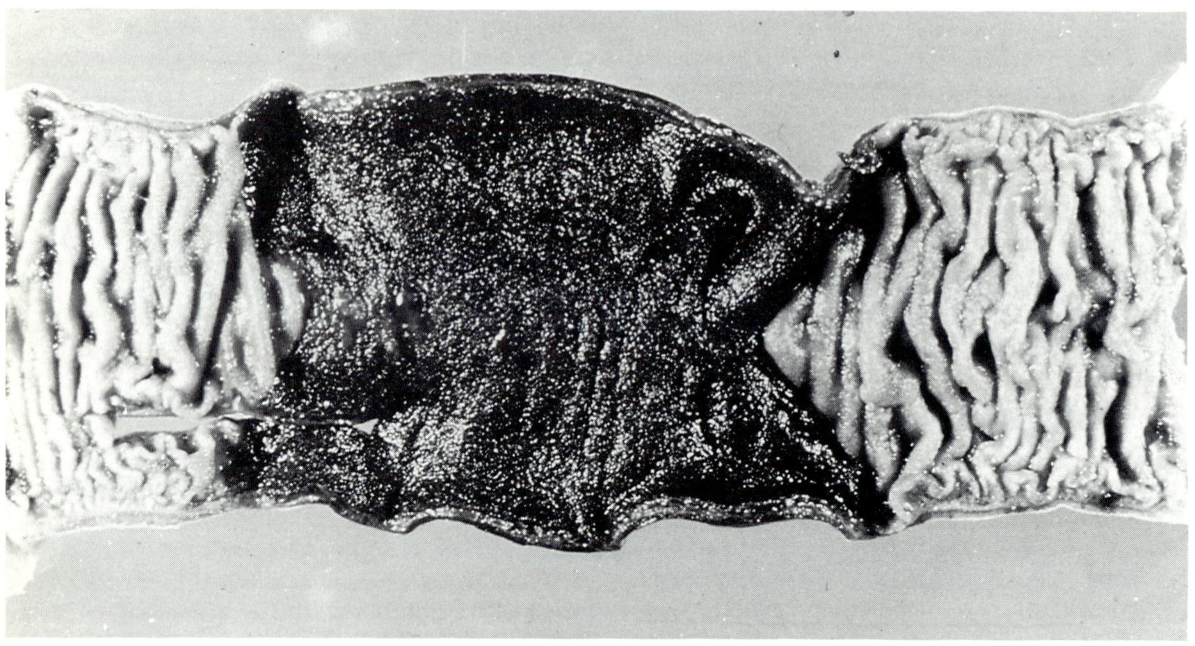

Fig. 9.1 Area of acute ischaemia caused by strangulated hernia. The bowel is viable but damaged, and if returned to the abdomen would probably give rise to a fibrous structure.

ulated hernia at which compromised, though viable, gut had been returned to the abdomen, developed symptoms of intestinal obstruction, and at a second operation was found to have a 20 cm long stenosis which was densely adherent to other loops of small bowel. The condition is still sometimes referred to as 'intestinal stenosis of Garré', and has been reported on many occasions since. Its frequency has undoubtedly decreased over recent years, partly due to the fact that inguinal herniae are now almost invariably treated at an early stage, before strangulation occurs, and also no doubt because attempted manual reduction of an obstructed hernia has become a discredited surgical manoeuvre.

Nevertheless, Cherney[8] discovered in the literature 82 authenticated cases of stenosis following surgery for strangulation, and Vowles,[9] and Cunningham and Regan[24] have reported further cases. As already mentioned, Raf[4] found 8 examples in his Swedish series, of which 4 were the result of reduction of non-viable bowel from a hernial sac, and 4 resulted from strangulation by fibrous bands.

There is usually an interval of weeks or months between the vascular insult to the bowel and the development of symptomatic stricture.

Traumatic stricture

Blunt trauma to the abdominal wall may cause a haematoma to accumulate in the mesentery, or may actually separate mesentery from bowel over a variable length. In either case, the result is severe local ischaemia. If a sufficient length of bowel is devascularized, it will become necrotic, and will perforate, leading to gross peritonitis. This may occur several days after an accident which initially appeared quite trivial. For this reason, among others, every patient with a closed injury to the abdomen must be suspected of having sustained serious damage, and minor complaints must be investigated with care in order to exclude the presence of a loop of infarcted bowel.

Less complete degrees of ischaemia may be followed by the development of a fibrous stricture, which may not become manifest until months or even years after the original accident, although the usual interval between trauma and the development of obstruction is 2–12 weeks. Such cases are rare. Although Gillet, Phillippe and Adloff[25] were able to collect 48 from the world literature, in Raf's series from Stockholm there was only 1 traumatic stenosis in 95 cases.

Haemodynamic causes

Because of the very efficient collateral circulation to the small bowel (see Chapter 1), it is practically unknown for spontaneous occlusion of small vessels to lead to gangrene. Focal gangrene, when it occurs, is usually the result of SMA occlusion. This is in contrast to what has been described above in relation to trauma, where a tear or a haematoma in the mesentery destroys the collateral network. However, ischaemic ulceration, stenosis and stricture are not uncommon, and are quite often found at autopsy in patients who suffered no alimentary symptoms during life. Additionally, a number of cases of acute small bowel obstruction are due to localized strictures, which histologically have all the characteristics of an infarction.

Again, a known vascular accident may later be followed by intestinal obstruction. In some reported cases,[12, 14, 26] a mesenteric embolus had been treated conservatively and, presumably due to the development of an adequate collateral circulation, did not result in the death of the patient. After an interval of up to 10 weeks, during which symptoms of the original abdominal crisis had passed off and the patient had recuperated, subacute small bowel obstruction developed as the fibrous tissue within the bowel wall began to organize and contract.

Apart from obstruction to the major arterial trunks, focal ischaemic damage can occur from small atheromatous emboli reaching the distal arteries. This situation has been produced in the laboratory by the use of microspheres[27] and by cholesterol suspensions,[28] and it can also take place spontaneously in human beings. The occurrence of atheromatous emboli has been recognized ever since the classic description by Panum[29] of a ruptured plaque in the coronary artery of the sculptor Thorvaldsen, which embolized into the mycoardium and caused his sudden death in a Copenhagen theatre. Gore and Collins[30] were the first to draw attention to the same process occurring in the alimentary tract, and there have been several recorded cases since.[31] Perhaps the best documented is that of Mulliken and Bartlett,[13] who resected a 17 cm length of fibrous obstructed ileum and demonstrated that the submucosal arteries were packed with the typical biconvex clefts left by cholesterol emboli.

Both the gross and the microscopic appearances of focal ischaemia of the bowel may closely resemble Crohn's disease. This was emphasized by Hawkins,[12] who described a stenosis of the proximal jejunum occurring in a 74-year-old man 3 months after a myocardial infarction which had been complicated by a mesenteric embolus. At subsequent laparotomy the appearance of the bowel was identical with that of Crohn's disease, although unfortunately the general condition of the patient did not allow for resection or biopsy, so no histological information was available. However, in a case report by Dingendorf, Swart and Haberich[32] there was a double embolus into the distal branches of the SMA (demonstrated angiographically), and operation showed congestion and absent pulsation over a 70 cm length of small intestine. No resection was carried out at that time but 3 months later, following the development of obstructive symptoms, a grossly abnormal 40 cm segment of ileum was removed. Careful histological study showed the typical appearance of Crohn's disease, with focal granulomata and epithelioid cells. This case is of some importance. No one would suggest that Crohn's disease is caused by ischaemia, but Dingendorf's observation draws attention to the fact that the histological behaviour of the bowel is not very versatile, and that the granulomatous response may be non-specific and may occur in the face of widely differing types of challenge, including that of ischaemia.

Most varieties of intestinal ischaemia are found in adults, but an interesting series of small bowel infarcts occurring in Thai children was described by Headington et al.[33] In their 5 patients (2 of whom died), whose ages ranged from 4 to 7, there was acute focal gangrene of the small intestine, with no associated arterial occlusion and no vasculitis. The authors were careful to exclude specific infection and, in particular, the presence of β-toxin-producing strains of *Clostridium perfringens* as are seen in 'pig-bel' (See Chapter 7). A striking feature in every case was gross enlargement of the mesenteric lymph nodes. The authors were unable to explain this finding. It is possible that the lesions were a variety of the neonatal enterocolitis described in Chapter 7, or perhaps were the result of non-occlusive ischaemia or infection by *Yersinia enterocolitica* III.[34] Certainly, fibrous stenosis of the small bowel can follow an episode of cardiogenic shock due to massive myocardial infarction,[5] and it is likely that dehydration could lead to the same effect.

Vasculitis

Many types of vascular disease, some of them extremely rare, can affect the gastrointestinal tract.

The subject has been well covered by Kumar and Dawson,[35] and the reader is referred to their review. The more important conditions in this category are:

Inflammatory conditions
Infective angiitis:
typhoid
tuberculosis
syphilis
leprosy
Specific arteritis of Crohn's disease
Buerger's disease (thromboangiitis obliterans)

Immune complex and collagen disorders
Systemic lupus erythematosus
Polyarteritis nodosa
Rheumatoid arthritis
Dermatomyositis
Sjögren's syndrome
Systemic sclerosis
Wegener's granuloma

Miscellaneous
Amyloidosis
Pseudoxanthoma elasticum
Ehlers–Danlos syndrome
Degos' disease (malignant papillitis)
Cogan's disease (non-syphilitic interstitial keratitis)

In most of these conditions the bowel lesion is either a terminal event or simply forms part of a widespread symptom complex involving many organs and systems. However, some patients with known connective tissue disease and recurrent small infarctions may survive for several years on maintenance treatment with corticosteroids. A specific arteriographic sign is 'beading' of the small mesenteric vessels (Fig. 9.2).

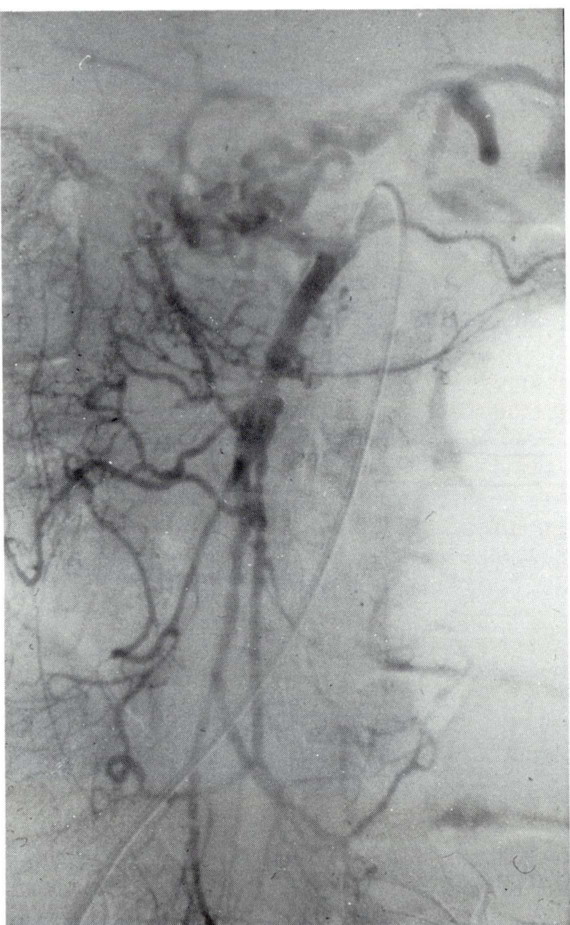

Fig. 9.2 Angiogram of the SMA in a case of polyarteritis nodosa (note 'beading' of the distal vessels).

Carcinoid tumours

One of the most common clinical manifestations of these tumours is paroxysmal abdominal pain; this has usually been ascribed to episodes of intestinal obstruction, although why these should occur is by no means clear, and supporting radiological evidence is not always found.[36] The tumours secrete 5-hydroxytryptamine (5-HT), which is known to stimulate small bowel motility, but elevation of free plasma 5-HT levels is rare during these attacks.[37] Anthony and Drury,[15] reviewing consecutive cases of ileal carcinoid at The Middlesex Hospital, noted elastic sclerosis of the mesenteric vessels and a high incidence of histological ischaemic changes, sometimes (4 of 25 cases) amounting to gangrene. The degree of narrowing of the vessels did not seem enough, however, to account for the severe ischaemia and it is thought that the vasospastic effect of 5-HT may be of equal or greater importance. The association of general and focal ischaemic lesions with these tumours is now well recognized,[16] and should always be suspected when abdominal pain occurs in patients with the carcinoid syndrome, particularly if the primary growth is in the terminal ileum.

Radiation enteritis

Fibrous stricture of the intestine secondary to radiotherapy for carcinoma of the pelvic organs was originally referred to by Jones in 1935,[18] and many thousands of cases have been reported since. The frequency of the complication varies from 1 to 12 per cent of the patients treated; although improved dosimetry and radiation techniques may decrease the incidence, some authorities take the view that the wider use of linear accelerators may have the opposite effect. Furthermore, if chemotherapy improves survival, slowly progressive disease will become apparent. The complication may appear from months to years after radiation. In some 75–90 per cent of cases the large intestine and rectum are affected following irradiation of uterine cancer. The most frequently affected zone of bowel is some 8–14 cm from the anus. Due to its mobility, the small intestine is less comonly affected, and the usual site of damage here is 6–10 cm from the ileocaecal valve. Jacobs[38] reported a lesion in the ileum developing 32 years after radiotherapy, but most cases appear very much sooner than this. Sometimes the damage occurs progressively over a long period, and it is not unknown for successive operations to be required for the repeated development of strictures in areas of bowel previously thought to be normal.[19]

Four syndromes have been described, the features of which may overlap.

1. *Acute necrotizing enteritis* occurs during therapy and presents with acute diarrhoea which may occasionally result in dehydration and collapse. This is due to a direct effect of the radiation on the mucosa, as the villi become progressively shorter following irradiation, until a completely flat mucosa is produced, resulting in malabsorption and exudative enteropathy. Recovery occurs by the formation of flattened ridges rather than the normal finger-like processes. The timing of the processes of destruction and recovery is very variable.

2. *Subacute segmental enteritis* comes on at the end of therapy and presents with nausea, vomiting, diarrhoea and abdominal pain. This may clear up completely, or may lead to chronic enteritis, described next.

3. *Chronic enteritis* is characterized by long-continued episodic diarrhoea.

4. *Focal intestinal strictures* may develop, which can lead to complete obstruction. This latter may be very difficult to distinguish from recurrent malignancy. Perforation, fistula, malabsorption and haemorrhage are further late stage complications of radiation damage.

Microscopically, a spectrum of changes is seen, beginning with an infiltration with inflammatory cells and proceeding eventually to necrosis of the specialized layers of the wall, even at times ending in perforation. The bowel in most cases becomes thick and fibrous, and vascular adhesions develop between it and neighbouring structures. Vascular damage is patchy and in general confined to the area of stenosis. The small vessels are most susceptible to injury and capillary occlusion precedes fibrosis. Although vessels in all layers of the bowel wall and mesentery are affected, by no means are all the vessels abnormal. The vascular changes vary from endothelial proliferation to focal medial necrosis or complete thrombotic occlusion. The characteristic change is the accumulation of large foam cells beneath the intima and on the intimal side of the elastic lamina. This appears to be a specific diagnostic feature.

Drugs

In 1964, Lindholmer, Nyman and Raf of Stockholm[39] were surprised to encounter, in a period of less than 1 month, 4 cases of annular stricture of the small intestine, leading to obstruction. In view of the known rarity of this condition, they suspected that this sudden increase might be drug induced, and set about investigating such a possibility. They discovered that the Stockholm hospitals had treated 16 similar patients during this period, making a total of 20, and further investigation showed that 17 of these patients had been taking tablets containing chlorothiazide and potassium. Two months later, Baker, Schrader and Hitchcock[40] published an identical observation from the USA. More reports followed[41, 42] which stimulated the interest of the Federal Food and Drug Administration in the problem. In a survey of 488 hospitals throughout the world, a total of 395 patients with small bowel ulceration were found, of whom 196 had been taking enteric-coated potassium chloride tablets and/or a thiazide diretic.

It was not known at this point whether it was the thiazide, the potassium or the enteric coat which was in fact responsible for the production of the lesion, and neither was it known how the damage occurred. Experimental work followed on the part of Lawrason et al.[43] who showed that intestinal ulceration could be produced in monkeys with thiazide and potassium chloride, but not with diuretic alone, and that the effect was probably dose related. Further studies[20] confirmed the damaging

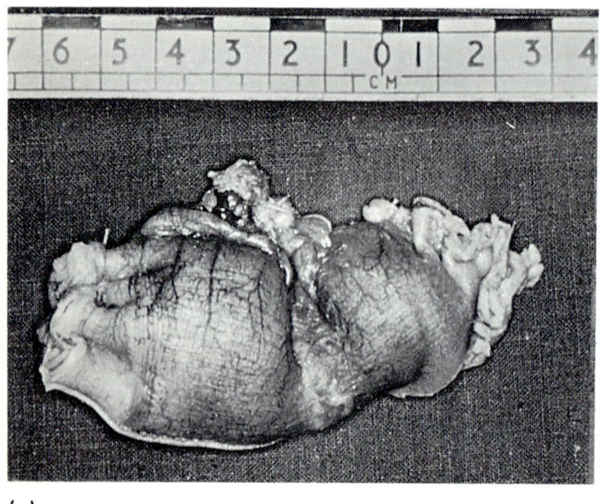

(a)

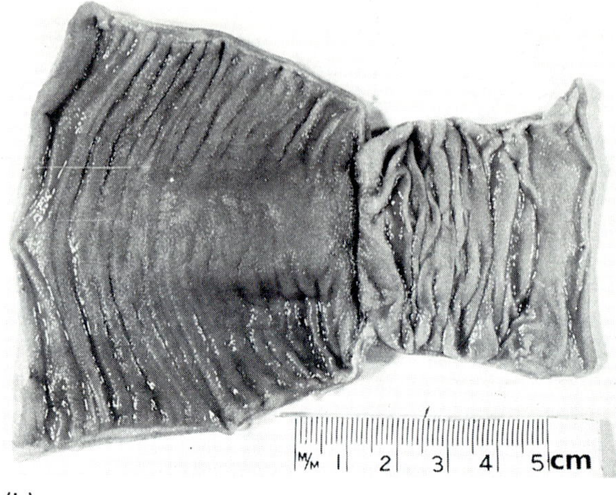

(b)

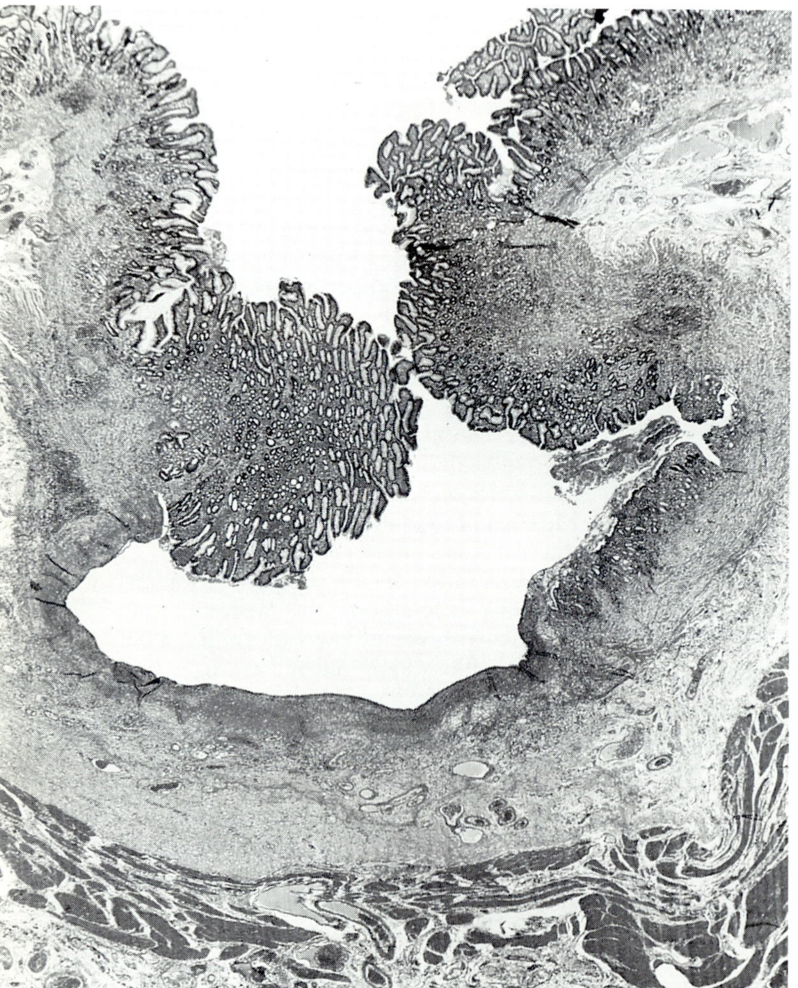

(c)

Fig. 9.3 (**a**) Stricture of the terminal ileum caused by enteric-coated potassium. The patient was a 57-year-old male hypertensive who developed subacute small bowel obstruction. (**b**) Solitary ulcer (KCl stricture) of the small intestine. The ulcer is annular and very narrow, with dilatation of the proximal bowel. (By courtesy of Dr B.C. Morson.) (**c**) Microscopic appearance of a potassium stricture of the small bowel (KCl ulcer of the small intestine). This is shallow and involves nothing deeper than the submucosal layer. The overhanging edges of intact mucous membrane are characteristic and explain why in some cases the ulcer is difficult to demonstrate macroscopically. (H&E, × 16) (By courtesy of Dr B.C. Morson.)

effect of high concentrations of potassium chloride, and showed that the effect is greatly enhanced if SMA flow is reduced by constriction of the arterial lumen. Of the many thousands of patients taking this sort of medication, only a small minority develop ulceration, and it appears very much as though for structural damage to occur there must be a combination of pre-existing ischaemia and a high local concentration of potassium (Fig. 8.3).

The work of Boley et al.[44] shed some light on the evolution of the process. It appears that the first effect of a strong solution of potassium chloride is to cause venous spasm followed by thrombosis, leading to oedema of the submucosa and capillary damage. The resulting ischaemia goes on to mucosal loss, bacterial invasion, deposition of fibrous tissue and stricture formation. On occasion, the lesion may actually perforate and present with peritonitis. The results of the animal studies were reproduced in humans by Myers, Brown and Deaver,[41] who injected hypertonic and isotonic solutions of potassium and sodium chloride into the intestinal lumen during resection procedures for colonic cancer.

Although the use of enteric-coated potassium tablets was undoubtedly responsible for the rapid increase in small bowel ulceration and stricture noted in the mid-1960s, this cannot be the whole story. The incrimination of potassium aroused much interest in the question of ulceration and stricture formation in the small bowel, and many cases were reported which otherwise would not have been brought to light. Davies and Brightmore[42] quoted 12 patients with strictures, 6 of whom had received no potassium but who had been medicated with phenobarbitone, reserpine, phenylbutazone and steroids. Other series of case reports[45, 46] have suggested similar implications. Whether or not the medication is relevant is a matter of debate, but from what has already been said (Chapter 2), the small bowel circulation is sensitive to a great number of pharmacological agents, and intestinal ischaemia must be watched for as a possible side effect of any newly introduced drug.

Oral contraceptive agents

Among the many cardiovascular problems associated with the use of oral contraceptives, acute ischaemia of the small bowel is one of the most familiar but most deadly. Hoyle et al.[47] reviewed 21 cases, of whom half perished and half required repeated surgery invovling extensive resection of bowel; blood group A.Rh+, hypertension and heavy smoking were additional risk factors. The lesions can also occur in the colon (see Chapter 10). The damage may be diffuse, but frequently a localized stricture results.

The subject has recently been reviewed by Cavin et al.,[21] who confirm the earlier findings. Abdominal pain occurring in patients taking high-oestrogen contraceptives should always prompt the suspicion of a small bowel infarction, particularly if other risk factors are present.

Clinical Features

Symptoms

The patient presents with the typical features of subacute small bowel obstruction; that is to say, colicky abdominal pain occurring usually some 2–3 hours after meals, and accompanied by nausea, occasional vomiting and distension. There may be episodes of diarrhoea. Fever, anorexia and gross loss of weight are unusual. Characteristically, the symptoms continue for a few weeks and months at a time and then regress, to return at a later period with rather more intensity. Untreated, the condition progresses either to frank perforation of the bowel wall or to complete intestinal obstruction, in either of which instances the patient will be admitted as a surgical emergency.

Naturally, a preceding history of strangulated hernia, ingestion of potassium tablets, episodes of ischaemia in other organs or radiation to the pelvis must be sought and carefully noted.

Physical signs

Physical examination of the abdomen is frequently quite normal, but may on occasion show a 'ladder pattern' of distension, with visible peristalsis and exaggerated bowel sounds. Except in very advanced cases, the serum biochemistry remains normal.

Radiological examination

X-ray examination will confirm the presence of dilated loops of jejunum with oedema of the wall and occasional fluid levels. A small bowel meal via the intubated duodenum is perhaps the most useful investigation, as it will on occasion delineate the position of the stricture as well as confirm the diagnosis.

Management

Fluid losses are replaced, and anaemia is corrected, before undertaking surgery for the obstructing lesion. In most cases the operation consists simply in resection of the stricture, with end-to-end anastomosis, and usually proceeds very simply along standard lines. Naturally, if there is any question of a pre-existing lesion in the SMA, particular care must be taken to check the vascularity of the ends of the bowel.

Different considerations apply to postirradiation cases, where tissue healing may be seriously impaired, and conservative treatment is preferred. If operation becomes necessary, it is probably better to bypass rather than to resect the lesion. Thus Swan, Fowler and Boronow,[19] in a review of the world literature and a study of their own cases, showed a significantly lower operative mortality and morbidity in those patients whose lesions were bypassed and a correspondingly higher incidence of fistulae in the resected group. If the bowel is so seriously damaged that it must be removed, then the resection must be wide because the abnormal area is always greater than appears on the surface. Anastomoses should, if possible, be wrapped in unirradiated tissue because vascular adhesions provide an important collateral blood supply to healing suture lines. If wounds made in normal rat intestine are wrapped in irradiated tissues, the incidence of dehiscence is high.[48] It is therefore wise to wrap anastomoses in vascular pedicles of omentum from outside the radiation field.

References

1 Garengoet, R.J.C. de *Traité Operations de Chirurgie*, 3rd edn. Paris: Huart, (1748) 246.

2 Vincent. Observations sur l'opération de Ramd'hor. *Journal de Medecine et Chirurgie et Pharmacologie* (1781) **56**: 151.

3 Bolognesi, G. De l'occlusion expérimentale des vaisseaux Mésentériques. *Zentralbl. Chir.* (1909) **36**: 1641–7.

4 Raf, L.E. Ischaemic stenosis of the small intestine. *Acta Chir. Scand.* (1969) **135**: 253–9.

5 Thaker, P., Weingarten, L., Friedman, I.H. Stenosis of the small intestine due to non-occlusive ischemic disease. *Arch. Surg.* (1977) **112**: 1216–17.

6 Avery, J. Almost complete obstruction of the small intestine from injury. *Trans. Pathol. Soc.* (1853) **4**: 156–7.

7 Maass, V. Über die Entstahung von Darmen Stenose nach Brucheinklemmerung. *Dtsch. Med. Wochenschr.* (1895) **21**: 365–7.

8 Cherney, L.S. Intestinal stenosis following strangulated hernia. *Ann. Surg.* (1958) **148**: 991–3.

9 Vowles, K.D.J. Intestinal complications of strangulated hernia: incidence of ischaemic strictures. *Br. J. Surg.* (1959) **47**: 189–92.

10 Beringuier, M. Rétrécissement fibreux de l'intestin grêle. *Bull. Soc. Anat. Paris* (1877) **2**: 86–8.

11 Küttner, H. Die Spätsschädigungen des Darmes nach Stumpfer Bauchverlätzung. *Ergeb. Chir. Orthop.* (1930) **23**: 205–37.

12 Hawkins, C.F. Jejunal stenosis following mesenteric artery occlusion. *Lancet* (1957) **ii**: 121.

13 Mulliken, J.B., Bartlett, M.K. Small bowel obstruction secondary to atheromatous embolization. *Ann. Surg.* (1971) **174**: 145–50.

14 Feller, E., Rickert, R., Spiro, H.M. Small vessel disease of the gut. In: Boley, S.J., ed., *Vascular Disorders of the Intestine.* New York, London: Appleton-Century-Crofts (1971) 483–509.

15 Anthony, P.P., Drury, R.A.D. Elastic vascular sclerosis of mesenteric vessels in argentaffin carcinoma. *J. Clin. Pathol.* (1970) **23**: 110–18.

16 Sworn, M.J., Reasbeck, P., Buchanan, R. Intestinal ischaemia associated with ileal carcinoid tumours. *Br. J. Surg.* (1978) **65**: 313–15.

17 Perkins, D.E., Spjut, H.J. Intestinal stenosis following radiation therapy. *Am. J. Radiol.* (1962) **88**: 993–6.

18 Jones, T.F. Intestinal complications resulting from prolonged irradiation damage to the ileum. *Am. J. Gynecol. Obstet.* (1935) **29**: 309–16.

19 Swan, R.W., Fowler, W.C., Boronow, R.C. Surgical management of radiation injury to the small intestine. *Surg. Gynecol. Obstet.* (1976) **142**: 325–7.

20 Mansfield, J.B., Schoenfeld, F.B., Suwa, M., Geurkinkre, R.E., Anderson, M.C. The role of vascular insufficiency in drug induced small bowel ulceration. *Am. J. Surg.* (1967) **113**: 608–14.

21 Cavin, R., Boumghar, M., Loosli, H., Saegesser, F. Les accidents digestifs aigües des contraceptifs oraux. *Chirurgie* (1982) **108**: 64–74.

22 Guignard, P.E. Du rétrécissement et de l'Oblitération de l'Intestin. Thesis. Paris University (1846).

23 Garré, C. Über eine eigenartige Form von narbiger Darmstenose nach Brucheinklemmerung *Beitr. Klin. Chir.* (1892) **9**: 187–97.

24 Cunningham, W.L., Regan, J.F. Fibrous stenosis of the small bowel and the role of ischemia. *Surgery* (1965) **58**: 488–96.

25 Gillet, M., Phillippe, E., Adloff, M. Les sténoses cicatricielles après contusion de l'abdomen. *J. Chir.* (1967) **93**: 469–77.

26 Corbett, C.R.R. Personal communication: ischaemic stricture (1981).

27 Boley, S.J., Krieger, H., Schultz, L., et al. Experimental aspects of peripheral vascular occlusion of the intestine. *Surg. Gynecol. Obstet.* (1965) **121**: 789–94.

28 Marston, A., Lundqvist, P., McCombs, R.L. Unpublished observation (1961).

29 Panum, P.L. Experimentale Beiträge zu Lehre von der Embolie. *Arch. Pathol. Anat.* (1862) **25**: 308–12.

30 Gore, I., Collins, D.P. Spontaneous atheromatous embolization. *Am. J. Clin. Pathol.* (1960) **33**: 416–18.

31 Saegesser, F., Borgeaud, J., Schnyder, P., Tabrizian, M., Richon, C.A. *Sténoses de l'Intestin Grêle d'origine Ischémique.* Paris: Expansion Scientifique (1975) 75–89.

32 Dingendorf, W., Swart, B., Haberich, H. Inkomplette Mesenterial gefässverschlüsse als mögliche Ursache der Enteritis regionalis Crohn. *Radiologe* (1971) **2**: 37–42.

33 Headington, J.T., Sathornsumathi, S., Simark, S., Sujatakond, W. Segmental infarcts of the small intestine and mesenteric adenitis in Thai children. *Lancet* (1967) **i**: 802–6.

34 Leino, R.E., Renvall, S.Y., Lipasti, J.A., Toivenen, A.M. Small-bowel gangrene caused by *Yersinia enterocolitica* III. *Br. med. J.* (1980) **280**: 1419.

35 Kumar, P.J., Dawson, A.M. Vasculitis of the alimentary tract *Clin. Gastroenterol.* (1972) **1**: 719–45.

36 Morgan, J.G., Marks, C., Hearn, D. Carcinoid tumors of the gastrointestinal tract. *Ann. Surg.* (1974) **180**: 720–27.

37 Isaac, P. Carcinoid syndrome. In: Walker, G., ed. *Ninth Symposium on Advanced Medicine*, London: Pitman Medical (1973): 173–81.

38 Jacobs, L.G. Unusual case of late irradiation damage to the ileum. *Radiology* (1963) **80**: 57–60.

39 Lindholmer, B., Nyman, E., Raf, L. Non-specific stenosing ulceration of the small bowel. *Acta Chir. Scand.* (1964) **128**: 310–11.

40 Baker, D.R., Schrader, W.H., Hitchcock, C.R. Small bowel ulceration apparently associated with thiazide and potassium therapy. *J.A.M.A.* (1964) **190**: 586–90.

41 Myers, K.N., Brown, C.E, Deaver, J.M. In vivo effect of potassium on small bowel. *Ann. Surg.* (1967) **166**: 693–703.

42 Davies, D.R., Brightmore, T. Idiopathic and drug-induced ulceration of small intestine. *Br. J. Surg.* (1970) **57**: 134–9.

43 Lawrason, F.D., Alpert, E., Mohr, F.L., McMahon, F.G. Ulcerative obstructive lesions of the small intestine. *J.A.M.A.* (1965) **191**: 641–5.

44 Boley, S.J., Schultz, S., Krieger, H., Schwartz, S., Elguezabal, A., Allen, A.C. Evaluation of thiazides and potassium as a cause of small bowel ulcer. *J.A.M.A.* (1965) **192**: 763–8.

45 Wayte, D.M., Helwig, E.B. Small bowel ulceration — iatrogenic or multifactorial origin? *Am. J. Clin. Pathol.* (1968) **49**: 26–39.

46 Danis, J., Fraxinos, J. Aspects étiopathogeniques des sténoses non-tumorales de l'intestin grêle. *Rev. méd. Toulouse* (1973) **9**: 277–88.

47 Hoyle, M., Kennedy, A., Prior, A.L., Thomas, G.E. Small bowel ischaemia and infarction in young women taking oral contraceptives. *Br. J. Surg.* (1977) **64**: 533–5.

48 Ormiston, M.C. A study of rat intestinal wound healing in the presence of radiation injury. *Br. J. Surg.* (1985) **72**: 56–8.

10

Vascular disease of the colon

Introduction

As was made plain in Chapter 2–5, the result of deprivation of blood supply to a loop of intestine can range from full-thickness necrosis to a transient invasion by bacteria and inflammatory cells which heals completely. Falls in blood flow which are insufficient to kill the bowel wall may result in permanent damage to the mucosal and muscle layers, which become replaced by scar tissue, resulting in the formation of a fibrous stricture.

These events occur more frequently in the colon than in the small bowel because of its relatively sparse collateral arterial supply (see Chapter 1) and also because of the infectivity of its contents. Short of gangrene, the changes produced by arterial insufficiency are those of inflammation, or 'colitis'. The concept of ischaemic colitis arose from the convergent experience of vascular surgeons, gastroenterologists and pathologists.

Causes of colonic ischaemia

Trauma

Blunt closed injury to the abdomen or stab injury involving the mesentery are increasingly important causes of intestinal arterial damage. The small bowel has the capacity to escape from such threats, but the colon, being in a more anatomically fixed position, is at greater risk. If the mesenteric tear or haematoma is parallel rather than perpendicular to the gut wall, the chance of mucosal damage is that much greater. The lesion may present early within days of the injury as necrosis, or later as an obstructing stricture.

Surgical interruption of the blood supply

Although the damaging effects of interference with the intestinal arterial supply had been recognized for many years the credit (if this is the right term to use for a surgical mistake!) is usually given to Lauenstein[1] as being the first to describe gangrene of the colon following a vascular accident. His patient developed a slough of the transverse colon after ligation of the middle colic artery in the course of a gastrectomy. With the development of radical surgery for cancer of the colon, surgeons became interested in high ligation of the arterial trunks so as to achieve wider clearance of the lymphatics, and the risk of devitalization of anastomoses and stomata became a major preoccupation. The first successful ligation of the inferior mesenteric artery was recorded by Treves in 1898,[2] and further reports followed by Kummel,[3] Hartmann[4] and Pope and Judd[5] who recommended that in excision of the rectum the artery should be divided below its first sigmoid branch. Later, 'high ligation' of the IMA (i.e. at its aortic origin) became standard practice, but a note of warning was sounded by Goligher[6] who described a 25 per cent incidence of devitalization of the terminal colon following this manoeuvre, and others[7] reported similar complications and disasters. It became apparent that a crucial factor in the preservation of the colonic blood supply was the marginal artery to the colon and that an arterial and lymphatic watershed existed at the splenic flexure where the middle and left colic arteries frequently fail to communicate[8] (see Chapter 1). A deficient marginal artery, an absent arteria anastomotica magna or unsuspected occlusive disease of the SMA may, either singly or in combination, imperil the blood supply of an anastomosis in the left colon.

More recently, attention has been directed to the relation between deficient blood supply and the behaviour of colostomies. Thomson and Hawley[9] and later Henry and Everett[10] pointed out the dangers of early closure, and this was investigated by Forrester, Spence and Walker[11, 12] who measured colonic mucosal–submucosal blood flow in colostomies using a washout technique with ^{125}I 4-iodantipyrine. This group showed that there was an early diminution in the microcirculation following construction of the stoma, which gradually improved, and that fistula formation was associated with premature closure during the ischaemic phase.

From quite another area, surgeons interested in cardiovascular disease were beginning, in the early 1950s, to reconstruct the lower aorta, which frequently involved sacrificing one or more of its visceral branches, in particular the IMA. The first major report along these lines came from Smith and Szilagyi,[13] who described 12 cases of ischaemia of the left colon in 120 aortic resections. Many cases have now been recorded and the incidence of colonic ischaemia following aortoiliac surgery varies from 3 to 15 per cent, according to the care with which it is sought. Not all cases proceed to gangrene — transient inflammation is common (Fig. 10.1) and fibrous strictures can also occur.[14]

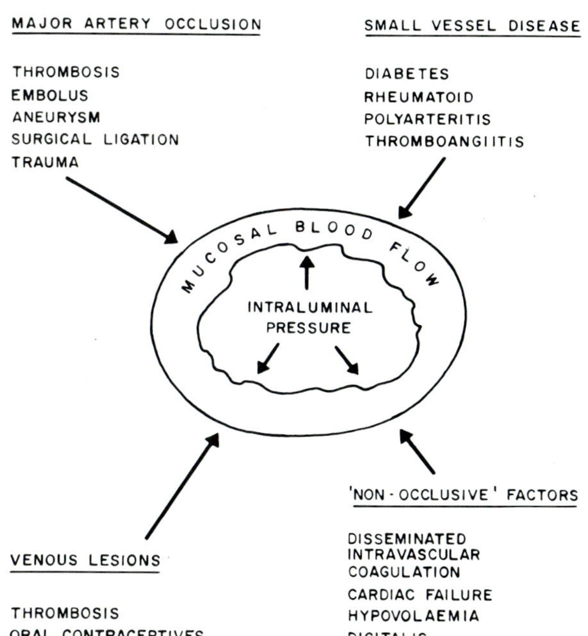

Fig. 10.1 Factors leading to ischaemia of the colon.

The IMA often requires to be ligated in operations on the lower aorta and the large bowel, and obviously this is quite safe if the vessel is already occluded. Before a *patent* IMA is tied, however, the surgeon must be sure of the integrity of the SMA and the marginal artery, and if doubt exists the vessel must be reimplanted into the prosthesis (Fig. 10.2). Necrosis of the colon following aortic surgery is highly lethal, and if reimplantation is not possible, it is probably wise to exteriorize and remove doubtful colon, accepting the undesirability of such a procedure in the presence of a vascular graft. The whole question of colonic damage following aortic reconstruction has been reviewed by Johnson and Nabseth[14] who found an overall incidence of 99 cases in 6100 patients at risk, (1.6 per cent) and by Ernst et al.[15]

Radiological injury

The colon can also be damaged following free or selective abdominal angiography. This was first reported by Joyeux et al.,[16] and was well reviewed by Killen, Sewell and Foster[17] who collected 15 cases from the literature, 3 of which exhibited inflammation only, the remaining 12 undergoing necrosis. Almost certainly the actual incidence at that time was higher as many milder cases would have passed unnoticed or unreported. It is not clear from this or other reports[18, 19] whether the contrast medium or the trauma of cannulation is to blame, or indeed whether the inferior mesenteric artery did not become blocked as a result of the angiography. Experimental work suggests that the gut is tolerant of concentrated angiographic media, and the more recently introduced of these agents are probably much more less toxic than those in use at the time of Killen's study.

Spontaneous thrombosis of major vessels

As already described (Chapter 1), the inferior mesenteric arterty is frequently narrowed or blocked at its origin by an atheromatous plaque,

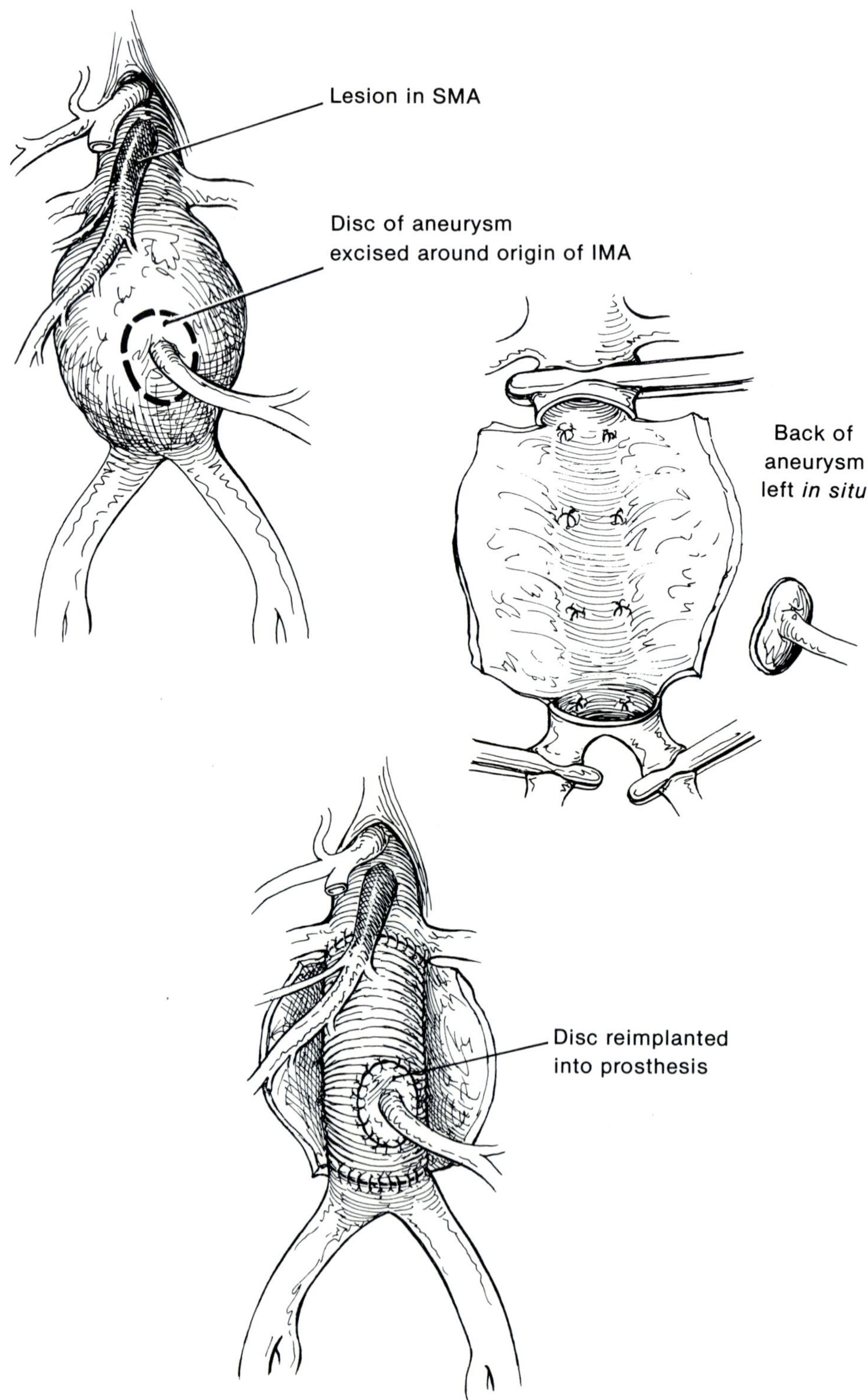

Fig. 10.2 Reimplanation of the IMA following resection of an aortic aneurysm.

[20, 21, 22] and this situation is usually well compensated for by the development of collateral pathways. If the compensatory mechanisms fail, the colon is damaged; there are many recorded examples of this occurring as a result of acute occlusion of the artery. The changes described vary from gangrene (and, understandably, the earlier series are exclusively concerned with this) to the more recently familiar changes of 'thumb-printing', mucosal ulceration and stricture formation (see below). These features have all been produced in the experimental laboratory (see Chapter 3).

Small vessel disease

Often, the causative lesion is at subradiological level, in the intramural vessels. As in the small bowel, any condition which produces inflammation of minor arteries may result in mucosal damage. These include primary vascular disorder such as polyarteritis and Buerger's disease, systemic lupus erythematosus, rheumatoid arthritis and dermatomyositis.[23] Also included in this group are Wegener's granuloma, anaphylactoid purpura and Degos' disease.[24] Once considered a terminal event in connective tissue disease, it is now appreciated that enteric and colonic ischaemia can be a chronic condition, which responds well to treatment with corticosteroids, and the eventual necrosis can be postponed by such suppressive therapy. Radiation colitis produces similar pathological changes, as may occur particularly following treatment of uterine carcinoma (see Chapter 9). Necrosis of the colon occasionally complicates renal transplantation, [25] presumably as an indirect effect of immune suppression.

Atheromatous emboli from the aorta, and intimal thickening occurring in diabetes, have also been incriminated. It seems entirely logical that such conditions should lead to colonic ischaemia, but the written work in this area is largely speculative and firm clinical reporting is hard to come by.

Low flow states

The colon is subject to all the factors contributing to intestinal ischaemia (see Chapter 5), and when its blood supply fails the resulting inflammatory damage will be more rapid and more metabolically harmful than a similar process in the small gut, due to the presence of pathogenic bacteria. Of particular importance in this connection are the clostridia, which can be found in the colons of 1 in 13 healthy human subjects. As in the small bowel, predisposing factors include cardiac failure (particularly in association with digitalis intoxication), hypertension, diabetes and any condition which might lead to intravascular coagulation (see Fig. 10.1). Colonic ischaemia has recently been described in association with sickle cell disease[26] in an 18-year-old male, and it would seem wise to bear this diagnosis in mind in patients with abdominal pain associated with a sickling crisis.

Obstruction to the lumen

Blood flow in the wall of the intestine is dependent on intramural pressure, radial muscle tension and diameter, quite apart from vascular influences (see Fig. 10.1). The characteristic radiological and pathological changes of ischaemia occur quite often in the segment of bowel immediately above an obstructing cancer,[27, 28] and there is some evidence that the microcirculation below the lesion can also be influenced. Sometimes the effects of the ischaemic lesion are so dramatic that they mask the presence of a tumour. Prolapse,[29] volvulus and adhesions can also give rise to vascular problems, and the relation to colostomy[11, 12] has already been discussed.

Venous occlusion

Laboratory studies[30] have shown that extensive venous thrombosis leads initially to oedema and haemorrhagic infarction, and later to fibrosis which may be indistinguishable from that arising from an arterial infarct. The clinician sees the lesion at a mature stage. By the time that a radiological and a pathological diagnosis become available, it is usually impossible to decide whether the original vascular accident was on the arterial or the venous side. Circumstantial evidence to incriminate the oral contraceptives[31, 32, 33] is not hard to come by, and they are known to have an effect on venous thrombosis elsewhere in the body, but at the time of writing it is difficult to prove that any colon has been directly damaged by such medication. The fact that the earlier reported series of ischaemic disease contained no premenopausal females, whereas subsequent ones did, is no more than suggestive, and the incidence of the condition among young men appears to be increasing.[34, 35]

The concept of ischaemic colitis

The situation in the mid-1960s was that it was known that arterial injury brought about by a surgeon or a radiologist, spontaneous thrombosis of major or minor arteries, low flow states, raised intraluminal pressure or blocked veins could produce a spectrum of colonic disorders which varied from mild transitory inflammation to gangrene. The radiological and pathological changes invoked by ischaemia were established, and were beginning to be reproduced in the experimental laboratory.[36] This prompted the suspicion that many unexplained cases of 'colitis' could perhaps be manifestations of arterial insufficiency.

For many years gastroenterologists had been aware that their classification of acute inflammatory disease of the colon was insufficient to accommodate all observed cases. Specific infections, such as bacillary and amoebic dysentery or infestation by parasites, were to an extent understood. Mechanical disorders resulting from stricture or bands or, as in the case of diverticular disease, muscle dysfunction, formed another well defined category. The causation of inflammatory bowel disease (i.e. ulcerative colitis and Crohn's disease) was not known, but this was a useful diagnostic label in terms of natural history, pathology and prognosis. Many examples of acute colitis had been reported which did not fit into any established clinical category and in which the pathology was quite unlike inflammatory bowel disease. These had been given various names such as 'regional colitis',[37] 'acute segmental colitis'[38] and 'fibrous stenosis'.[39] Some authors had in fact suggested a vascular basis for their cases, in particular Boley et al.[40] who, in an important paper, described 5 patients presenting with abdominal pain and rectal bleeding, whose barium enemas showed 'thumb-printing' around the splenic flexure, exactly as is seen following deliberate or spontaneous occlusion of the IMA. His patients recovered without specific treatment and were interpreted as having developed reversible vascular occlusions.

In 1966 our group[41] described a series of 16 patients with an illness whose clinical, radiological and pathological features were identical to those produced by known vascular insufficiency in the colon. From a study of this and of previous material, we concluded that a large number of hitherto obscure cases of colitis were in fact varieties of infarction. We developed the term 'ischaemic colitis' to describe this situation, and suggested a classification of the disease into gangrenous, stricturing and transient forms, according to the severity of the ischaemia, at the same time laying down its clinical, radiological and pathological features. This concept became generally accepted, and many reports of cases of ischaemic colitis have appeared in world literature during the subsequent decade.

The clinical, radiological and pathological features are now well established and have been reproduced in the experimental laboratory by varying degrees of interruption of the arterial supply to the colon[36, 42] (see Chapter 3). To diagnose ischaemic colitis is to make a statement of quite a different order from a diagnosis of ulcerative colitis or Crohn's disease, because an underlying aetiology is implied. The difficulty is that angiograms by no means always demonstrate a vascular occlusion. This state of affairs is of course to be expected, in view of the known fact that approximately one-third of fatal intestinal infarcts occur in the absence of a defined vascular pathology (Chapter 5). Nevertheless, when ischaemic colitis is diagnosed (as it often is) on the basis of a clinical history and a barium enema, without the opportunity of examining histological material, the clinician is open to the challenge that whatever has happened in the colon is not in fact the result of deficient blood flow. The situation is rather analogous to that of a myocardial infarct which is diagnosed on the evidence of the patient's symptoms, physical signs and electrocardiograph, but without a coronary angiogram.

Angiography in both these situations is not justified as a routine procedure, both because it is an invasive investigation which will not in itself influence treatment policy and because a normal arteriogram in no way disproves the diagnosis. There are, however, many cases reported[43, 44, 45] in which the underlying arterial lesion has been confirmed on an angiogram or a pathological specimen. Some of the best examples of supraselective angiography demonstrating ischaemic lesions of the colon have been produced in the University of Strasbourg,[46] and are reproduced with permission here (Figs. 10.3–10.5). However, attempts to demonstrate occlusion in the distal circulation may be inappropriate, for, as occurs elsewhere in the body, the response to ischaemia is vasodilatation. This has been shown in the colon experimentally.[47]

Williams and Wittenberg[48] emphasized this aspect of the problem in their study of 55 patients confidently diagnosed as having ischaemic colitis on clinical and conventional radiographic grounds. Of

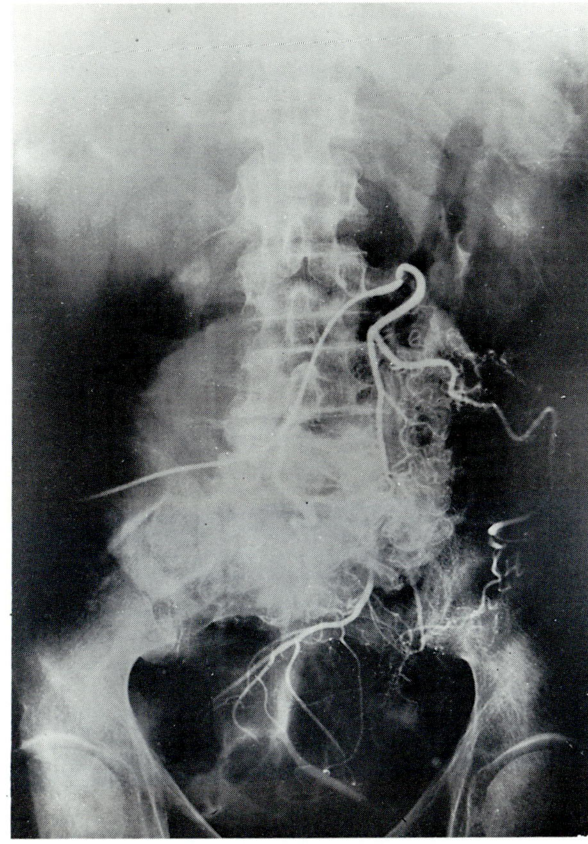

(a)

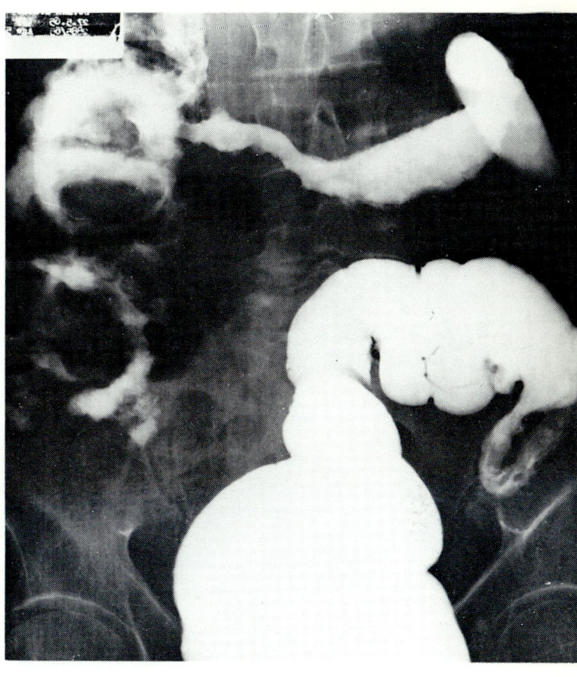

(b)

Fig. 10.3 Arterial lesion involving the colonic circulation (**a**), with corresponding barium study (**b**).

11 patients submitted to detailed angiography, 5 demonstrated an expanded vascular bed, which emphasizes that fine vessel angiography gives a better idea of the volume of blood within a vascular bed than of the flow taking place through it. Williams and Wittenberg question whether the pathogenesis of spontaneously occurring 'ischaemic colitis' in fact includes ischaemia. Clearly, in the absence of a direct method of measuring blood flow in the wall of the living human colon, the question must remain valid. Furthermore in the non-occlusive cases, the actual time during which blood flow to the colon falls off may in fact be quite brief, occurring perhaps during a transient episode of low cardiac output, so that the opportunity for making instrumental measurements at this point may never arrive. The consequences of vascular impairment in the colon are amply documented; when these features are seen in a patient the simplest explanation is that of ischaemia, if they closely resemble those where the arterial lesion has been imaged — and there is abundant evidence that this is possible. Ischaemic colitis is a concept which has become embedded in clinical literature on the basis of extensive clinical and laboratory work, and there now seems little reason to abandon it.

Classification of colonic ischaemia

Our 1966[41] classification described three forms of the disease graded according to severity:

1. *Gangrene of the colon* — including the previously categorized ischaemic infarction,[49] ischaemic enterocolitis[50] and gangrene.[18, 51]

2. *Ischaemic stricture.* These cases had been previously labelled as regional colitis,[37] stenosis,[39, 52] benign stricture[53] and fibrosis,[22] and in our view represented an intermediate state of affairs whereby the fall in arterial supply damaged the oxygen-sensitive specialized layers of the gut (mucosa and submucosa) but left the outer coats relatively intact. The result was the formation of a fibrous stricture.

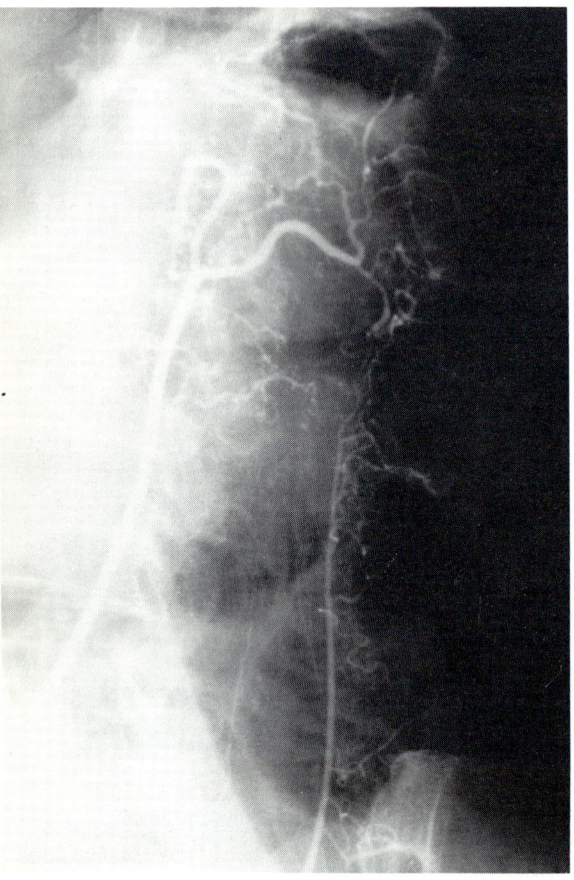

(a)

3. *Transient ischaemic colitis.* In these cases, which had previously been described as 'reversible vascular occlusion',[40] a relatively minor episode of ischaemia brought about a bacterial invasion of the ischaemic inner layers, followed by complete healing.

This classification, which was to an extent artificial because it was based on pathological data not available to the clinician on the spot, has now been abandoned. There are in fact only two clinical manifestations of colonic ischaemia. The first of these is *gangrene* which is part of the spectrum of acute intestinal ischaemia discussed in Chapter 5 and is usually associated with small bowel involvement. This condition is undiagnosable clinically, but is found at operation, and its presentation and management have already been discussed above. By *ischaemic colitis* is meant an inflammatory disorder, caused by a vascular accident, but which does not involve complete death of tissue. In practice, the fate of the ischaemic colon appears to be decided early in that the colitis almost never proceeds to frank gangrene (2 cases out of 180 in our experience).

Ischaemic colitis

By 'ischaemic colitis' we now mean the non-gangrenous form of the disease, which may vary

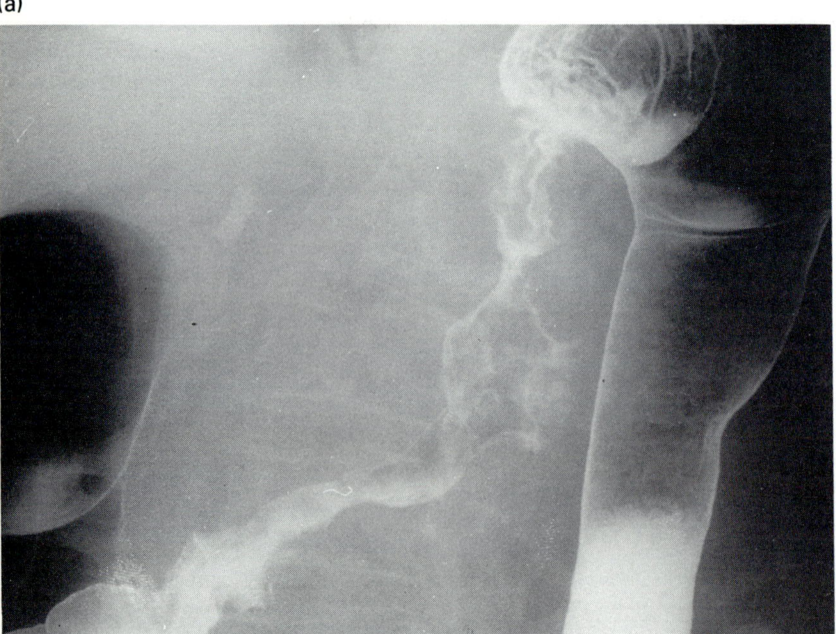

(b)

Fig. 10.4 Arterial lesion involving the colonic circulation (**a**), with corresponding barium study (**b**). (By courtesy of Dr J.J. Wenger and Professor L. Tongio, and by kind permission of Expansion Scientifique, Paris.)

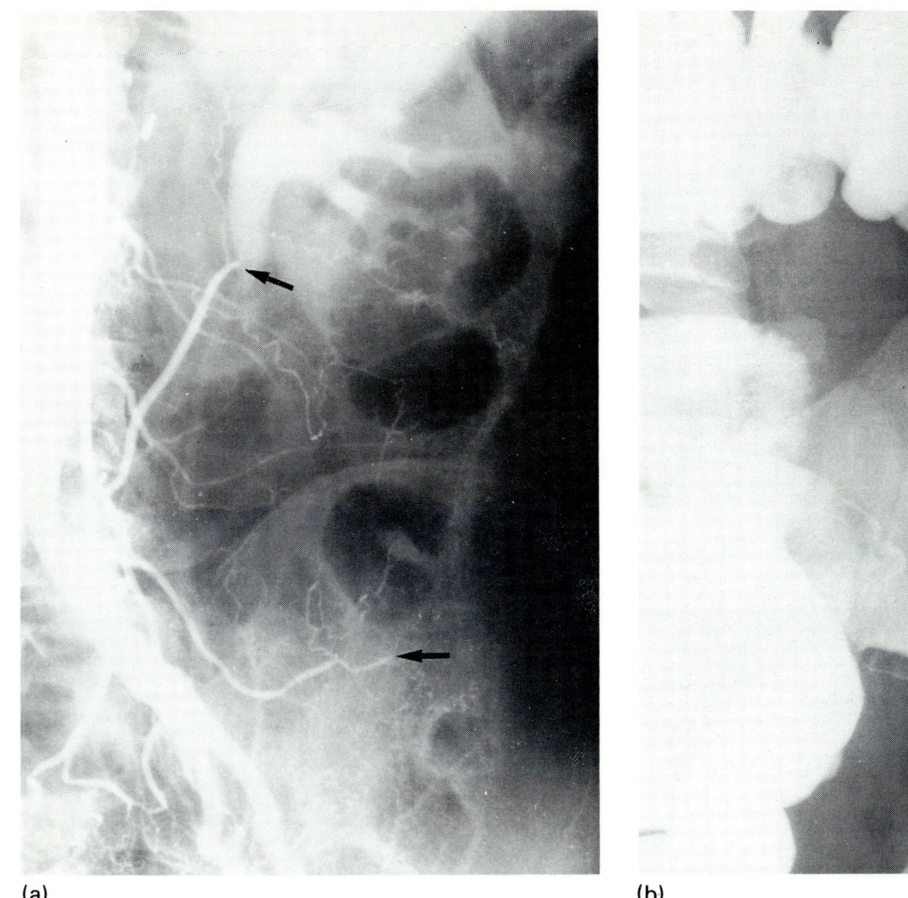

(a)

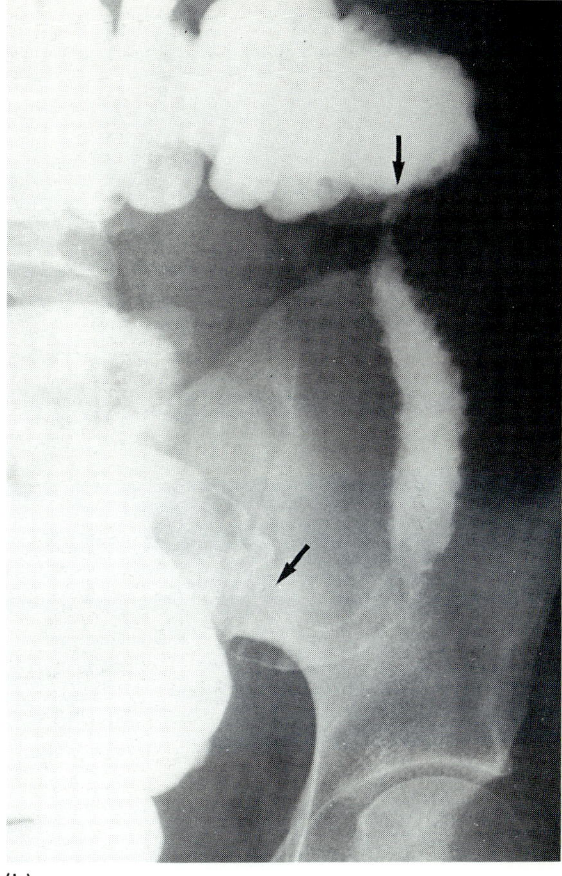

(b)

Fig. 10.5 Arterial lesions involving the colonic circulation (**a**), with corresponding barium study (**b**). (By courtesy of Dr J.J. Wenger and Professor L. Tongio, and by kind permission of Expansion Scientifique Francaise, Paris.)

from a transient episode of inflammation to massive fibrous stricture of the bowel causing complete obstruction.

Clinical Picture

This is a disease of the middle aged and elderly, as would be expected in any condition whose causation is diminished arterial blood supply (Fig. 10.6). There is usually a background of ischaemic heart disease or peripheral arterial insufficiency, collagen disorder or local colon pathology. The typical presentation is of acute pain in the left iliac fossa, early nausea and vomiting. This is followed by the passage of one or two loose motions which characteristically contain dark blood and clots.[47] On examination, the patient does not appear grossly ill or shocked, although the temperature and pulse are raised. The constant abdominal finding is of extreme tenderness in the left iliac fossa and in the pelvis, with dark blood on the fingerstall following rectal examination.

Endoscopy

Conventional rigid sigmoidoscopy does not usually bring the lesion into view, as the area affected lies above the reach of the instrument. However, there are a few reports in the literature[54] where the disgnosis has been made by this means. The appearances described are of irregular heaped-up bluish-purple mucosa, with oedema and contact bleeding. They closely resemble the changes found in the colon of the experimental animal following

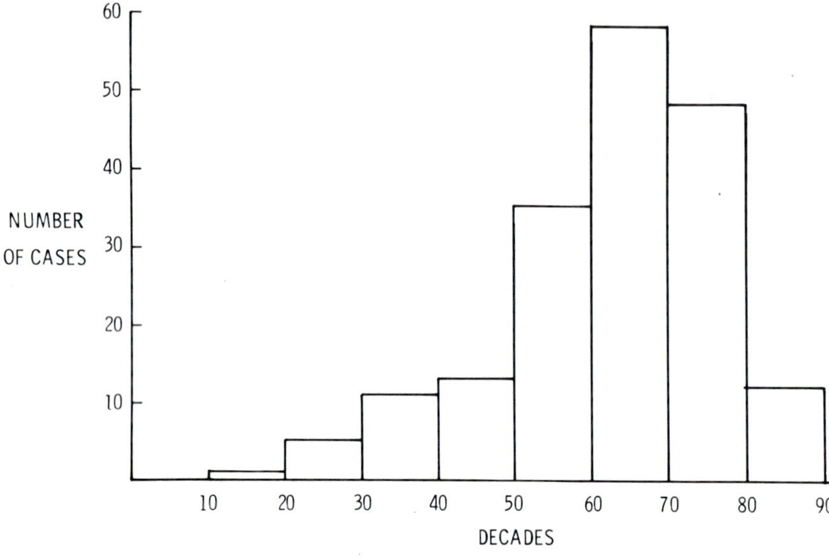

Fig. 10.6 Age incidence of ischaemic colitis.

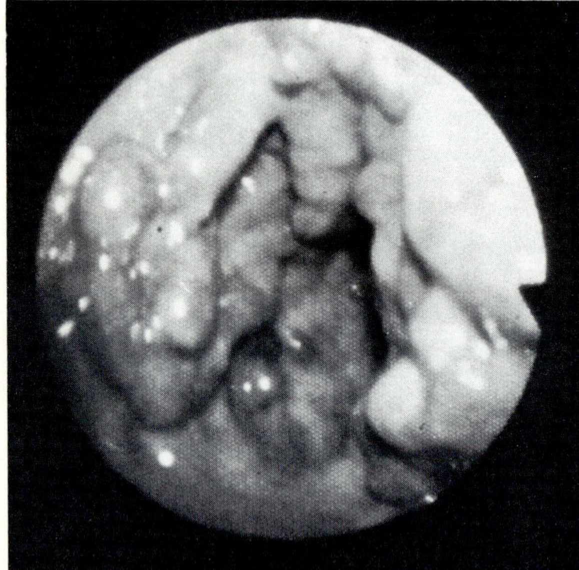

Fig. 10.7 Ischaemic colitis — colonoscopic appearances. Early stage showing 'thumb-prints'.

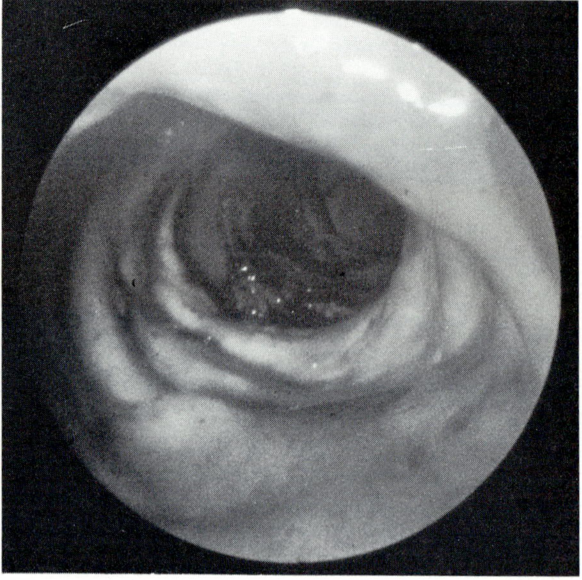

Fig. 10.8 Ischaemic colitis — colonoscopic appearances. Late stage showing ulceration.

vascular ligation (Chapter 3). Colonoscopy has proved an extremely useful diagnostic method in the early diagnosis of the disease and appears safe.[47] As yet, no complications or disasters have been reported from its use.

The appearances on colonoscopy (Figs. 10.7 and 10.8) confirm those found on rigid instrumentation. According to the timing of the examination, findings vary between oedematous blebs, surface ulceration and rigid strictures which prevent onward passage of the instrument.

Laboratory investigations

Early leucocytosis is the rule. Serum enzymes move in an unpredictable and inconstant fashion. The early promise of raised levels of serum phosphate concentration[55, 56] as a diagnostic pointer has not as yet been confirmed, but it seems likely that they will be unhelpful, as rises are found only in massive overwhelming ischaemia such as occurs in SMA embolus (see Chapter 5).

Radiological findings

Plain films

This simple, cheap and totally non-invasive investigation is always worthwhile. If thumb-prints outlined by bowel-gas shadows (Figs. 10.9 and 10.10) are seen, the diagnosis is made.

Barium studies

The barium enema has undoubtedly been the most useful tool in the diagnosis of ischaemic colitis. The appearances have been studied in detail by many radiologists, and are now well established.[41, 47, 57]

Unless the patient is very ill, the bowel is prepared by a standard technique such as an oxyphenisatin enema to clear it of faeces. The colon is filled with barium under the image intensifier, and the usual series of posteroanterior and oblique views are taken, followed by postevacuation and air insufflation films.

The changes seen on the contrast enema depend, naturally, upon the timing of the examination. They are as follows.

1. *Thumb-printing* is the earliest change seen on the barium enema, and has been observed as early as 3 days after the onset of the symptoms. The term was originally suggested nearly twenty years ago by Boley and his group,[40] and in spite of other suggestions ('pseudopolyposis', 'polypoid change', 'scalloping') has stood the test of time. It is illustrated in Figs. 10.10–10.12) and can also be created experimetnally (Chapter 3). The sign

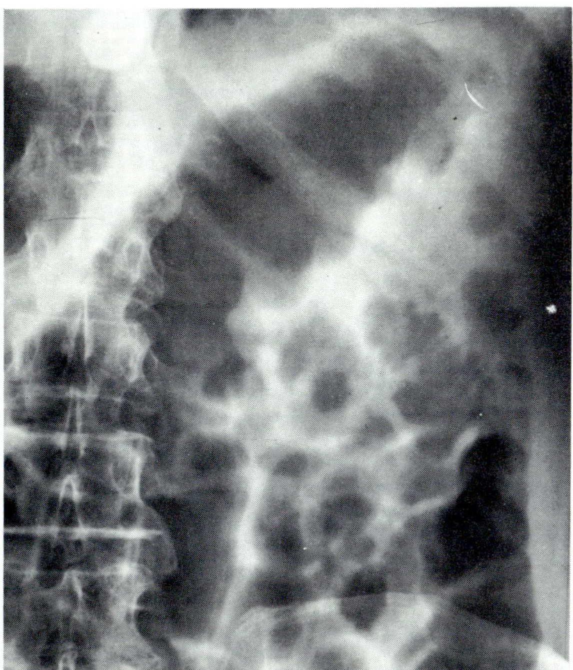

Fig. 10.9 Ischaemic colitis. Plain film showing 'thumb-prints' in the region of the splenic flexure. (By courtesy of Dr Michael Lea Thomas.)

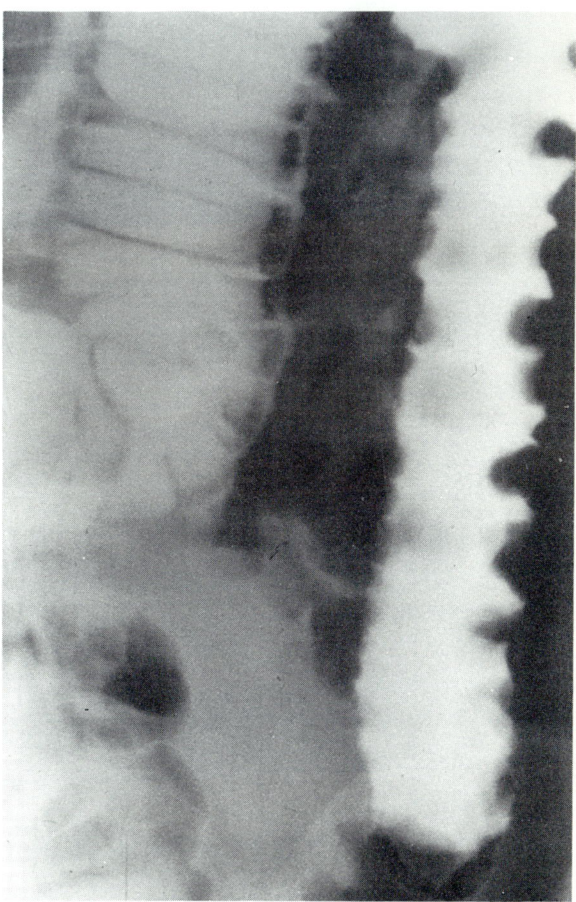

Fig. 10.10 The same patient as in Fig. 10.9 — colon outlined with barium. (By courtesy of Dr Michael Lea Thomas.)

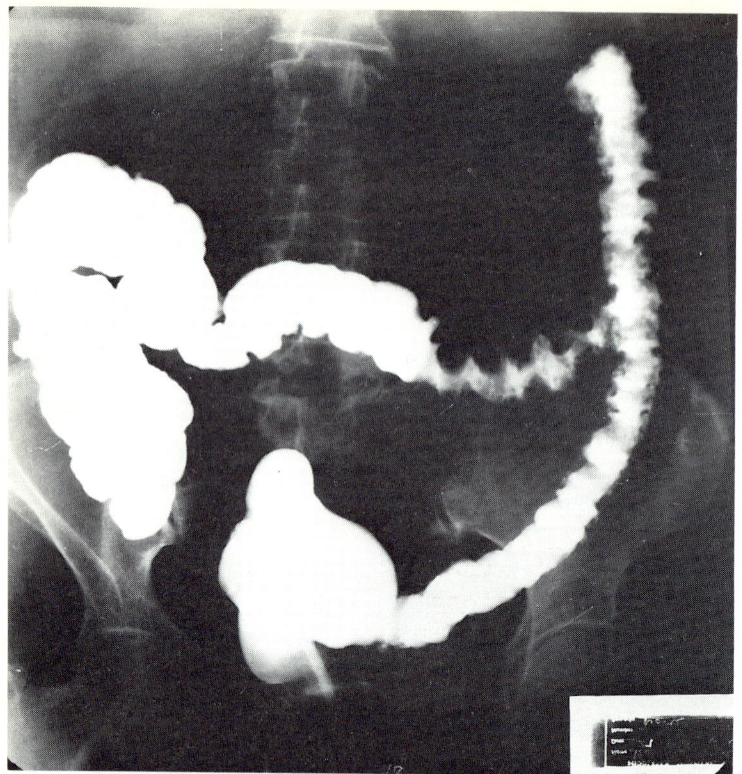

Fig. 10.11 Ischaemic colitis. Barium studies showing 'thumb-prints' around the splenic flexure.

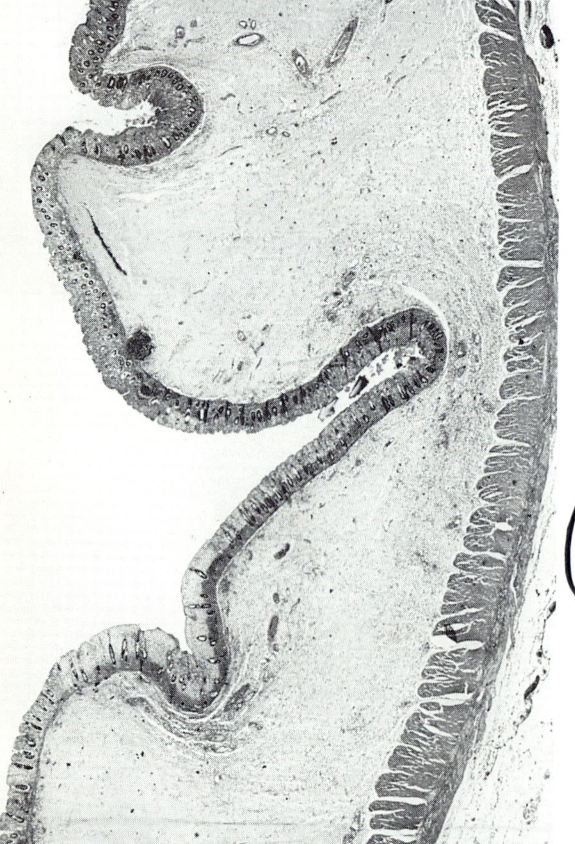

Fig. 10.12. Ischaemic colitis. Acute necrosis of the mucous membrane of the colon with pronounced submucosal oedema. This is the histology of the radiological sign of thumb-printing. (×9) (By courtesy of Dr B.C. Morson.)

consists of a series of blunt semi-opaque projections into the intestinal lumen, with a margin of half-shadowing, and once experienced is quite unmistakable. Correlation with endoscopic findings in the experimental animal[36] leaves little doubt that the large thumb-prints are due to submucosal oedema and haemorrhage. Although they are seen most frequently in the region of the splenic flexure, they may occur anywhere from the caecum to the pelvirectal junction.

Thumb-printing is an early change, and has been recorded as disappearing at an interval as short as 48 hours. It may, however, persist for several weeks.[41, 47]

2. *Mucosal irregularity*. During the days or weeks following the onset of the illness, the radiological appearances may alter in two directions. In many instances, the original thumb-printing clears completely and the outline of the bowel returns to normal (Fig. 10.13). However, depending on the degree of vascular insult, the appearance may progress to the next phase, namely that of mucosal ulceration and irregularity (Fig. 10.14). The ulcers

(a)

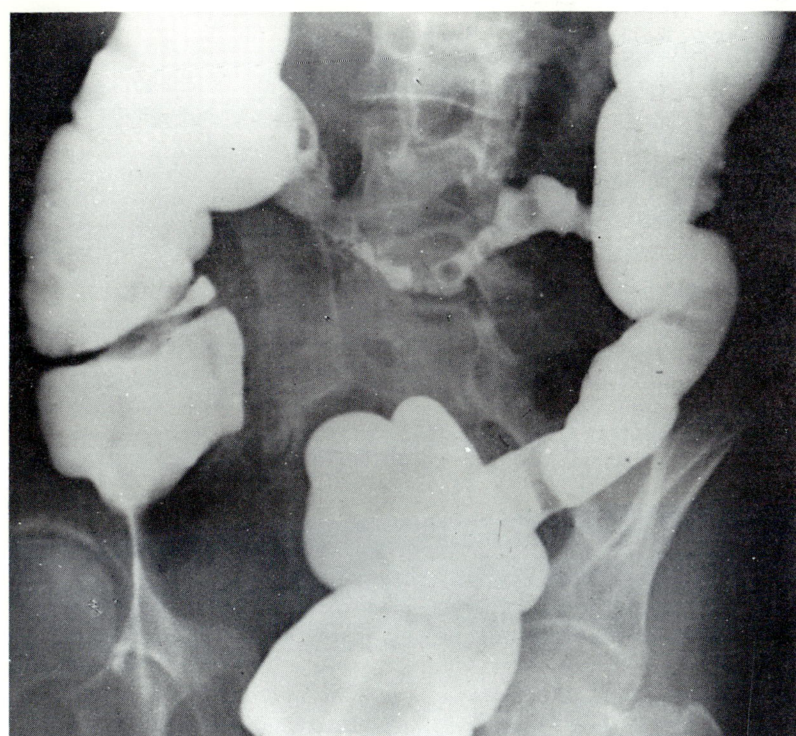

Fig. 10.13 Ischaemic colitis. Segmental infarction of the transverse colon (a) Initial appearance; (b) 4 months later.

(b)

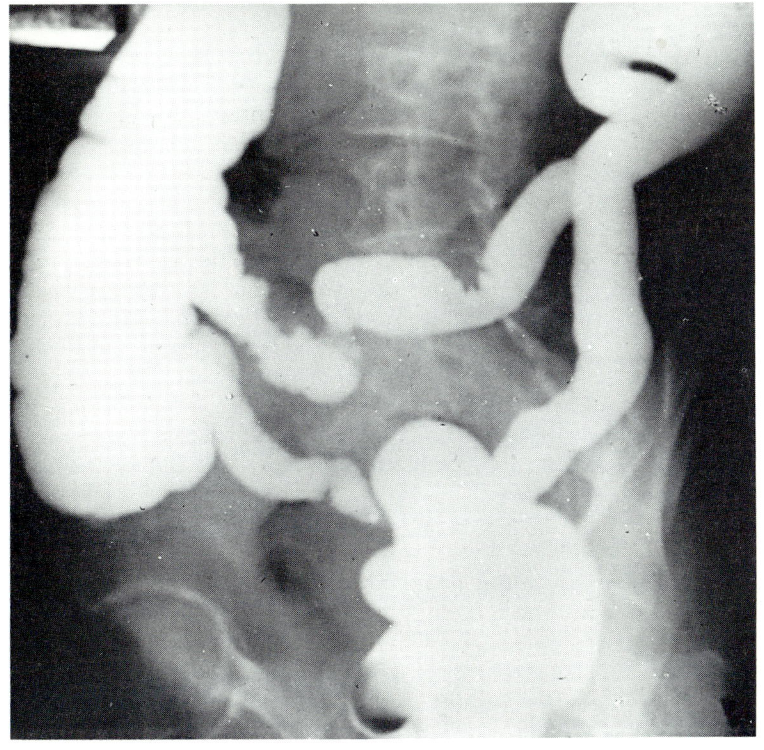

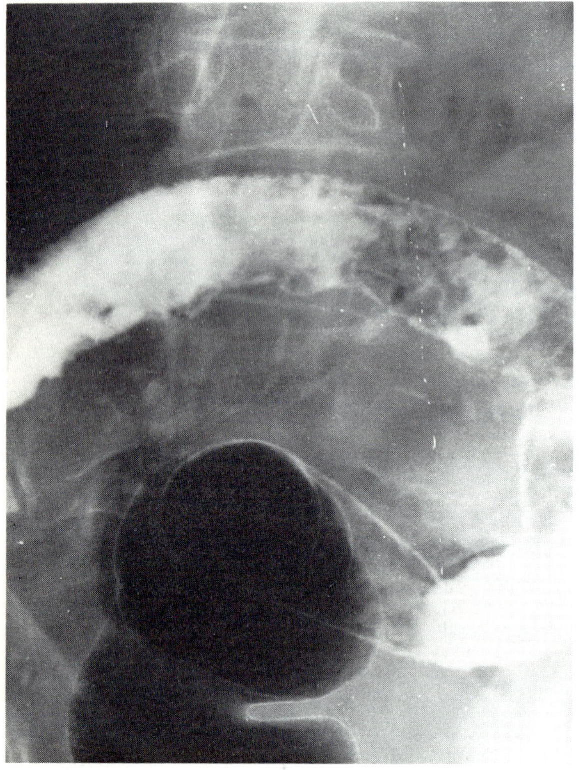

Fig. 10.14 Ischaemic colitis. Ulceration occurring 10 days after aortic resection.

are of varying size and depth and are quite irregular in their disposition around the circumference of the bowel. A barium enema taken at this stage may produce changes reminiscent of those of ulcerative colitis, and confusion with the transmural fissures seen in Crohn's disease may also occur.

In ulcerative colitis, however, rectal involvement is invariable, and the colon shows loss of haustration and a uniform abolition of mucosal pattern. In Crohn's disease the deep transmural fissures give a 'rose thorn' appearance, and the lesions are characteristically separated by areas of normal bowel. None of these features appears in ischaemia.

3. Once again, the changes can be reversible or progress to irreversibility. In the latter event, the next phase of radiological change is the formation of a *stricture* of varying length extending from a few centimetres in the splenic area (Fig. 10.15) to complete obliteration of the transverse and descending colon. No other process than ischaemia will produce such dramatic contraction (or even, at times, obliteration) of the colonic lumen over a period of a few weeks (Figs. 10.3 and 10.16). *Sacculation* (Fig. 10.17) is a late change, usually irreversible, which is the result of uneven deposition of fibrous tissue in the submucosa.

On occasion the narrowing occurs over a very limited segment of the bowel. This appearance gives rise to diagnostic difficulty because any localized stricture must of course be regarded as malignant until proven otherwise. A differentiating feature here is the appearance, which Lea Thomas[32, 47] has termed 'funnelling' (see Fig. 10.15a), which presents a smooth graduated beginning and end to the stricture, quite different from the irregular 'shoulders' or 'apple core' appearance associated with an ulcerating malignant tumour.

The timing of the barium enema. There is no evidence that an early barium enema has ever harmed a patient with ischaemic colitis. Obviously, when the colon is gangrenous, such an examination would be very dangerous, but this is not a practical clinical situation. In the absence of immediate facilities for colonoscopy, there is no question but that an early barium enema is a most valuable and safe adjunct to the management of any case of acute colonic inflammation.

The place of angiography

If facilities for early angiography are available, such an examination may help to confirm the diagnosis. Digital subtraction techniques are acceptably non-invasive, but do not at present provide enough resolution on which to base surgical decisions. From the practical point of view, arterial imaging is not needed for the management of the patient. However, the elegant studies from Strasbourg[46] represented in Figs. 10.4 and 10.5 demonstrate what can be achieved in this field.

Management

This will depend on the phase of the illness at which the patient is seen.

The emergency case

When the patient has been assessed as described above, it then becomes possible to draw a fairly accurate distinction between what is probably ischaemic colitis, where continued observation is justified, and what is probably some form of inflammation, perforation or other intra-abdominal

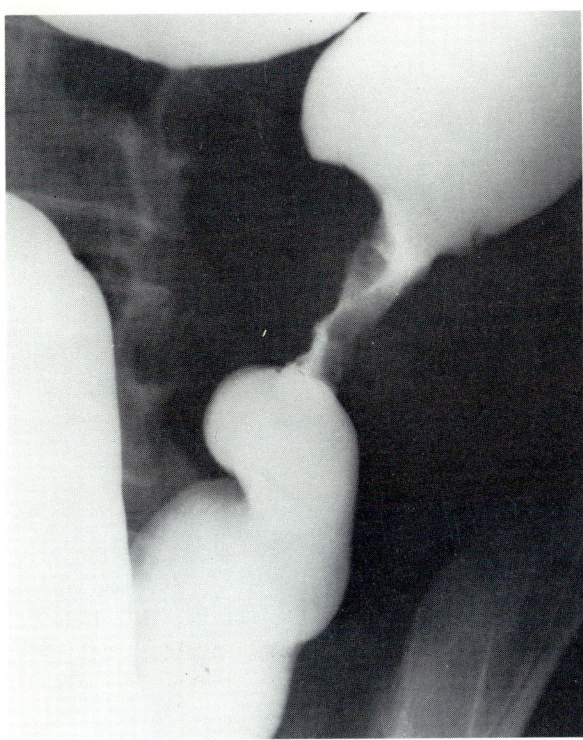

(a)

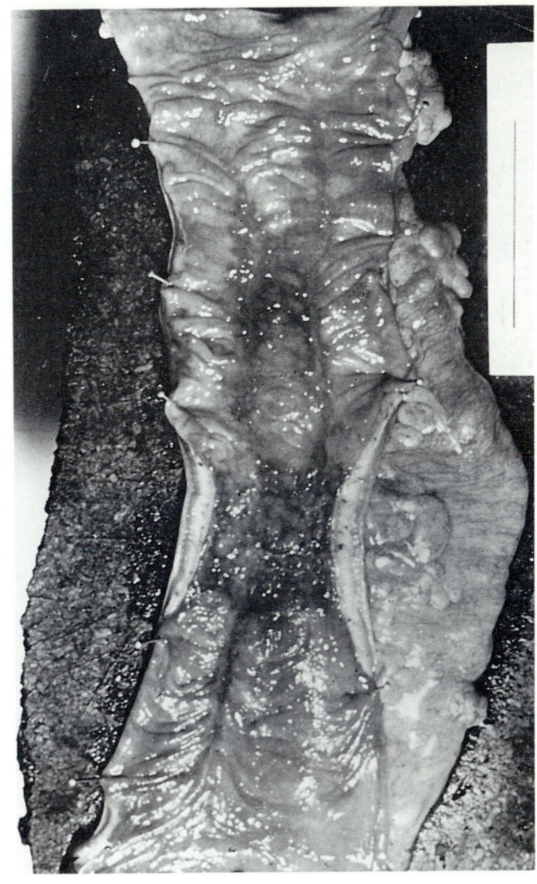

(b)

Fig. 10.15 Ischaemic colitis. A localized ischaemic stricture: (**a**) barium study (by courtesy of Dr Michael Lea Thomas); (**b**) the operative specimen.

crisis, which demands immediate surgery. The crucial diagnostic step is to obtain a barium enema at the earliest opportunity, because the appearances are so characteristic. Experience with fibrendoscopy is as yet limited for its role to be defined, but with the new generation of short flexible instruments which require little specialist training and cause the patient minimal discomfort, this examination may well come to be the procedure of choice.

Once the diagnosis has been established, treatment should in almost every case be expectant. This is to say, the patient is rested in bed, nourished either intravenously or by oral fluids, acccording to the degree of peritoneal irritation, and monitored by daily leucocyte counts and haematocrit readings. It is our practice to give an aminoglycoside and cephalosporin, rather on *a priori* grounds, as it has been established in the experimental laboratory that systemic antibiotics mitigate the effect of colonic ischaemia (see Chapter 3), but it must be admitted that the logic behind this therapy is uncontrolled, and it may in fact be unnecessary. Anticoagulants, here as in other situations of acute arterial occlusion, are unlikely to influence the pathological process, and are not indicated. Indeed, it is possible that their use might exacerbate bleeding in what is, after all, a haemorrhagic infarct. Needless to say, there is no place whatever for the use of corticosteroids.

On this expectant regimen, there are three possible sequelae:[41, 47]

1. Progression to gangrene.
2. Resolution (transient ischaemic colitis).
3. Stricture formation.

For a patient with acute non-gangrenous ischaemic colitis to develop gangrene of the colon is, fortunately, extremely rare.[41] In our personal series[58] it occurred only twice in 174 cases. The usual course of events is for the pain, bleeding and diarrhoea to settle rapidly over the course of a few days, or perhaps a week or two, and for a subse-

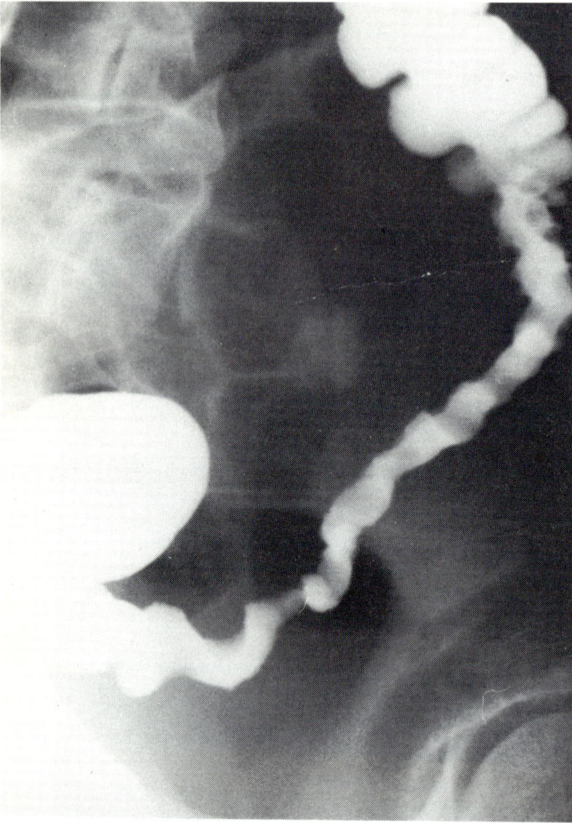

Fig. 10.16 Ischaemic colitis. An extensive stricture.

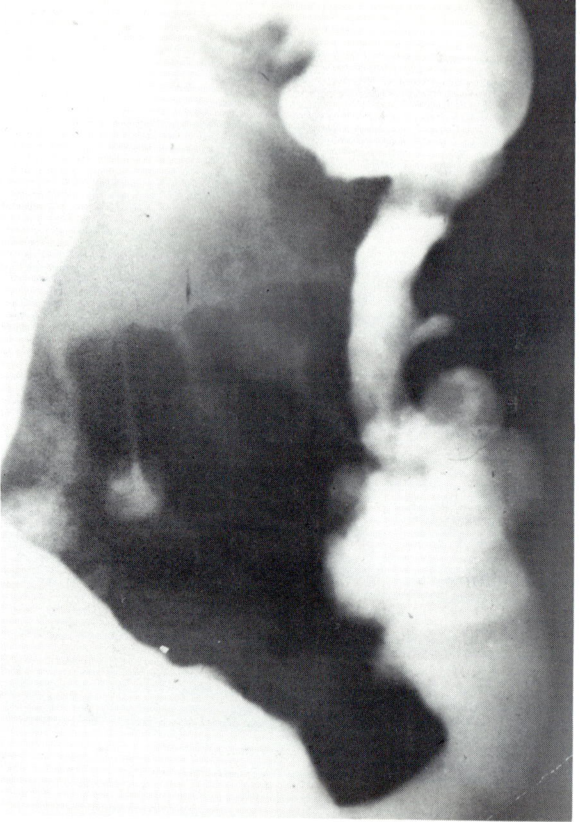

Fig. 10.17 Ischaemic colitis. Late case showing sacculation on the antimesenteric aspect of the bowel.

quent barium enema to show a normal colon, or one with minimal involvement (see Fig. 10.14). Sometimes, probably in about one-third of all cases, a fibrous stricture develops, but this is frequently quite asymptomatic and does not in itself require treatment.

Urgent surgery is required in:

1. Gangrene (rare).
2. Persistent bleeding due to deep ulceration.
3. Obstruction.

The elective case

Note every patient presents at an early stage of the disease. Quite commonly, there is a history of several weeks' (or even months') disturbance of bowel habit, with mucus, diarrhoea and bleeding, and a barium study shows mucosal ulceration or stricture formation. It is, of course, possible that, had an earlier study been carried out, thumb-prints would have been seen, but this is a question of surmise. The differential diagnosis here, of course, is between ischaemia, inflammatory bowel disease and cancer, as is illustrated in Tables 10.1 and 10.2. In any event, there is no urgency for surgery, and time will normally allow the symptoms to subside, paralleled by a return to normality of the endoscopic and x-ray appearances.

Elective surgery is thus required for:

1. An obstructing stricture.
2. A short stricture (see Fig. 10.15a) which cannot be differentiated from carcinoma.

Operative treatment and results

There is no particular difficulty in resecting ischaemic strictures of the colon, provided that the ordinary operative rules are respected.

The patient is positioned in the abdominoperineal (Lloyd-Davies) position so as to allow access to all parts of the large bowel including the splenic flexure, and the peritoneum opened via a long

Table 10.1 Clinical differential diagnosis of ischaemic colitis

	Ulcerative colitis	Crohn's disease	Ischaemic colitis
Age at onset	10–30	30–40	60+
Course	Chronic, relapsing; tendency to malignancy	Chronic	Acute episodes
Associated conditions	Iritis, arthritis, pyodermia	Megaloblastic anaemia, fistulae	Arterial disease, collagen disease, diabetes
Site	Left-sided or total, rectum always involved	Anywhere. rectum usually involved	Splenic flexure, rectum almost never involved
Radiology	Shortening, loss of haustration	Fissures, skip areas	Polypoid change, tubular narrowing, sacculation

midline or left paramedian incision. Clearly, special care must be taken with the vascularity of the resected ends, but, provided that the mucosa bleeds freely and the anastomosis is made without tension, there is no particular difficulty and leakage is rare.

In our series of 174 patients we carried out 51 operations for 78 strictures; 4 patients died in the perioperative period.[58] However, the figures are skewed in that the series includes a large number of cases seen in the 1960s who nowadays would not be operated upon, given our increased understanding of the disease. Furthermore, we do not have accurate follow-up statistics for either the operative or the non-operative group.

Pathology of ischaemic colitis

For detailed pathological appearances, the reader is referred to the writings of Morson[59] and Morson and Dawson.[60] The main findings are as follows.

Table 10.2 Pathological differential diagnosis of ischaemic colitis

	Ischaemic colitis	Crohn's disease	Ulcerative colitis
Depth of inflammation	Transmural	Transmural	Mucosal submucosal (except in fulminating colitis)
Submucosa	Widened	Widened	Normal width or reduced
Focal aggregates of lymphocytes	Absent or very few	Always (often transmural)	Sometimes (restricted to mucosa and submucosa)
Crypt abscesses	Few	Few	Very common
Goblet cell population of mucosa	Reduced (acute phase). Normal (ischaemic stricture)	Normal or slight reduction	Much reduced in active disease
Paneth cell metaplasia	Uncommon	Uncommon	Common
Sarcoid granulomas	Absent	Present about 60%	Absent
Fissuring	Absent	Common	Absent
Precancerous epithelial changes	No	Rare	Yes
Mucosal necrosis	Yes (acute phase)	No	No
Intravascular platelet thrombi	Yes (acute phase)	No	No
Submucosal oedema	Yes (acute phase)	Yes	Usually absent
Vascularity	Yes (acute phase)	Not prominent	Very prominent, particularly in active disease
Fibrosis	Usually very pronounced (ischaemic stricture)	Moderate or absent	None
Secondary vasculitis	Yes	Rare	Rare
Haemosiderin-laden macrophages	Yes	No	No
Hyalinization of connective tissue in submucosa	Yes	Never	No
Muscle necrosis	Common	Never	Only in toxic megacolon
Muscle fibrosis	Common	Never	Never

Reproduced from *Vascular Disorders of the Intestine* (1971; ed. by S.J. Boley), by kind permission of Dr B.C. Morson and the publishers, Appleton-Century-Crofts, New York. (Amended by Dr Morson, 1984.)

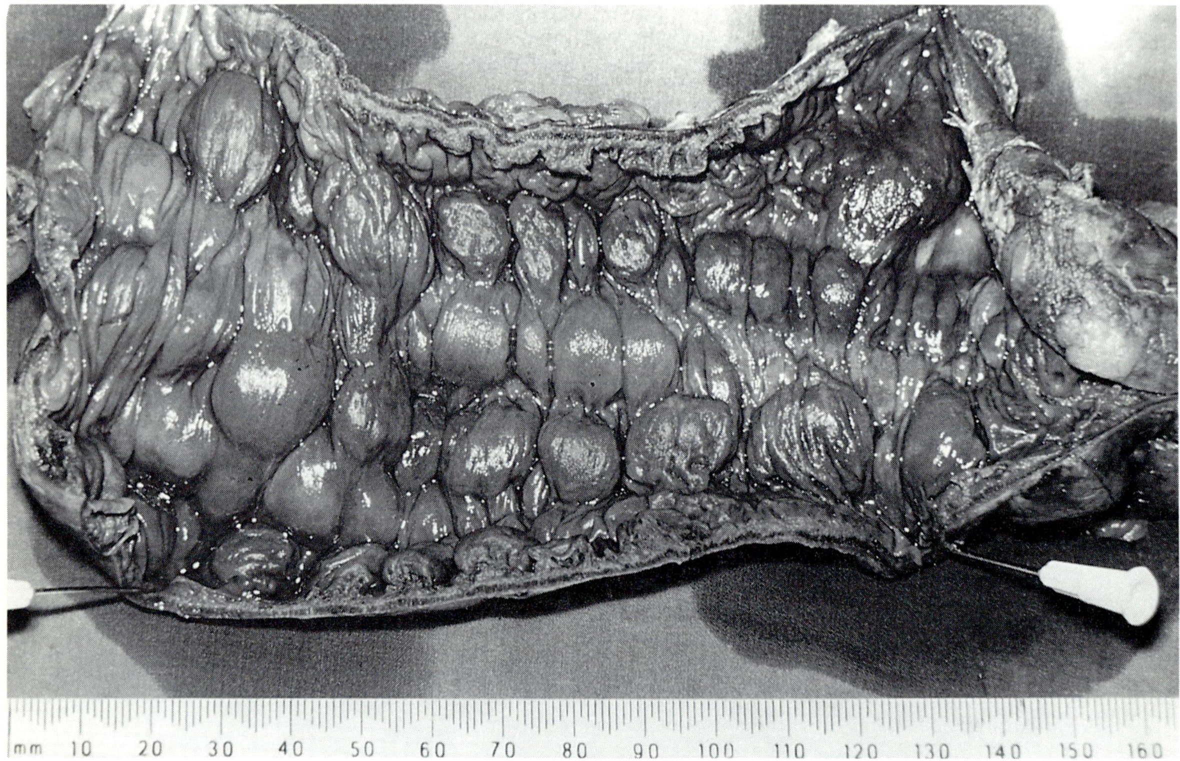

Fig. 10.18 Gangrene of the colon.

Gross appearances
In gangrene of the colon (Fig. 10.18) the bowel appears green or even black, dilated and thinned, with absent mucosa, gross ulceration and sometimes frank perforation. The major supplying vessels are usually open.

In ischaemic colitis the colon appears thickened and rigid and resembles the picturesquely described 'eel in rigor mortis', seen in Crohn's disease. The exact appearances will depend on the stage in the illness at which the specimen was taken. Early change (coinciding with the radiological appearance of thumb-printing) will appear as coarse, 'cobblestoning' of the mucosa, with linear ulceration and surface haemorrhage. The length of bowel involved may be from 5 to 25 cm, and on occasion can involve the entire colon. Where there is a limited stricture, the gross appearance is quite different from that of a carcinoma in that the mucosa is ulcerated in a shallow pattern, and there is a heavy deposition of thick white fibrous tissue in the submucosa, easily appreciated by the naked eye (see Fig. 10.20). Frequently there is an associated thickening of the serosal coats, with condensation of the surrounding fatty tissue, namely in the appendices epiploicae, and in the mesentery.

Microscopic appearances
In gangrene the appearances are the same as those shown in Figs. 3.6 and 3.7, with respect to the terminal stages of acute small bowel ischaemia. If the mucosa has sloughed, there is an intense infiltration of inflammatory cells into the deeper layers, and the muscle layers show severe destruction of their fibres, with vacuolation of the cytoplasm and pyknosis of the nuclei.

In ischaemic colitis there is full-thickness loss of mucosa in the ulcerated areas, whose base is composed of congested granulation tissue. There may be some epithelial regeneration at the edges. Between the ulcers the mucosa shows patchy atrophy and irregularity, with splaying of the muscle fibres of the muscularis mucosae. The most striking changes are found in the submucosal layers (Figs. 10.19 and 10.20), which are greatly thickened and filled with proliferating fibroblasts, oedema and

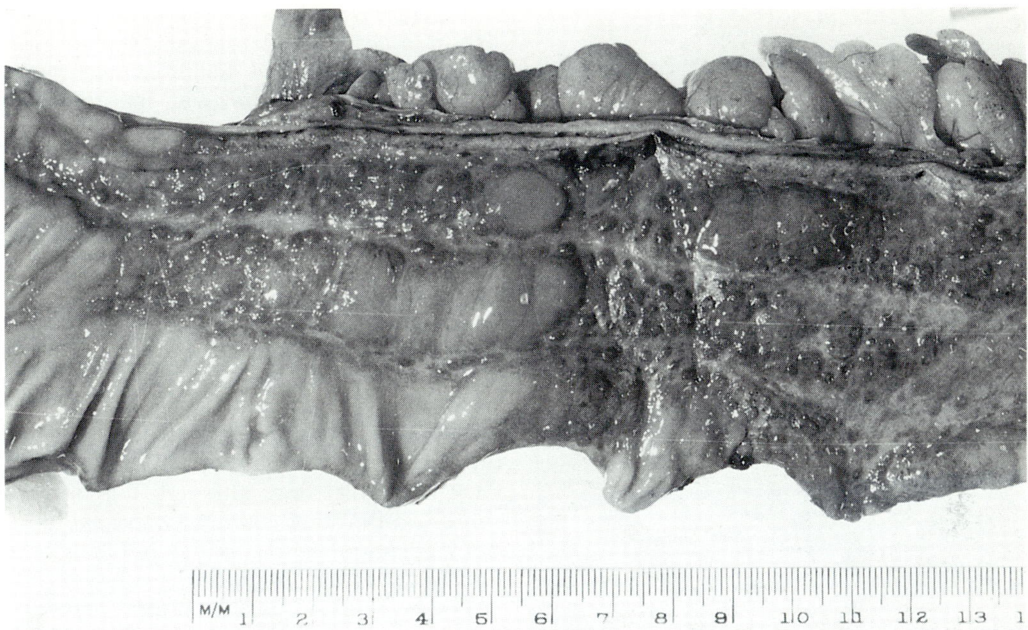

Fig. 10.19 Ischaemic stricture of the colon. The bowel wall is thickened and the lumen narrowed. There is mucosal ulceration with characteristic linear streaking. Patches of normal mucosa between areas of ulceration are a usual feature. (By courtesy of Dr B.C. Morson.)

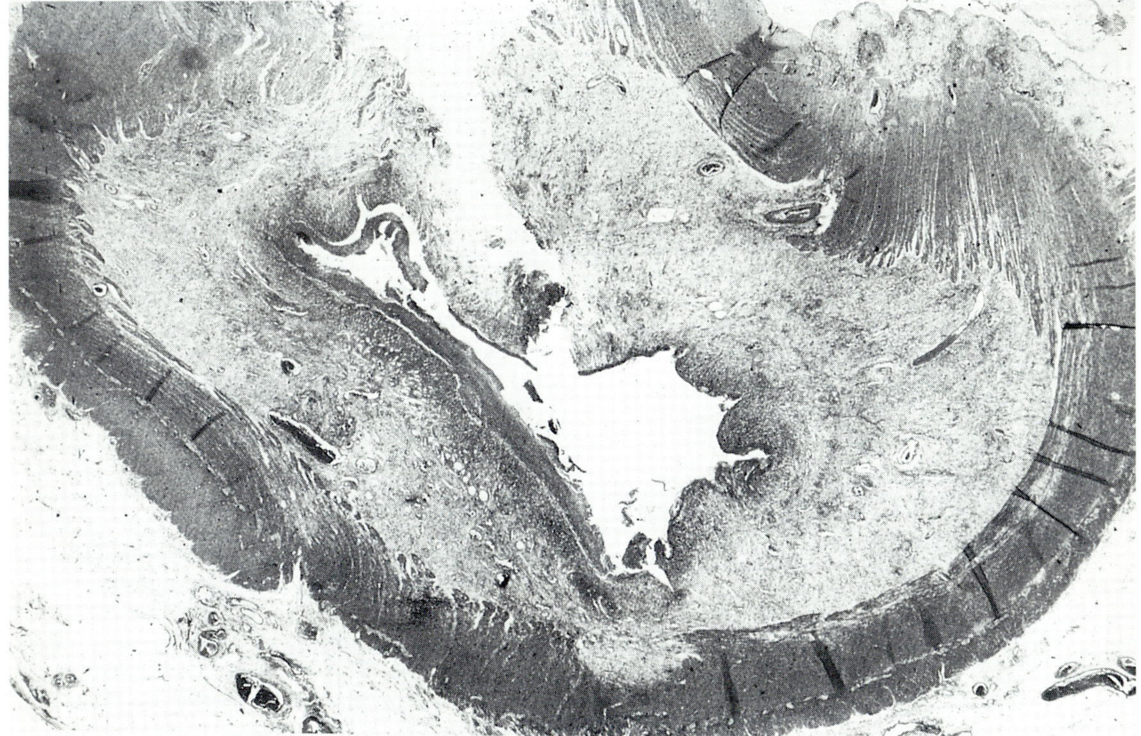

Fig. 10.20 Ischaemic stricture of the colon. There is mucosal loss with widening of the submucosal layer which is filled with granulation tissue. There is some patchy fibrosis of the muscular layer. ($\times$ 16)

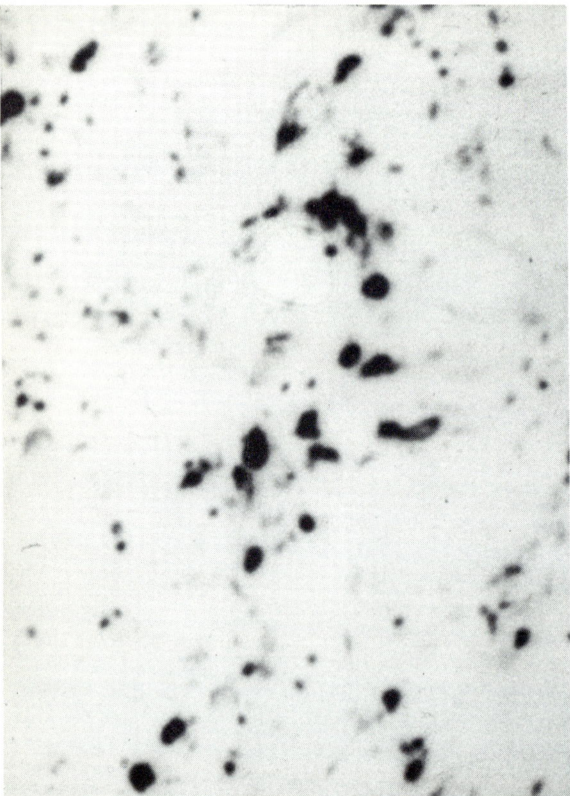

Fig. 10.21 Ischaemic colitis. Iron-laden macrophages in the submucosa.

inflammatory cells including lymphocytes, eosinophils and plasma cells. A characteristic finding common to both the clinical and the experimentally produced specimens is the presence of haemosiderin-laden macrophages, much as are found in a resolving myocardial infarct. For this reason, it is a wise policy to examine with Perls' Prussian blue method any resected specimen of colon whose pathological appearances are not wholly typical (Fig. 10.21).

Differential diagnosis

In a typical case presenting as an emergency the diagnosis should be fairly straightforward, particularly if there is associated rectal bleeding. The main conditions with which it tends to be confused are:

1. Infective gastroenteritis.
2. Acute diverticular disease, including ruptured pericolic abscess, and perforation of the colon.
3. Acute large bowel Crohn's disease, or exacerbation of chronic inflammatory disease.
4. Perforation of a hollow viscus such as the stomach or duodenum with peritonitis tracking down the left side of the abdomen.
5. Acute pancreatitis.
6. Left-sided renal colic.
7. Leading abdominal aortic aneurysm.

It is quite likely that many episodes of abdominal pain and diarrhoea, particularly in the older age groups, which are diagnosed as gastroenteritis or diverticular disease are in fact transient ischaemic episodes. There is no way to prove this point but common sense would suggest that such is the case. The feature which distinguishes ischaemia from other conditions is the presence of the characteristic dark rectal bleeding, although this occurs only in some two-thirds of cases.[41] Often, the diagnosis is not made immediately, but comes to light only with endoscopy or barium enema.

When seen later in the course of the illness, the condition may closely resemble Crohn's disease or ulcerative colitis. The main distinguishing features are set out in Tables 10.1 and 10.2. The most important of these are the characteristic age range of the patients, the association with degenerative cardiovascular disease and the distinctive radiological and pathological appearances.

Ischaemic proctitis

Our initial impression was that ischaemic disease never attacked the rectum. This finding was not unexpected in view of the rich collateral supply which arrives to the lower bowel from the pelvic vessels (see Chapter 1). However, later experience has shown that, particularly in patients with occlusive disease of the internal iliac arteries, ischaemic proctitis can indeed occur, and lead to confusion with other varieties of rectal inflammation.[61] Thus Weaver[62] reported on a case of a 77-year-old man with a past history of stroke and myocardial infarction, who developed spontaneous gangrene of the whole of the bowel from the rectosigmoid junction to the pectinate line, with thrombosis of the terminal branches of the inferior mesenteric vessels. Other authors[63] have reported similar events. Just as in the proximal colon, degrees of infarction of the rectum can occur which fall short of gangrene and lead to a haemorrhagic inflammation or to the formation of a fibrous stricture. It appears[64] that ischaemic proctitis can occur also as a result of fibromuscular hyperplasia of the rectal arteries.

Summary and conclusions

Gangrene of the colon may occur from various causes but is clinically part of the spectrum of acute intestinal ischaemia, and is not usually an isolated event. Its recognition and management have been discussed in earlier chapters. The condition of (non-gangrenous) ischaemic colitis is a well recognized clinical entity, which may occur spontaneously following interference with the vasculature of the colon or as a result of other disease processes. The illness presents as an acute left-sided peritonitis, usually associated with diarrhoea and rectal bleeding, which can safely be treated expectantly. About half the patients managed in this way will go on to form a fibrous stricture in the colon, but only a minority of these develop symptoms which are bad enough to need an operation. When required, the surgery presents little difficulty and the results are comparable with those of colonic resection for other indications.

References

1 Lauenstein, C. Ein unerwarteter Ereignis nach der Pylorusresektion. *Zentralbl. Chir.* (1882) **9**: 137–41.

2 Treves, F. Idiopathic dilation of the colon. *Lancet* (1898) **i**: 276–9.

3 Kummel, H. Uber Resektion des Colon descendens und Fixation des Colon Transversum in den Analimen. *Arch. Kiln. Chir.* (1899) **59**: 555–8.

4 Hartmann, H.A. Some considerations upon high amputations of the rectum. *Ann. Surg.* (1909) **50**: 1091–7.

5 Pope, C.E., Judd, E.S. The arterial blood supply of the sigmoid, rectosigmoid and rectum. *Surg. Clin. North Am.* (1929) **9**: 957–60.

6 Goligher, J.C. The adequacy of the marginal blood supply to the left colon after high ligation of the inferior mesenteric artery during excision of the rectum. *Br. J. Surg.* (1954) **41**: 351–8.

7 Harrison, A.W., Croal, A.E. Left colon ischemia following occlusion or ligation of the superior mesenteric artery. *Can. J. Surg.* (1962) **5**: 293–8.

8 Morgan, C.N., Griffiths, J.D. High ligation of the inferior mesenteric artery during operations for carcinoma of the distal colon and rectum. *Surg. Gyecol. Obst.* (1959) **108**: 641–50.

9 Thomson, J.P.S., Hawley, P.R. Results of closure of loop transverse colostomies. *Br. Med. J.* (1972) **3**: 459–62.

10 Henry, M.M., Everett, W.G. Loop colostomy closure. *Br. J. Surg.* (1979) **66**: 275–7.

11 Forrester, D.W., Spence, V.A., Walker, W.F. The measurement of colonic mucosal/submucosal blood flow in man. *J. Physiol.* (1980) **299**: 1–11.

12 Forrester, D.W., Spence, V.A., Walker, W.F. Colonic mucosal/submucosal blood flow and the incidence of faecal fistula formation following colostomy closure. *Br. J. Surg.* (1981) **68**: 541–4.

13 Smith, R.F., Szilagyi, D.E. Ischemia of the colon as a complication in the surgery of the abdominal aorta. *Arch. Surg.* (1960) **80**: 806–21.

14 Johnson, W.C., Nabseth, D.C. Visceral infarction following aortic surgery. *Ann. surg.* (1974) **180**: 312–18.

15 Ernst, C.B., Hagihara, P.F., Daugherty, M.E., Sachatello, C.R., Griffen, W.O. Ischemic colitis: incidence following abdominal aortic resection. A prospective study. *Surgery* (1976) **80**: 417–21.

16 Joyeux, R., Courty, A., Biscaye, A., Carli, G., Lisbonne, M. Une complication grave et inédite de l'aortographe. *Sem. Hôp. Paris* (1950) **26**: 152–6.

17 Killen, D.A., Sewell, R., Foster, J.H. Colonic injury resulting from angiographic contrast media. *Am. J. Surg.* (1967) **114**: 904–9.

18 Wald, M. Gangrene of the distal two thirds of transverse colon, left colon, rectum and anal canal due to superior mesenteric vascular insufficiency. *Dis. Colon Rectum* (1964) **7**: 303–5.

19 Padhi, R.K. Fatal infarction of the descending colon after lumbar aortography. *Can. Med. Ass. J.* (1960) **82**: 199–201.

20 Gambee, L.P. Occlusion of the inferior mesenteric vessels. *West. J. Surg.* (1937) **45**: 105.

21 Gibson, W.E., Pearce, G.W., Creech, O. Infarction of the left colon due to primary vascular occlusion. *Disc. Colon Rectum* (1969) **12**: 323–6.

22 Hannan, J.R., Jackson, B.F., Pipik, P. Fibrosis and stenosis of the descending colon following occlusion of the inferior mesenteric artery. *Am. J. Roentgenol.* (1964) **91**: 826–32.

23 Mogadam, M., Schuman, B.M., Duncan, H., Patton, R.B. Necrotizing colitis associated with rheumatoid arthritis. *Gastroenterology* (1969) **57**: 168–72.

24 Feller, E., Rickert, R., Spiro, H.M. Small vessel disease of the gut. In: Boley, S.J., ed. *Vascular Disorders of the Intestine*, New York, London: Appleton-Century-Crofts (1971) 483–509.

25 Powis, S.J.A., Barnes, A.D., Dawson-Edwards, P., Thompson, H. Ileocolonic problems after cadaveric renal transplantation. *Br. Med. J.* (1972) **1**: 99–101.

26 Gage, T.P., Gagnier, J.M. Ischemic colitis complicating sickle cell crisis. *Gastroenterology* (1983) **84**: 171–4.

27 Herrman, J.W., Paine, J.R., Stubbe, N.J. Acute obstruction with gangrene of the colon secondary to carcinoma of the sigmoid. *Surgery* (1965) **57**: 647–50.

28 Ambruoso, V.N., Ferrari, F. Massive gangrene of the colon due to distal obstruction. *Surgery* (1967) **61**: 228–30.

29 Kawarada, Y., Satinsky, S., Matsumoto, T. Ischemic colitis following rectal prolapse. *Surgery* (1974) **76**: 340–43.

30 Marcuson, R.W., Stewart, J.O., Marston, A. Experimental venous lesions of the colon. *Gut* (1972) **13**: 1–7.

31 Kilpatrick, Z.M., Silverman, J.F., Betancourt, E., Farman, J., Lawson, J.P. Vascular occlusion of the colon and oral contraceptives. *N. Engl. J. Med.* (1968) **278**: 438–40.

32 Cotton, P.B., Thomas, M.L. Ischaemic colitis and contraceptive pill. *Br. Med. J.* (1971) **3**: 27–9.

33 Cavin, R., Boumghar, M., Loosli, H., Saegesser, F. Les accidents digestifs aigüe des contraceptifs oraux. *Chirurgie* (1982) **108**: 64–71.

34 Archibald, R.B., Burnstein, A.V., Knackstedt, V.E., Tolman, K.G., Holbrook, J.H. Ischemic colitis in a young adult due to inferior mesenteric vein thrombosis. *Endoscopy* (1980) **12**: 140–43.

35 Duffy, T.J. Reversible ischaemic colitis in young adults. *Br. J. Surg.* (1981) **68**: 34–7.

36 Marston, A., Marcuson, R.W., Chapman, M., Arthur, J.F. Experimental study of devascularisation of the colon. *Gut* (1969) **10**: 121–30.

37 Brownlee, T.J. Regional colitis as an acute abdominal emergency. *Br. J. Surg.* (1951) **38**: 507–9.

38 Kellock, T.D., Acute segmental ulcerative colitis. *Lancet* (1957) **ii**: 660–3.

39 Corbett, R. Stenosed segment of descending colon associated with trauma. *Proc. R. Soc. Med.* (1957) **50**: 271–2.

40 Boley, S.J., Schwartz, S., Lash, J., Sternhill, V. Reversible vascular occlusion of the colon. *Surg. Gynecol. Obst.* (1963) **116**: 53–60.

41 Marston, A., Pheils, M.T., Thomas, M.L., Morson, B.C. Ischaemic colitis. *Gut* (1966) **7**: 1–10.

42 Matthews, J.G.W., Parks, T.G. Ischaemic colitis in the experimental animal. 1. Comparison of the effects of acute and subacute vascular occlusion. 2. Role of hypovolaemia in the production of the disease. *Gut* (1976) **178**: 671–6; 677–84

43 Shippey, S.H., Acker, J.J. Segmental infarction of the colon demonstrated by selective inferior mesenteric angiography. *Am. J. Surg.* (1965) **109**: 671–5.

44 Reuter, S.R., Kanter, I.E., Redman, H.C. Angiography in reversible colonic ischemia. *Radiology* (1970) **97**: 371–5.

45 Haddad, H. Clinical features of ischemic bowel disease. *Can. J. Surg.* (1974) **17**: 434–46.

46 Wenger, J.J., Kempf, F., Tongio, J. *Les Ischémies Intestinales Aigües.* Paris: Expansion Scientifique Francaise (1980).

47 Reeders, J.W.A.J., Tytgat, G.N.J., Rosenbusch, G., Gratama, S. *Ischaemic Colitis*, The Hague: Martinus Nijhoff (1984).

48 Williams, L.F., Wittenberg, J. Ischemic colitis; a useful clinical diagnosis, but is it ischemic? *Ann. Surg.* (1975) **182**: 439–48.

49 Payan, H., Levine, S., Bronstein, L., King, E. Subtotal ischemic infarction of colon simulating ulcerative colitis. *Arch. Path.* (1965) **80**: 530–33.

50 McGovern, V.J., Goulstone, S.G. Ischaemic enterocolitis. *Gut* (1965) **6**: 213–20.

51 Lister, E., Jungmann, H. Gangrene of the colon. *Br. J. Radiol.* (1956) **29**: 341–3.

52 Mays, E.T., Noer, R.J. Colonic stenosis after trauma. *J. Trauma* (1966) **6**: 316–29.

53 Boreham, P. Benign strictures of the colon. *Proc. R. Soc. Med.* (1957) **50**: 601–4.

54 Scowcroft, C.W., Sanowski, R.A., Kozarek, P.A. Colonoscopy in ischemic colitis. *Gastronintestinal Endoscopy* (1981) **27**: 156–61.

55 Jamieson, W.G., Lozon, A., Durand, D., et al. Changes in serum phosphate levels associated with intestinal infarction and necrosis. *Surg. Gynecol. Obst.* (1975) **140**: 19–21.

56 Jamieson, W.G., Marchuk, S., Rowson, J., Durand, J. The early diagnosis of massive acute intestinal ischaemia. *Br. J. Surg.* (1982) **69**: Suppl. S52–S53.

57 Farman, J. The radiologic features of colonic vascular disease. In: Boley, S.J., ed. *Vascular Disorders of the Intestine*, New York, London, Appleton-Century-Crofts. (1971) 229–42.

58 Marcuson, R.W. Ischaemic colitis. *Clin. Gastroenterol.* (1972) **1**: 745–63.

59 Morson, B.C. The pathology of ischaemic colitis. *Clin. Gastroenterol.* (1972) **1**: 765–6.

60 Morson, B.C., Dawson, I.M.P. *Gastrointestinal Pathology*, 2nd edn. Oxford: Blackwell Scientific (1979) 594–5.

61 Parks, T.G., Johnston, C.W., Kennedy, T.L., Gough, A.D. Spontaneous ischaemic proctocolitis. *Scand. J. Gastroenterol.* (1972) **7**: 241–6.

62 Weaver, R.M. Atherosclerotic infarction of the rectum. *Br. Med. J.* (1984) **288**: 684.

63 Nelson, R.L., Schuler, J.J. Ischemic proctitis. *Surg. Gynecol. Obstet.* (1982) **154**: 27–33.

64 Quirke, P., Campbell, I., Talbot, I.C. Ischaemic proctitis and adventitial fibromuscular dysplasia of the superior rectal artery. *Br. J. Surg.* (1984) **71**: 33–8.

11

Miscellaneous conditions

Trauma

The visceral arteries are among the most deeply placed and inaccessible structures in the body, and lie in close relation to many vital organs. For practical purposes, therefore, injury to them occurs only in association with major and widespread trauma from which the patient often succumbs before reaching hospital. Thus in a review of 126 civilian arterial injuries, Bole et al.[1] quoted only 1 case each of injury to the hepatic, superior mesenteric and inferior arteries. Clearly, however, management of the visceral circulation will be a major preoccupation in the repair of injuries of the lower thoracic and upper abdominal aorta, although the arterial trunks themselves may have remained unscathed. More recently, Lucas et al.[2] report 15 cases treated at Louisville between 1957 and 1979, again almost all associated with widespread multiple trauma. These authors advise a retroperitoneal approach to the vessels, and emphasize the importance of seeking and correcting any lesion of the superior mesenteric or portal veins.

There is little information on the maximum tolerable period of interruption of the SMA in the healthy young adult, although from animal experiments and from the analogy of mesenteric embolus, some degree of recovery would be expected to follow restoration of flow up to as much as 24 hours following the injury. Even if reconstruction is technically unsuccessful, collateral circulation may develop and be sufficient to nourish the bowel. Thus Ledgerwood and Lucas[3] have reported the case of a 19-year-old heroin addict who underwent resection of 2 cm of the SMA following a gunshot wound of the upper abdomen. This was followed by a prolonged period of mucosal necrosis and consequent malabsorption, but eventually there was good recovery. Aortography carried out at 10 weeks and at 2 years following the injury showed complete occlusion of the SMA with hypertrophy of the colonic circulation. The patient was found to be well at a follow-up examination 39 months after the original injury. There have been two other reports in the literature of prolonged survival following traumatic thrombosis of the SMA[4, 5] and, bearing in mind the astonishing capacity of the visceral circulation to develop a collateral supply, it would seem probable that this injury occurs much more frequently than is generally suspected.

Arteriovenous fistula

There appear to be three varieties of this condition.

1. Spontaneous arteriovenous fistulae occur between the SMA and the portal vein, in the region of the porta hepatis. This condition was first recorded by Goodhart,[6] whose patient was a 49-year-old woman with a history of abdominal pain and melaena. She was found at autopsy to have a fistulous communication between the splenic vessels, which had resulted in gross venous congestion of the colon. This was certainly the first case recorded of venous lesion of the colon leading to hypoxic damage. There have been several other cases reported since,[7, 8] and the subject was reviewed by Stone et al.,[9] who collected 38 examples from the literature, some of them spontaneous and some of traumatic origin.

2. Gunshot wounds of the abdomen occasionally lead to arteriovenous communications of the

mesenteric vessels, which usually pass unnoticed at the time of the emergency operation but become manifest later whether because of intestinal symptoms, because of bleeding varices or because of the chance observation of an abdominal bruit.[10]

3. Iatrogenic fistulae occasionally follow intestinal resection, particularly if mass ligatures have been applied to the vessels at the root of the mesentery. They may be symptomless or may cause epigastric pain, melaena or an uncomfortable 'buzzing' sensation in the abdomen.[8, 11] Repair of the fistula, with or without additional resection of bowel, is usually a straightforward surgical exercise (Table 11.1), but it has recently been suggested[12] that the lesion is better managed by embolization.

Aneurysms

Two-thirds of all splanchnic arterial aneurysms occur in the splenic artery[13] and usually present as catastrophic abdominal haemorrhage. Provided that the patient can be brought in time to the operating theatre, splenectomy with excision of the aneurysm is usually a straightforward matter. Whether excision should be advised for the asymptomatic splenic aneurysm which presents as a calcified shadow on a plain abdominal x-ray is more doubtful, except in the case of young women (especially in pregnancy), where operation is indicated.

Aneurysms of the coeliac axis and SMA are comparatively rare. Thus Stanley, Thompson and Fry[13] who reviewed the literature in 1970, found only 9 cases of coeliac axis aneurysm (including 2 of their own) and 89 cases of superior mesenteric aneurysm (including 2 of their own). The authors advise an aggressive surgical approach to these lesions, particularly when they occur in association with bacterial endocarditis. They also draw attention to the occurrence of small, previously asymptomatic, aneurysms of the jejunal and colic vessels, which may present as acute abdominal haemorrhage ('abdominal apoplexy').

There have been a number of cases of successful excision of complicated visceral aneurysms, including the pioneer report by Haimovici et al.[14] of an aortic reconstruction which involved reimplantation of the left gastric, hepatic, splenic, right and left renal and inferior mesenteric arteries. Isolated aneurysms of the IMA are a much simpler problem and can often be resected without difficulty,[15] even when ruptured.[16] Graham et al.[17] have recently reported two cases.

Aneurysms of the distal vessels have been reviewed by McNamara and Griska,[18] who found and reported the incidence of 12 jejunal, 9 ileal, 11 midcolic and 7 unspecified such lesions. Unless they rupture and exsanguinate the patient, they can usually be treated by resection of the mesentery.

The detailed techniques of reconstruction of these aneurysm are beyond the scope of this work, and will not be discussed further. The point should be made that dilatation of the coeliac and superior mesenteric arteries is very often a manifestation of widespread degenerative arterial disease, and the patient's fate and prognosis will then usually be determined by factors outside the visceral circulation.

External compression

Just as the coeliac axis may be compressed by fibres of the median arcuate ligament of the diaphragm, so the occurrence of fibrous bands which narrow the ostium of the SMA has also been reported.[19, 20] It is doubtful whether such structures have any physiological or surgical significance.

A note on sickling

Acute abdominal pain is a well recognized complication of sickle cell disease, particularly in the homozygous form,[21] and florid ischaemic colitis has been recorded as a complication.[22, 23]

Whether or not most of the abdominal crises seen in sickle cell disease are in fact manifestations of intestinal ischaemia remains undecided, and certainly associated gallstones, splenic infarction and peptic ulcer account for many cases.[22] However, the report by Gage and Gagnier[23] suggests very strongly that intravascular coagulation within the gut is an important manifestation. From the practical point of view, it follows that any patient with the ethnic or genetic likelihood of carrying the sickle cell gene, presenting with abdominal pain, must be considered as having a possible intestinal infarction. If, moreover, there is associated dyspnoea and chest pain, life-threatening respiratory failure may develop.[24] Treatment is along standard lines and involves rehydration and the administration of bicarbonate; surgery is not often required.

References

1. Bole, P.F., Purdy, R.T., Munda, R.T., Moallem, S., Devanesan, J., Clauss, R.H. Civilian arterial injuries. *Ann. Surg.* (1976) **183:** 13-23.
2. Lucas, A.E., Richardson, J.D., Flint, L.M., Polk, H.C. Traumatic injury to the proximal superior mesenteric artery. *Ann. Surg.* (1981) **193**: 30–34.
3. Ledgerwood, A., Lucas, A.E. Survival following proximal superior mesenteric artery occlusion from trauma. *J. Trauma* (1974) **14:** 622–5.
4. Fry, W.J. In: Strandness, D.E., ed. *Collateral Circulation in Clinical Surgery*, Philadelphia, London: W.B. Saunders (1969) 508–9.
5. Kleitsch, W.P., Connors, E.K., O'Neill, T.J. Surgical operations on the superior mesenteric artery. *Arch. Surg.* (1957) **75:** 752–5.
6. Goodhart, J.F. Arteriovenous aneurysm of splenic vessels with thrombosis of mesenteric veins and acute colitis. *Trans. Pathol. Soc. Lond.* (1889) **40:** 67–70.
7. Wheeler, H.B., Warren, R. Duodenal varices due to portal hypertension from arteriovenous aneurysm. *Ann. Surg.* (1957) **146:** 229–38.
8. Metzger, D.G., Hamilton, R.F., Stephenson, D.V. Mesenteric arteriovenous fistula. *Am. J. Surg.* (1972) **124:** 767–9.
9. Stone, H.H., Jordan, W.D., Acker, J.D., Marton, J.D. Portal arteriovenous fistula: review and case report. *Am. J. Surg.* (1965) **109:** 191–6.
10. Spellman, M.S., Manda, L., Freeman, H.D., Massumi, R.A. Successful repair of an arteriovenous fistula between the superior mesenteric vessels secondary to a gunshot wound. *Ann. Surg.* (1967) **165:** 458–63.
11. Paloyan, D., Collins, P.A., Washburn F.P. Superior mesenteric arteriovenous fistula. *Am. J. Surg.* (1974) **40:** 481–4.
12. Capron, J.P., Gineston, J.L., Redmond, A., et al. Inferior mesenteric artery arteriovenous fistula associated with portal hypertension and acute ischemic colitis. *Gastroenterology* (1984) **86:** 351–5.
13. Stanley, J.C., Thompson, N.W., Fry, W.J. Splanchnic artery aneurysms. *Arch. Surg.* (1970) **101:** 689–97.
14. Haimovici, H., Steinman, C., Bosniak, M., Spiegler, E. Excision of a saccular aneurysm. *Ann. Surg.* (1964) **159:** 368–74.
15. Vidal-Barraquer, F., Martinez Cercos, R., Puncernau, J., Lisbona, C., Castro, F., Munné, A. Aneurysm of the inferior mesenteric artery. *J. Cardiovasc. Surg.* (1983) **24:** 677–80.
16. Saint-Julien, J., Hamon, M., Cazenove, J.C., Abgrall, J. Aneurysme de làrtère mésentérique inférieure. *Chirugie* (1083) **109**: 113–115.
17. Graham, L.M., Hay, M.R., Cho, K.J., Stanley, J.C. Inferior mesenteric artery aneurysms. *Surgery* (1985) **97:** 158–63.
18. McNamara, M.F., Griska, L.B. Superior mesenteric branch aneurysms. *Surgery* (1980) **88:** 625–71.
19. Gautier, R., Barrié, J., Sarrazin, R. Les angors abdominaux non-athéromateux. *Lyon Chir.* (1965) **61:** 893–4.
20. Lawson, J.D., Ochsner, J.L. Median arcuate ligament syndrome with severe two vessel involvement. *Arch. Surg.* (1984) **119:** 226–8.
21. Tomlinson, W.J. Abdominal crises in sickle cell anemia: a clinical-pathological study of eleven cases. *Am. J. Med. Sci.* (1945) **209:** 722–41.
22. Platt, O., Nathan, D.G. Sickle cell disease. In: Nathan, D.G., Oski, F.A., eds. *Hematology in Infancy and Childhood*, Philadelphia: W.B. Saunders (1981) 703.
23. Gage, I.P., Gagnier, J.M. Ischemic colitis complicating sickle cell crisis. *Gastroenterology* (1983) **84:** 171–4.
24. Brownell, A.I., Menzies Gow, N., Win, A.A., Brozowic, M. (abstract). *Br. J. Haematol.* (1985) In press.

12

Summary and conclusions

The experimental evidence shows that low blood blow in the intestine, whether this arises from local causes or from a diminished cardiac output, leads to physiological disturbances which at first are subtle and hard to detect, but later become gross and unmanageable. Almost certainly, this must have a clinical parellel. However, in terms of day-to-day experience, cases of manifest intestinal ischaemia are rare, and the average doctor may not see such a patient during his professional lifetime. Some would say that the condition is common but unrecognized, but this is to beg the question. Special pleading has in the past been advanced for many 'diseases' which are no longer acknowledged to have a firm basis in pathology.

Quite apart from its being rare, mesenteric vascular disease predominantly affects the elderly, and it must be asked whether in a world whose main medical problems derive from malnutrition and overpopulation it is justifiable to devote any attention at all to such a condition.

In a symposium on the subject in 1976 I put this question to three leading surgeons with particular interest in mesenteric arterial disease, and here are their replies.

G.W. Taylor (London): 'Although mesenteric vascular disease is rare, it does not always affect the elderly; a significant number of our patients have been women in their middle 40s with well localized aortic disease. I certainly think this syndrome should be kept in mind in any patient with otherwise unexplained postprandial abdominal pain, nutritional disturbance, weight loss and abdominal arterial bruit.'

R. Kieny (Strasbourg): 'The question is essentially philosophical, and one needs to be precise about what constitutes an "elderly person". I would agree that intestinal ischaemia is quite often encountered in patients in their 40s. Furthermore, the bad reputation that treatment of lesions of the mesenteric artery has acquired is by no means justified. Early operation, before infarction has occurred, can have very satisfactory results. For instance, we reported 1 operative death in 35 reconstructions, and several 10-year survivals. Of the rest, 4 patients died within 3 years of operation, and 7 later. Causes of death were myocardial infarction (4 patients), cerebrovascular accident (5 patients), and renal failure (1 patient). Considering that the patients for the most part suffered from widespread degenerative vascular disease, these figures are not too bad.'

D.E. Szilagyi (Detroit): "Offhand, I do not see the connection between the therapeutic problems of my elderly patients and the regrettable problems of malnutrition in many countries in which the rich eat too much and the poor eat too little, or in which the available meager public funds go into the building of atomic weapons rather than into sensible programs of public assistance for the hungry poor. Moreover, I do not see the relevance of being elderly and sick to the question of overpopulation. Obviously, the elderly do not contribute to the population explosion. Your question would be relevant if ischemic gut disease affected mostly, or only, the reproductive young. Then, if one were worried about overpopulation, one might let the young with ischemic bowel disease die. One might— but I would not. Overpopulation will not be corrected by euthanasia.'

For my own part, I cannot pretend to be unbiased, but I nevertheless feel that continued interest in the area of mesenteric vascular insufficiency is justified, both for the reasons given above and because laboratory and clinical research into the problems of this very large compartment of the circulation must in the long term have an impact on clinical thinking. At present, the gap between physiologist and clinician is broad, but it is one that only the clinician can bridge.

Acute intestinal ischaemia

Acute intestinal ischaemia is a condition whose causation, let alone treatment, we do not understand, although the development of the concept of countercurrent exchange in the villus has helped to clarify the situation. Once the mucosal defences have been breached and bacteria are invading the bowel wall, a chain of events is set up which it seems almost impossible to reverse. Recovery in established intestinal failure is at present virtually unknown, but this does not mean that the situation need be quite hopeless. There must surely be patients in whom the process is initiated and then resolves spontaneously without being diagnosed, and others whose lives are saved by supportive treatment given for different clinical indications. What is needed, is, on the one hand, a high index of suspicion for early cases (and a method of identifying them) and, on the other, a realization of the measures we can take to prevent the process starting. At the same time it is probable that there is an irreducible mortality rate in that necrosis of the alimentary tract is often rather a mode of dying than a cause of death, and represents the end-stage of multisystem failure.

Chronic intestinal ischaemia

The problem of chronic intestinal ischaemia, due to surgically correctable lesions of the major arteries, has preoccupied vascular surgeons and gastroenterologists ever since arteriography became possible. Over the years, however, the impression which has been borne in upon most of us working in this field is that the patient whose abdominal pain is demonstrably due to arterial disease is exceedingly hard to identify. The criteria must be strict. It is not enough to observe a stenosis on an arteriogram, to reconstruct it surgically and to accept thanks from the patient. The history of surgery is littered with operations which have been judged on such uncontrolled grounds and are now deservedly forgotten. For a surgical procedure to be proved successful, it is necessary for there to be a quantifiable abnormality which correlates with the symptoms and which, following the operation, is shown to be abolished while at the same time the symptoms are relieved. Very few reported operations for supposed chronic intestinal arterial disease have met these criteria. This applies with particular force to the concept of the coeliac axis compression syndrome. However, as Dunphy originally suggested and as others have subsequently shown, intestinal infarction is almost always preceded by a warning period, during which an elective arterial reconstruction should be life saving. The technique of the reconstruction is important, which is why it was discussed in detail in the text. But how to select the patient with this type of disease remains our great problem, particularly as the resting intestinal blood flow will almost certainly be normal. It may even be that, before surgeons have devised an answer, their efforts will have been rendered obsolete by discoveries in the biochemical control of atheroma, so that chronic arterial obstruction to the gut, as in other parts of the body, will no longer require operation.

Focal intestinal ischaemia

Of less interest to the vascular purist, but of great significance to the gastroenterologist and general clinician, are the peripheral effects of focal intestinal ischaemia, whether in the small bowel or in the colon. The concepts of ischaemic enteritis and colitis have become firmly established, and are important not only because they differ in causation and behaviour from the granulomatous diseases but also because they are curable. We now, for instance, know a great deal about the natural history and management of ischaemic colitis, and have learned how rarely it is necessary to operate in this condition. But is the whole idea wrong? Is what we clinically recognize and categorize as ischaemic colitis in fact anything to do with deficient blood flow? The pathological appearances are reminiscent of infarction, but it is unjust to the pathologist to expect him to define the cause of a newly documented disease process with his microscope, in the absence of hard clinical data. After all, we do not know what (except under very abnormal conditions) the blood flow in millilitres per minute to the normal human colon should be, and still less are we able to document low flow during an attack of ischaemic colitis. The major blood vessels are often seen to be open on angiography. These questions need to be asked, and are valid. Nevertheless, there is a very strong body of circumstantial evidence both from the laboratory and from clinical experience that the changes in the gut wall are consistent with oxygen lack, whether mediated through large vessel occlusion or at microcirculatory level. Until another such hypothesis is put forward which fits the facts better than does the present one, it is pragmatically useful to regard patients with these now familiar syndromes as suffering from intestinal infarction. This implies a conservative approach to treatment as regards both drugs and operations, and, indeed, when viewed and managed in this way, most of these patients get better.

Postscript

The number of international conferences, symposia, research projects and published papers devoted to the subject of intestinal blood flow, its measurement and its disturbances has probably been exaggerated. Nevertheless, the fact remains that vascular accidents do occur in the alimentary tract, and that they are potentially lethal and certainly underdiagnosed. The purpose of this work, which has now extended over twenty-five years, has been an attempt to put the subject in perspective.

Further reading

Marston, A., Kieny, R., Szilagyi, D.E., Taylor, G.W. Intestinal ischaemia—a panel by correspondence. *Arch. Surg.* (1976) **111:** 107–12.

Marston, A., Clarke, J.M.F., Garcia Garcia, J. Intestinal function and intestinal blood supply. *Gut* (1985) **26**: 656–66.

Index